Cardiac Anatomy

Robert H. Anderson and Anton E. Becker

This book has been developed in
association with the Slide Atlas of
Cardiac Anatomy presented by the
American College of Cardiology
Heart House Learning Center and
ACCEL Program in conjunction with
Stuart Pharmaceuticals, Division of
ICI Americas Inc.

Further information concerning the
Slide Atlas of Cardiac Anatomy
is available from the
American College of Cardiology
Heart House,
9111 Old Georgetown Road,
Bethesda, MD 20014

Cardiac Anatomy

An Integrated Text and Color Atlas

Robert H. Anderson and Anton E. Becker

Robert H. Anderson
B.Sc., M.D., M.R.C.Path.

Joseph Levy Reader in Cardiac Morphology
Cardiothoracic Institute
Brompton Hospital
London UK

Anton E. Becker
M.D.

Professor of Pathology
Wilhelmina Gasthuis
University of Amsterdam
The Netherlands

With a contribution from:

Sally P. Allwork
M.Phil., Ph.D.

Licensed Teacher of Anatomy
Department of Surgery
Royal Postgraduate Medical School
University of London
London UK

Photography by:

Wilfried P. Meun
Ruud E. Verhoeven

Wilhelmina Gasthuis
Amsterdam The Netherlands

Foreword by:

John W. Kirklin,
M.D.

Charles and Faye Kerner Professor of Surgery
University of Alabama Medical College
Birmingham
Alabama USA

Gower Medical Publishing · London

STUART

Stuart Pharmaceuticals, Division of ICI Americas Inc., Wilmington, DE 19897

Distributed in Canada by:
ICI Pharmaceuticals
6299 Airport Road
Mississauga
Ontario L4V 1N3

Distributed in Japan by:
Nankodo Company Limited
42-6, Hongo 3-chome
Bunkyo
Tokyo 113

Distributed in all countries except
USA, Canada, and Japan by:
Churchill Livingstone
Medical Division of Longman Group
Robert Stevenson House
1/3 Baxter Place
Edinburgh AH1 3AF

ISBN 0-906923-00-X

British Library Cataloguing in Publication Data:

   Anderson, Robert H.
      Cardiac anatomy.
      1. Heart – Anatomy
      I. Title   II. Becker, Anton E.
      611′.12   QM181

Printed by Smeets Offset, Weert, The Netherlands

Foreword

The previous publications of the authors of this remarkable book on cardiac anatomy have established throughout the world the clarity of their analyses of morphology and the usefulness of the concepts that they have derived. Therefore, it will surprise no one that this textbook is indispensable to all surgeons, cardiologists, pathologists, radiologists, and others who must be seriously interested in the details of cardiac anatomy and morphology. The superb color plates and the lucid descriptions will make this text, for me at least, a prized possession.

John W. Kirklin, M.D.

Preface

At a time when gross anatomy as a whole is generally becoming curtailed in the medical curriculum, it is paradoxical that cardiac anatomy should be undergoing a renaissance of interest and significance. Following the excellent and detailed monograph on cardiac anatomy produced by Tandler in 1913 and a similar volume published by Walmsley in 1929, books devoted solely to cardiac anatomy have been rare. Even in the past decade, with the thirst for detailed knowledge of cardiac morphology coming from cardiac surgeons, physicians, echocardiographers, angiographers and scintigraphers, publications devoted solely to satisfy these needs have been scanty. That is not to deny the production of some excellent studies of cardiac anatomy during this period, for example, the detailed and beautiful volume of McAlpine (1975). However, this book requires considerable study together with some degree of prior knowledge before surrendering the information which abounds within its pages. In our book, therefore, we have tried to present cardiac anatomy in a reasonably brief but hopefully meaningful fashion. To this end, we have followed the lead of Walmsley and Watson (1978) and presented our material as far as possible with the heart in its *in situ* position. It is our firm belief that cardiac anatomy is done a great disservice by the all-too-popular habit amongst morphologists of describing and illustrating the heart as if it stood on its apex, with the atria above the ventricles in St. Valentine's fashion! We have used color photographs of human hearts to illustrate our concepts, supplementing this where appropriate with histological and clinical material. Finally, we have concluded with a chapter of simple (perhaps even simplistic!) embryology, since it is axiomatic that knowledge of the development of the heart considerably facilitates the understanding of its morphology.

R.H.A.
A.E.B.

v.

Acknowledgements

It would not have been possible to write this book without help, assistance and constructive criticism from so many of our friends and colleagues. We express our particular thanks to our contributor, Dr. Sally Allwork, for so readily putting her own special expertise at our disposal. We are also indebted to Dr. Koert Dingemans of Wilhelmina Gasthuis, Amsterdam, Dr. Jorgen Tranum-Jensen of Copenhagen University, Denmark and Professor J. A. Gosling and Dr. J. Dixon of the University of Manchester, United Kingdom, for providing us with illustrative material for Chapter 9.

The whole project would have been impossible without the photographic skills and innovations of Wilfried Meun and Ruud Verhoeven, who worked far beyond the call of duty in producing the illustrative material. To Yen Ho we are grateful for her continuing immaculate artwork and technical assistance, while further technical help was provided instantly when required by Inike Dijk and Ernst Heeren.

We are indebted to Professor C. A. Wagenvoort for his encouragement and for placing so many facilities at our disposal, and to Rinus Klaver and Marsha Schenker for aiding us in other technical and clerical aspects. As we have already indicated, our thanks and gratitude are due to all our friends who have advised, criticized, cajoled and sworn at us with regard to our concepts and their illustration, but in particular to Carlo Marcelletti. Finally, without the love and support of our wives, Christine and Mies, nothing would have been possible.

R.H.A.
A.E.B.
Amsterdam

References

Allwork, S. P. (1979) Apropos de la distribution normale des artères coronaires du coeur chez l'homme. *Anatomia Clinica*, **1**, 311-319.

Allwork, S. P. & Anderson, R. H. (1979) Developmental anatomy of the membranous part of the ventricular septum in the human heart. *British Heart Journal*, **41**, 275-280.

Anderson, K. R., Ho, S. Y. & Anderson, R. H. (1979) The location and vascular supply of the sinus node in the human heart. *British Heart Journal*, **41**, 28-32.

Anderson, R. H. (1972) The disposition, morphology and innervation of cardiac specialised tissues in the guinea pig. *Journal of Anatomy*, **111**, 453-468.

Anderson, R. H. & Becker, A. E. (1978) Anatomy of conducting tissues revisited. *British Heart Journal*, **40 supplement**, 2-16.

Anderson, R. H., Ho, S. Y., Becker, A. E. & Gosling, J. A. (1978) The development of the sinuatrial node. In *The Sinus Node*, edited by F. I. M. Bonke, pp 166-182. The Hague: Martinus Nijhoff.

Anderson, R. H. & Taylor, I. M. (1972) Development of atrioventricular specialised tissue in the human heart. *British Heart Journal*, **34**, 1205-1214.

Anderson, R. H., Wilkinson, J. L., Arnold, R. & Lubkiewicz, K. (1974) Morphogenesis of bulboventricular anomalies. (1) Consideration of embryogenesis in the normal heart. *British Heart Journal*, **36**, 242-256.

Asami, I. (1969) Beitrag zur Entwicklung des Kammerseptums in menschlichen Herzen mit besonderer Berucksichtigung der sogenannten Bulbusdrehung. *Zeitschrift fur Anatomie und Entwicklungsgeschichte*, **128**, 1-17.

Bargeron, L. M., Elliott, L. P., Soto, B., Bream, P. R. & Curry, G. C. (1977) Axial angiography in congenital heart disease. Section I – technical and anatomical considerations. *Circulation*, **56**, 1075-1083.

Baron, M. G., Wolf, B. S., Steinfield, L. & Van Mierop, L. H. S. (1968) Angiocardiographic diagnosis of subpulmonic ventricular septal defect. *American Journal of Roentgenology*, **103**, 93-103.

Becker, A. E. (1979) Normal variations in the morphology of the mitral valve. *British Heart Journal*. In press.

Becker, A. E. & Anderson, R. H. (1976) Morphology of the human atrioventricular junctional area. In *The Conduction System of the Heart – Structure, Function and Clinical Implications*, edited by H. J. J. Wellens, K. I. Lie & M. J. Janse, pp 263-286. Philadelphia: Lea & Febiger.

Becu, L. (1971) Case cited in Van Praagh, R. (1971) Transposition of the great arteries – II Transposition clarified. *American Journal of Cardiology*, **28**, 739-741.

Becu, L., Somerville, J. & Gallo, A. (1976) Isolated pulmonary valve stenosis as part of more widespread cardiovascular disease. *British Heart Journal*, **38**, 472-482.

Benninghoff, A. (1923) Uber die beziehungen des Reizleitungssystems und der papillarmuskeln zu der Konturfasern des Herzschlauches. *Anatomischer Anzeiger*, **57**, 185-208.

Bruins, C. L. D. (1973) De arteriele pool van het Hart *(thesis)*. Leiden: Drukkerij Groen en Zoon.

Bulkley, B. H. (1977) Idiopathic hypertrophic subaortic stenosis afflicted: idols of the cave and marketplace. *American Journal of Cardiology*, **40**, 476-479.

Congdon, E. D. (1922) Transformation of the aortic arch system during the development of the human embryo. *Contributions to Embryology*, **14**, 65-70.

de la Cruz, M. V., Sanchez Gomez, C., Manuel Arteaga, M. & Arguello, C. (1977) Experimental study of the development of the truncus and conus in the chick embryo. *Journal of Anatomy*, **123**, 661-686.

Feizi, O., Farrer-Brown, G. & Emanuel, R. (1978) Familial study of hypertrophic cardiomyopathy and congenital aortic valve disease. *American Journal of Cardiology*, **41**, 956-964.

Ferrans, V. R., Morrow, A. G. & Roberts, W. C. (1972) Myocardial ultrastructure in idiopathic subaortic stenosis – a study of operatively excised left ventricular outflow tract muscle in 14 patients. *Circulation*, **45**, 769-792.

Finlay, M. & Anderson, R. H. (1974) The development of cholinesterase activity in the rat heart. *Journal of Anatomy*, **117**, 239-249.

Gittenberger de Groot, A. C. & Wenink, A. C. G. (1978) The specialized myocardium in the foetal heart. In *Embryology and Teratology of the Heart and Great Arteries*, edited by L. H. S. Van Mierop, A. Oppenheimer-Dekker & C. L. D. Bruins, pp 15-24. Boerhaave Series No. 13. The Hague: Leiden University Press.

Goor, D. A., Dische, R. & Lillehei, C. W. (1972) The conotruncus – 1) its normal inversion and conal absorption. *Circulation*, **46**, 375-384.

Gorlin, R., Klein, M. D. & Sullivan, J. M. (1967) Prospective correlative study of ventricular aneurysm. *American Journal of Medicine*, **42**, 512-531.

Hackensellner, H. A. (1956) Aksessorische Kranzgefassanlagen der Arteria pulmonalis unter 63 menschlichen Embryonenserien mit einer grossten Lange von 12 bis 36 mm. *Mikroskopischanatomische Forschung*, **62**, 153-161.

Hudson, R. E. B. (1967) Surgical pathology of the conducting system of the heart. *British Heart Journal*, **29**, 646-670.

James, T. N. (1963) The connecting pathways between the sinus node and the A-V node and between the right and left atrium in the human heart. *American Heart Journal*, **66**, 498-508.

James, T. N. (1970) Cardiac conduction system – fetal and postnatal development. *American Journal of Cardiology*, **25**, 213-226.

Janse, M. J. & Anderson, R. H. (1974) Internodal atrial specialized pathways – fact or fiction? *European Journal of Cardiology*, **2**, 117-137.

Kent, A. F. S. (1893) Researches on the structure and function of the mammalian heart. *Journal of Physiology*, **14**, 233-241.

Kent, A. F. S. (1913) Observations on the auriculo-ventricular junction of the mammalian heart. *Quarterly Journal of Experimental Physiology*, **7**, 193-195.

Kent, K. M., Epstein, S. E., Cooper, T. & Jacobowitz, D. M. (1974) Cholinergic innervation of the canine and human ventricular conducting system – anatomic and electrophysiologic correlation. *Circulation*, **50**, 948-956.

Koch, W. (1909) Weiter Mitteilungen uber den Sinusknoten des Herzens. *Verhandlung der Deutschen Pathologischen Gesellschaft*, **13**, 85-92.

Kramer, T. C. (1942) The partitioning of the truncus and conus and the formation of the membranous portion of the interventricular septum in the human heart. *American Journal of Anatomy*, **71**, 343-347.

Krehl, L. (1891) Beitrage zur Kenntnisse der Fullung und Entleerung des Herzens. *Abhandlungen der mathematische-physischen Klasse der Koniglichen Sachsischen Gesellschaft der Wissenschaften*, **17**, 341-362.

Lev, M., Liberthson, R. R., Eckner, F. A. O. & Arcilla, R. A. (1968) Pathologic anatomy of dextrocardia and its clinical implications. *Circulation*, **37**, 979-999.

Lev, M., Liberthson, R. R., Golden, J. G., Eckner, F. A. O. & Arcilla, R. A. (1971) The pathology of mesocardia. *American Journal of Cardiology*, **28**, 428-435.

Lev, M. & Simkins, C. S. (1956) Architecture of the human ventricular myocardium. *Laboratory Investigation*, **5**, 396-409.

Liberthson, R. R., Hastreiter, A. R., Sinha, S. N., Bharati, S., Novak, G. M. & Lev, M. (1973) Levocardia with visceral heterotaxy – isolated levocardia: pathologic anatomy and its clinical implications. *American Heart Journal*, **85**, 40-54.

Los, J. A. (1968) Embryology. In *Paediatric Cardiology*, edited by H. Watson, pp 1-29. London: Lloyd-Luke.

Ludwig, C. (1849) Ueber den Bau und die Bewegungen der Herzventrikel. *Zeitschrift fur Rationelle Medizin*, **7**, 189-220.

McAlpine, W. A. (1975) *The Heart and Coronary Arteries*. Berlin: Springer Verlag.

MacCallum, J. B. (1900) On the muscular architecture and growth of the ventricles of the heart. *Bulletin of the Johns Hopkins Hospital*, **9**, 307-335.

Mall, F. P. (1911) On the muscular architecture of the ventricles of the human heart. *American Journal of Anatomy*, **11**, 211-266.

Masson-Pevet, M., Bleeker, W. K., Mackay, A. J. C., Gros, D. & Bouman, L. N. (1978) Ultrastructural and functional aspects of the rabbit sinoatrial node. In *The Sinus Node*, edited by F. I. M. Bonke, pp 195-211. The Hague: Martinus Nijhoff.

Masuda, M. O. & Paes de Carvalho, A. (1975) Sinoatrial transmission and atrial invasion during normal rhythm in the rabbit heart. *Circulation Research*, **37**, 414-421.

Neufeld, H. N. (1974) Studies of the coronary arteries in children and their relevance to coronary heart disease. *European Journal of Cardiology*, **1**, 335-518.

Odgers, P. N. B. (1938) The development of the pars membranacea septi in the human heart. *Journal of Anatomy*, **72**, 247-259.

Partridge, J. B., Scott, O., Deverall, P. B. & Macartney, F. J. (1975) Visualization and measurement of the main bronchi by tomography as an objective indicator of thoracic situs in congenital heart disease. *Circulation*, **51**, 188-196.

Perloff, J. K. & Roberts, W. C. (1972) The mitral apparatus – functional anatomy of mitral regurgitation. *Circulation*, **46**, 227-239.

Pexieder, T. (1978) Development of the outflow tract of the embryonic heart. In *Morphogenesis and Malformation of the Cardiovascular System*, edited by G. C. Rosenquist & D. Bergsma, pp 29-68. Birth Defects Original Article Series 14.

Raphael, M. J. & Allwork, S. P. (1974) Angiographic anatomy of the left ventricle. *Clinical Radiology*, **25**, 95-105.

Raphael, M. J. & Allwork, S. P. (1976) Angiographic anatomy of the right heart. *Clinical Radiology*, **27**, 265-272.

Raphael, M. J., Hawtin, D. R. & Allwork, S. P. (1979) Angiographic anatomy of the coronary arteries. *British Journal of Surgery*. In press.

Robb, J. S. & Robb, R. C. (1942) The normal heart – anatomy and physiology of the structural units. *American Heart Journal*, **23**, 455-467.

Rosenbaum, M. B., Elizari, M. V. & Lazzari, J. O. (1970) *The Hemiblocks*. Oldsmar, Florida: Tampa Tracings.

Rosenquist, G. C., Clark, E. B., Sweeney, L. S. & McAllister, H. A. (1977) The normal spectrum of mitral and aortic valve discontinuity. *Circulation*, **54**, 298-301.

Spach, M., King, T. D., Barr, R. C., Booz, D. E., Marrow, M. N. & Giddens, S. H. (1969) Electrical potential distribution surrounding the atria during depolarization and repolarization in the dog. *Circulation Research*, **24**, 857-873.

Streeter, G. L. (1945) Developmental horizons in human embryos — description of age group XIII, embryos about 4 or 5 millimetres long, and age group XIV, period of indentation of the lens vesicle. *Contributions to Embryology*, **31**, 27-64.

Tajik, A. J., Seward, J. B., Hagler, D. J., Mair, D. D. & Lie, J. T. (1978) Two dimensional real time ultrasonic imaging of the heart and great vessels. *Mayo Clinic Proceedings*, **53**, 271-303.

Tandler, J. (1913) *Anatomie des Herzens*. Jena: Gustav Fischer.

Tawara, S. (1906) *Das Reizleitungssystem des Saugetierherzens*. Jena: Gustav Fischer.

Thane, G. D. (1894) The heart. In *Quain's Elements of Anatomy, 10th Ed., Vol. 2, Part II*, edited by A. Schafer & G. D. Thane. London: Longmans, Green & Co.

Tranum-Jensen, J. (1975) The ultrastructure of the sensory end-organs (baroreceptors) in the atrial endocardium of young mini-pigs. *Journal of Anatomy*, **119**, 255-275.

Tranum-Jensen, J. & Bojsen-Moller, F. (1973) The ultrastructure of the sinuatrial ring bundle and of the caudal extension of the sinus node in the right atrium of the rabbit heart. *Zeitschrift fur Zellforschung und Mikroskopische Anatomie*, **138**, 97-112.

Van Mierop, L. H. S., Alley, R. D., Kausel, H. W. & Stranahan, A. (1963) Pathogenesis of transposition complexes — 1) embryology of the ventricles and great arteries. *American Journal of Cardiology*, **12**, 216-225.

Van Mierop, L. H. S. & Gessner, I. H. (1972) Pathogenetic mechanisms in congenital cardiovascular malformations. *Progress in Cardiovascular Disease*, **15**, 67-85.

Verduyn Lunel, A. A. (1972) Significance of annulus fibrosus of heart in relation to AV conduction and ventricular activation in cases of Wolff-Parkinson-White syndrome. *British Heart Journal*, **34**, 1267-1271.

Vollebergh, F. E. M. G. & Becker, A. E. (1977) Minor congenital variations of cusp size in tricuspid aortic valves — possible link with isolated aortic stenosis. *British Heart Journal*, **39**, 1006-1011.

Walmsley, R. & Watson, H. (1978) *Clinical Anatomy of the Heart*. Edinburgh: Churchill Livingstone.

Walmsley, T. (1929) The heart. In *Quain's Elements of Anatomy, 11th Ed., Vol. 4, Part III*, edited by E. Sharpey Schafer, J. Symington & T. H. Bryce. London: Longmans, Green & Co.

Wenink, A. C. G. (1974) La formation du septum membranaceum dans le coeur humain. *Bulletin de l'Association des Anatomistes*, **58**, 163-166.

Wenink, A. C. G. (1976) Development of the human cardiac conducting system. *Journal of Anatomy*, **121**, 617-631.

Yamauchi, A. (1969) Innervation of the vertebrate heart as studied with electron microscope. *Archivum Histologicum Japonicum*, **31**, 83-117.

Contents

Foreword   v

Preface   v

Acknowledgements   vi

References   vii

1 The Heart Within the Body   1.1

The Relationships of the Heart   1.2
The Heart in Situ   1.10
    Position of the Heart within the Thorax   1.10
    Cardiac Chambers Relative to the Silhouette   1.13

2 The Atria   2.1

The Morphologically Right Atrium   2.2
The Morphologically Left Atrium   2.12
The Interatrial Septum   2.18
    Differences between Morphologically Right and Left Atria   2.22

3 The Ventricles I   3.1

Introduction   3.2
The Morphologically Right Ventricle   3.12
    The Tricuspid Valve   3.20

4 The Ventricles II   4.1

The Morphologically Left Ventricle   4.2
    The Mitral Valve   4.5
    Differentiation of Morphologically Right and Left Ventricles   4.19
The Interventricular Septum   4.20

5 The Cardiac Skeleton and Musculature   5.1

The Fibrous Skeleton of the Heart   5.2
The Orientation of Fibres within the Ventricular Mass   5.14

6 Cardiac Sub-systems   6.1

The Coronary Circulation   6.2
    The Coronary Arteries   6.2
    The Coronary Veins   6.11
    Histology of Coronary Arteries   6.14
The Conduction System   6.15
    The Sinus Node   6.16
    The Atrioventricular Conduction Tissues   6.19
The Nervous System   6.30
    The Parasympathetic and Vagus Systems   6.30
    The Cardiac Plexus   6.31

7 Clinical Cardiac Anatomy I   7.1
by Sally P. Allwork

Angiographic Anatomy   7.2
    The Angiographic Anatomy of the Coronary Arteries   7.4
    General Morphology   7.4
    Dominance   7.6
    Coronary Anatomy in Radiological Projections   7.7

8 Clinical Cardiac Anatomy II   8.1

Echocardiographic Anatomy   8.2
Scintigraphic Anatomy   8.9
Cardiac Anatomy for the Surgeon   8.12

9 Histology and Ultrastructure   9.1

    Light Microscopy   9.3
    Electron Microscopy   9.5
    Microscopic Innervation   9.11

10 The Development of the Heart   10.1

    Early Formation of the Heart Tube   10.3
    Septation of the Atria   10.7
    Development and Septation of the Ventricles   10.12
    Formation of the Great Arteries   10.19
    Development of the Coronary Arteries   10.22
    Development of the Conduction System and Fibrous Skeleton   10.23

1 The Heart Within the Body

The Relationships of the Heart
The Heart in Situ

The Relationships of the Heart

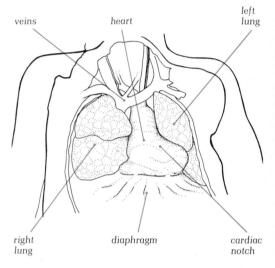

Fig. 1.1 *Removal of the anterior chest wall including the rib cage showing the in situ position of the heart and its relation to the lungs.*

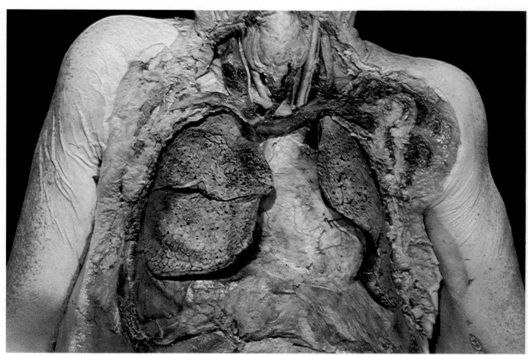

The heart lies in the mediastinum with its long axis orientated from the hypogastrium towards the right shoulder. It is covered on its anterior surface by the overlapping right and left lungs contained in their pleural sacs, apart from a small bare area *(fig. 1.1)*, the whole being contained within the thoracic cavity. The heart is described as having a base and an apex *(fig. 1.2)*. The base is formed by the atria and great arteries which lie in the mediastinum between the lung hila. The apex extends out towards the left hypogastrium *(fig. 1.2)*. The heart is tethered to adjacent structures at its base by the arteries and veins which leave and enter its chambers. It is enclosed in a fibrous sac, the pericardium, which is firmly attached to the diaphragm, providing further anchorage for the ventricular mass of the heart *(fig. 1.2)*.

When viewed from its apex, the ventricular mass is seen to be pyramidal in shape. Its surfaces are the anterior sternocostal surface, the inferior diaphragmatic surface and the more rounded superior surface which abuts against the lingula of the left lung. The edge between sternocostal and diaphragmatic surfaces is sharp *(fig. 1.3)* and is termed the acute margin. The edge between the sternocostal and pulmonary surfaces is much more rounded, and is termed the obtuse margin *(figs. 1.2 & 1.3)*. The ventricular mass extends out into the left hemithorax, indenting the left lung *(fig. 1.1)* and being separated from it by the pericardial cavity.

At the base of the heart, the two great veins descend and ascend anteriorly and to the right to enter the right atrium. The intrathoracic

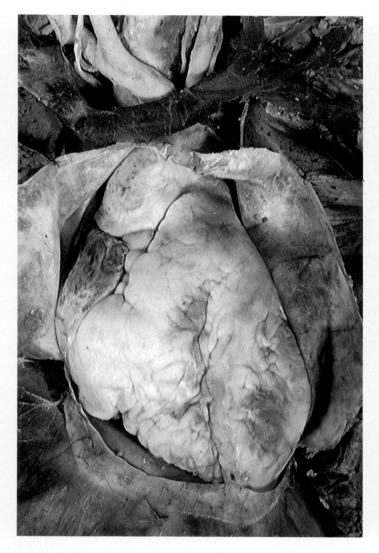

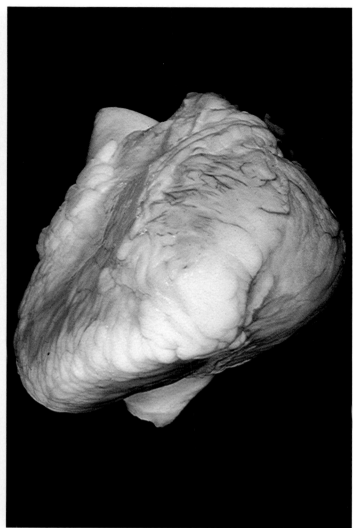

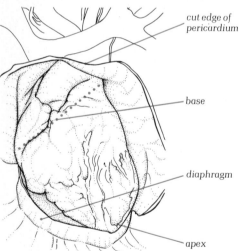

cut edge of
pericardium

base

diaphragm

apex

Fig. 1.2   The pericardial cavity shown in
fig. 1.1 opened to show the orientation of the
heart.

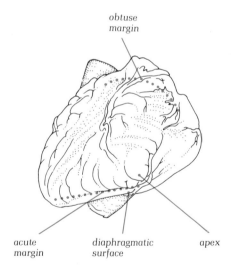

obtuse
margin

acute
margin

diaphragmatic
surface

apex

Fig. 1.3   The isolated heart viewed from its
apex showing the acute and obtuse margins.

segment of the inferior vena cava is a
short channel, ascending from the
substance of the liver to pierce the
diaphragm and enter the floor of the
right atrium (fig. 1.2). The superior
vena cava is a much longer channel,
being formed by the union of right
and left brachiocephalic veins before
descending (fig. 1.4), receiving the
azygos vein en route, to reach the
upper margin of the right atrium
(fig. 1.5).

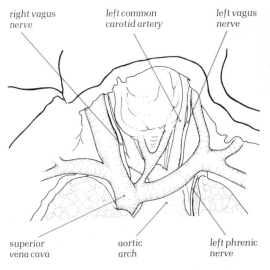

right vagus nerve

left common carotid artery

left vagus nerve

superior vena cava

aortic arch

left phrenic nerve

Fig. 1.4   Dissection of the root of the neck showing the anterior venous structures, the deeper arterial structures and the important nerves.

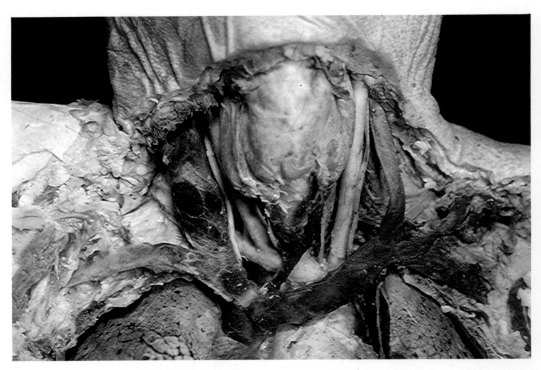

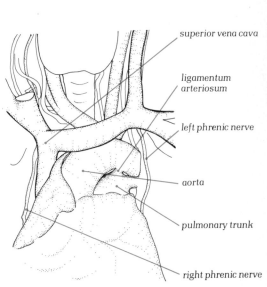

superior vena cava

ligamentum arteriosum

left phrenic nerve

aorta

pulmonary trunk

right phrenic nerve

Fig. 1.5   Dissection showing the junction of veins and arteries of the heart and the relationships of the phrenic nerves. Note that the aorta is to the right of the pulmonary trunk.

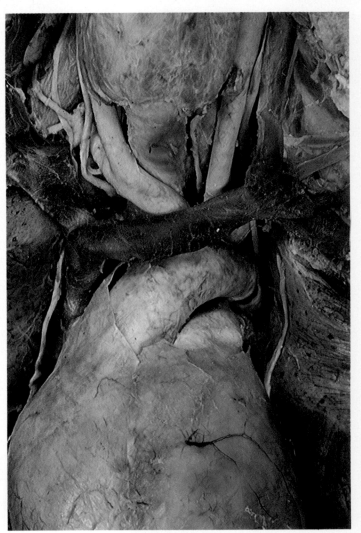

The great arteries leave the left side of the cardiac base, the pulmonary trunk being anterior and left-sided in relation to the aorta (fig. 1.5). Having emerged from the ventricular mass, the trunk passes posteriorly, dividing into right and left pulmonary arteries which pass into the lung hila. The right pulmonary artery gives rise to an artery to the upper lobe of the right lung before embedding itself within the lung hilum. This does not occur on

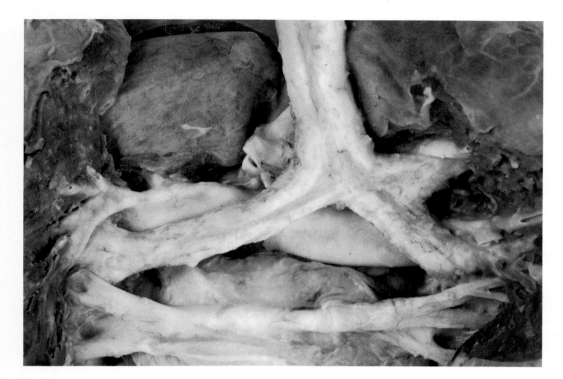

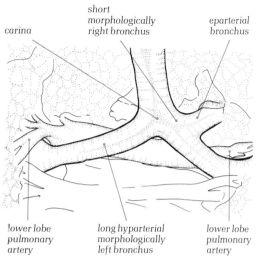

Fig. 1.6   *Posterior view of the bronchi showing their relationship to the pulmonary arteries. The morphologically right main bronchus (to the right as viewed here) is half the length of the morphologically left bronchus.*

the left. The aorta swings upwards from the midportion of the cardiac base, and as it ascends it curves at first to the right, then inclines upwards, leftwards and backwards to cross over the right side of the pulmonary bifurcation before descending to the left of the vertebral column and passing down through the thorax to exit between the crura of the diaphragm. As the arch of the aorta swings backwards it gives off the arterial branches to the head and neck, namely the brachiocephalic trunk (which soon divides into right subclavian and common carotid arteries), the left common carotid and left subclavian arteries. The arteries ascend lying posterior to their companion veins (*fig. 1.5*), the veins running in towards the heart to join the brachiocephalic veins.

Extending down into the thorax behind the head and neck arteries is the trachea, which bifurcates into the right and left bronchi at the level of the aortic arch. The two bronchi run down towards the lung hila, curling beneath the branches of the pulmonary artery as they do so. There is an important difference in the morphology of the bronchi which relates to the different branching pattern of right and left pulmonary arteries (*fig. 1.6*). The right main

bronchus gives off its first main branch to the upper lobe of the right lung before it is crossed by the right pulmonary artery extending into the lung to supply the middle and lower lobes. The bronchus to the upper lobe therefore arises above and posterior to the main right pulmonary, and is termed an eparterial (above the artery) bronchus. It is accompanied to the upper lobe by an early-rising branch from the right main pulmonary artery. In contrast to this arrangement, the left main pulmonary artery crosses over the left main bronchus before it divides into upper and lower lobe bronchi. The bronchus to the left upper lobe is consequently an hyparterial (below the artery) bronchus. Because of this asymmetric branching pattern, the morphologically left bronchus is a long bronchus, being approximately twice the length of the morphologically right main bronchus. This provides a radiological sign of considerable significance in children with congenital heart disease, since it permits the determination of atrial *situs*, the position of the atrial chambers (*Partridge et al., 1975*). Having branched, the bronchi run into the lung hila between the more anterior branches of the pulmonary arteries and the posterior branches of the pulmonary veins (*fig. 1.6*).

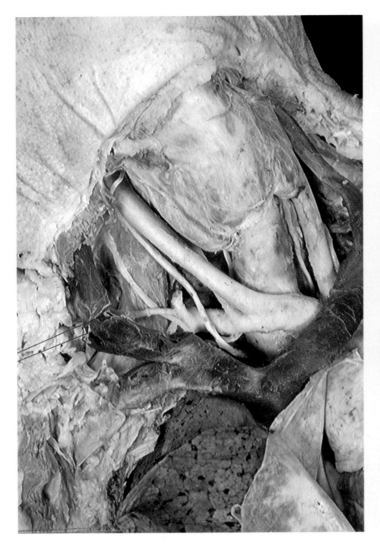

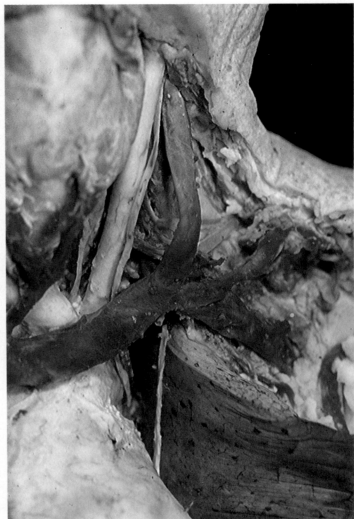

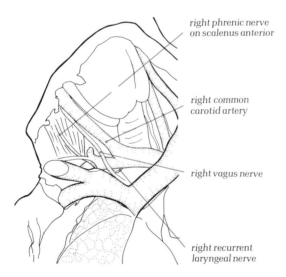

right phrenic nerve
on scalenus anterior

right common
carotid artery

right vagus nerve

right recurrent
laryngeal nerve

Fig. 1.7   The right side of the root of the neck
showing the phrenic nerve and the right
recurrent laryngeal nerve passing round the
right subclavian artery.

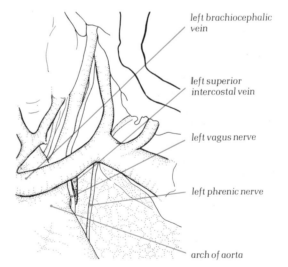

left brachiocephalic
vein

left superior
intercostal vein

left vagus nerve

left phrenic nerve

arch of aorta

Fig. 1.8   The left side of the root of the neck
showing the relationships of the left vagus
nerve and the left phrenic nerve to the arch of
the aorta and the superior intercostal vein.

The pulmonary veins run inwards from the hila to enter the posterior aspect of the cardiac base. Branches from upper and lower lobes of right and left lungs pass centripetally to enter the four corners of the posterior left atrium. Also running through the thorax, posterior to the trachea and to the right of the aortic arch and descending aorta, is the oesophagus. Immediately below the tracheal bifurcation the oesophagus is related to the posterior wall of the left atrium, running behind this chamber to enter the abdomen through the right crus of the diaphragm.

Also running down through the mediastinum and bearing important relationships to the arterial channels and the heart are two pairs of important nerves, the phrenic nerves and the vagus nerves. The phrenic nerves, branches of the cervical plexus, originate in the neck and enter the thoracic inlet on the surface of the scalenus anterior muscle (figs. 1.7 & 1.8) lying behind the prevertebral

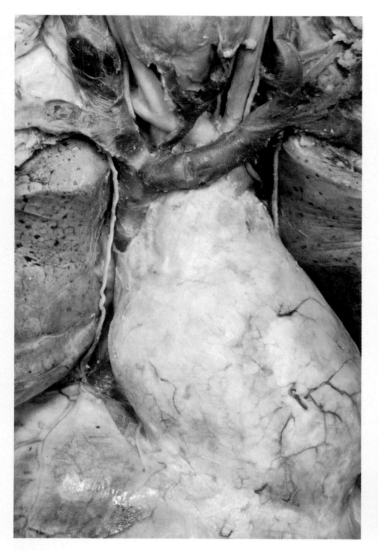

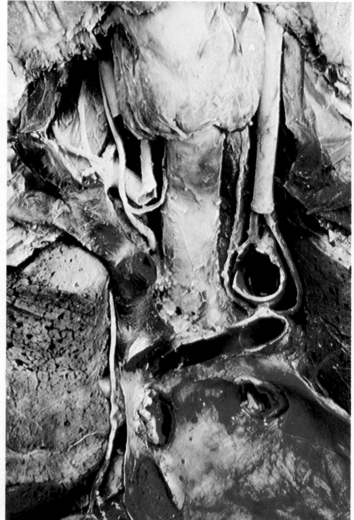

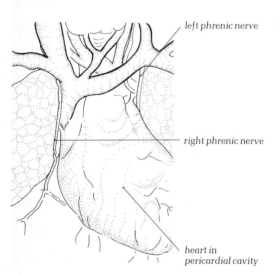

left phrenic nerve

right phrenic nerve

*heart in
pericardial cavity*

Fig. 1.9   *View of the heart in situ showing
the relationships of the right and left phrenic
nerves to the pericardium.*

right vagus nerve

*right subclavian
artery*

*right recurrent
laryngeal nerve*

*left recurrent
laryngeal nerve*

left vagus nerve

*ligamentum
arteriosum*

Fig. 1.10   *The relationships of the recurrent
laryngeal nerves. The right nerve recurs
round the subclavian artery whereas the left
nerve recurs round the ligamentum arteriosum.*

fascia. The right phrenic nerve then runs along the right brachiocephalic vein and the superior vena cava, and extends across the pericardium on the right margin of the heart to reach the diaphragm *(fig. 1.9)*. The left phrenic nerve passes behind the left subclavian vein as it enters the thorax and crosses behind the internal mammary artery to run over the aortic arch and pulmonary artery before passing over the left margin of the pericardial sac to reach the left cupula of the diaphragm. The vagus nerves, the tenth cranial nerves, are more intimately related to the arteries of the head and neck. The right vagus nerve enters the thoracic cavity on the anterior surface of the right common carotid artery and immediately gives off the right recurrent laryngeal nerve, which passes beneath the right subclavian artery and ascends to pass back up into the neck *(fig. 1.7)*. Also recurring around the right subclavian artery is the ansa subclavia, an important autonomic

1.7

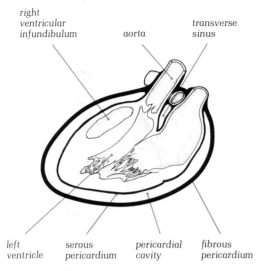

Fig. 1.11 Diagram showing the disposition of the fibrous and serous layers of the pericardium.

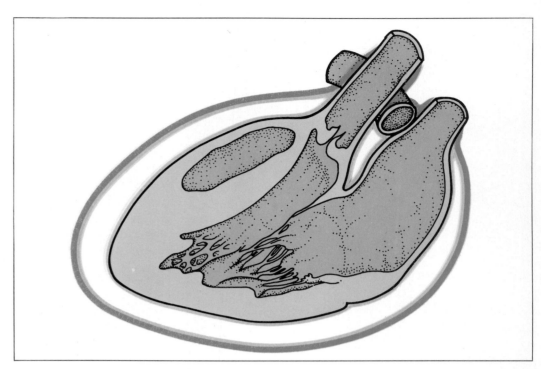

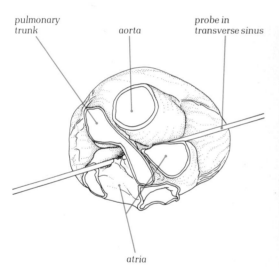

Fig. 1.12 The isolated heart removed from the dissection shown in figs. 1.10 and 1.13. The transverse sinus in the inner heart curvature is indicated by the probe.

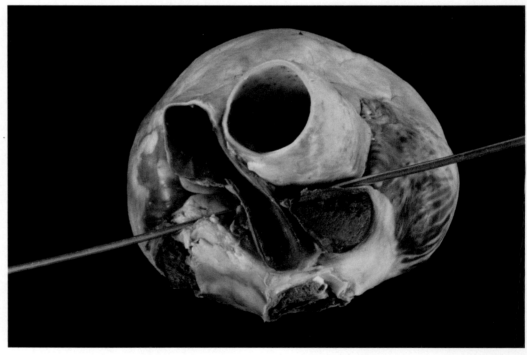

nerve loop from the stellate ganglion which conveys sympathetic fibres to the head, particularly the iris. The right vagus nerve, having given off the recurrent laryngeal nerve, passes along the brachiocephalic trunk and behind the union of right and left brachiocephalic veins (fig. 1.10). It then angles backwards across the trachea and runs onto the oesophagus behind the pulmonary hilum, intermingling with the left vagus to

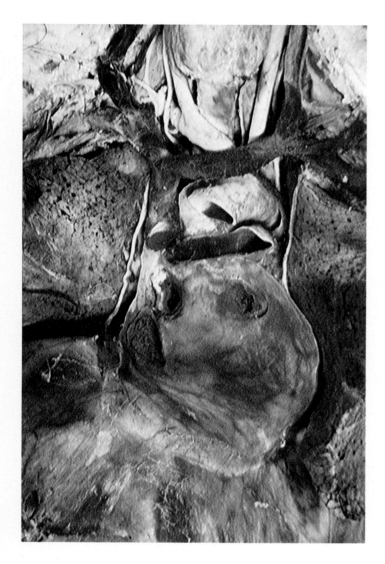

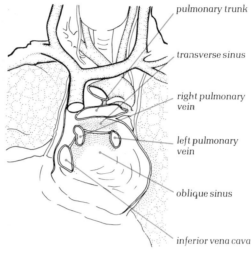

pulmonary trunk

transverse sinus

right pulmonary vein

left pulmonary vein

oblique sinus

inferior vena cava

Fig. 1.13 Dissection of the bed of the pericardium showing the relationship of the oblique and transverse sinuses.

form the pulmonary plexus. From there it extends backwards over the lung hilum, running along the pericardium and continuing down the oesophagus, with which structure it passes through the diaphragm. The left vagus nerve enters the thoracic cavity between the left common carotid and subclavian arteries, close to the phrenic nerve (fig. 1.8). As the phrenic nerve runs down towards the pulmonary trunk, the left vagus angles back towards the pulmonary hilum, the left superior intercostal vein passing between the nerves as it crosses the aortic arch (fig. 1.8). The vagus then continues backwards to pass behind the pulmonary hilum and joins the oesophagus. As it passes the lower edge of the aortic arch, it gives off the left recurrent laryngeal nerve, which recurs round the ligamentum arteriosum, passing round the aorta as well, to reascend through the thoracic inlet (fig. 1.10).

As indicated, the heart in its mediastinal position is enclosed in a firm fibrous sac, the fibrous

pericardium, which contains a much thinner inner sac, the serous pericardium. The fibrous pericardium clothes the apex of the heart like a bag and encloses it up to the base, where it merges with the arterial vessels entering and leaving the heart, clothing these vessels for about 1-2 cms before merging with their walls (fig. 1.2). The fibrous pericardium clothing the diaphragmatic surface of the heart is firmly attached to the diaphragm in the area of the central tendon, otherwise diaphragm and pericardium are connected only by loose fibroareolar tissue. The sac is also attached to the posterior surface of the sternum by superior and inferior sternopericardial ligaments. Elsewhere, the pericardium is covered by the pleural cavities, apart from the bare area where the pericardium abuts directly against the anterior chest wall (fig. 1.1.). The serous pericardium is a much thinner double envelope which encloses the heart as a double film, the pericardial

fluid being present between the two serous surfaces. The inner layer of the serous pericardium is densely adherent to the surface of the cardiac chambers and is the epicardium. The outer, parietal layer is attached to the fibrous pericardium. Thus, effectively, the pericardial fluid circulates between fibrous pericardium and heart wall, except that each of these is covered by a layer of the serous pericardium (fig. 1.11). The two layers of serous pericardium are continuous with each other at the entrances and exits of the vessels; but because of the arrangement of the vessels, two recesses or sinuses are present within the pericardial cavity. One, the transverse sinus, is in the inner curvature of the heart (fig. 1.12) and is between the anterior surface of the atrial chambers and the posterior surface of the great arteries. The other recess, the oblique sinus, is behind the left atrium and is limited by the reflection of pericardium off the four pulmonary veins and the inferior vena cava (fig. 1.13).

The Heart in Situ

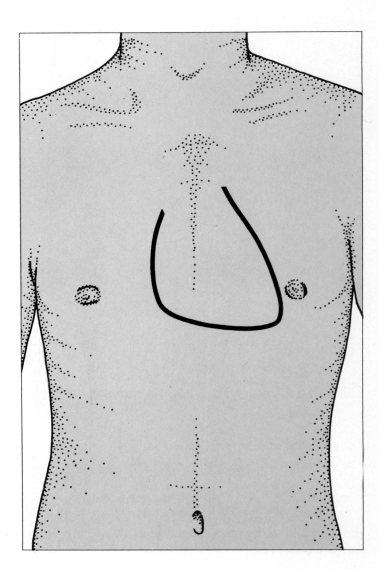

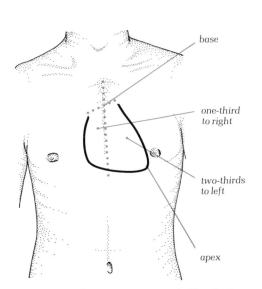

Fig. 1.14   The position occupied by the heart within the mediastinum. Note that two-thirds of the heart is to the left and one-third to the right of the midline.

One of the major hurdles to the understanding of cardiac anatomy and to relating it to clinical situations is the penchant of morphologists to illustrate and describe the heart sitting upright on its apex. To be of most value to the clinician and the echocardiographer, the heart must be described as it lies in the body. If described in this position, information should also be of value to the surgeon; since, although cardiac surgeons tend to view the heart from somewhat non-anatomic angles, they are restricted in their approach by the fact that the heart is tethered by the adjacent organs – a feature which need not and does not curtail the morphologist! Therefore, we will first describe the positions the heart may occupy relative to the surface markings of the thorax, then describe the relationship of cardiac chambers within the cardiac silhouette. Finally, we will consider the detailed anatomy of the heart in relation to the mediastinum and describe its own landmarks.

Position of the Heart within the Thorax

In its normal position, the heart occupies the inferior part of the mediastinum with two-thirds of its bulk to the left of the midline (fig. 1.14). Although usually described in terms of a triangle, the cardiac silhouette is more trapezoidal in shape. Its lower border lies on the diaphragm; its upper border, termed the base, lies behind the sternum. Its right margin is more or less vertical but its left margin projects in point-like fashion towards the left hypogastrium and is termed the apex (fig. 1.14). The ribs provide good markers for charting the silhouette, and give some guide as to whether or not cardiac position is 'normal'. The base of the heart is at the level of the second and third costal cartilages, hidden behind the sternum. The second costal cartilage is easily

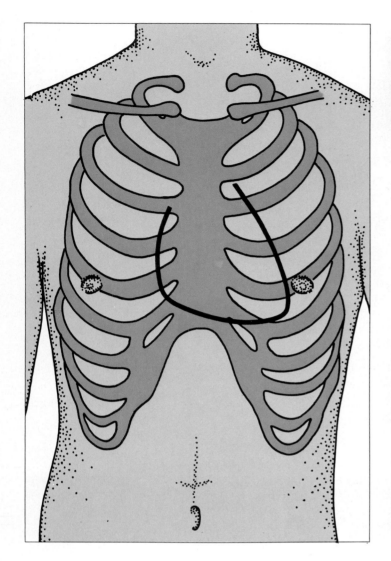

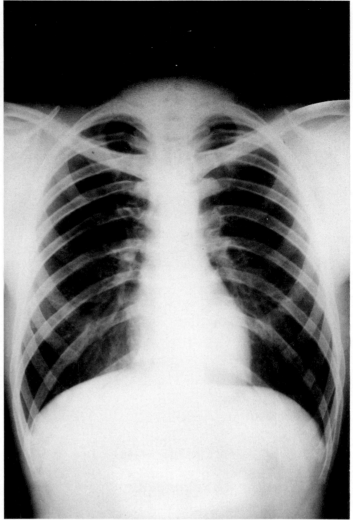

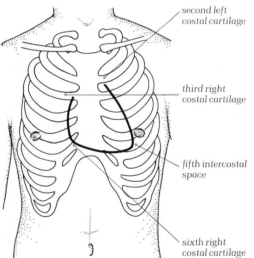

second left
costal cartilage

third right
costal cartilage

fifth intercostal
space

sixth right
costal cartilage

Fig. 1.15   The position of the heart with
reference to the ribs and sternum.

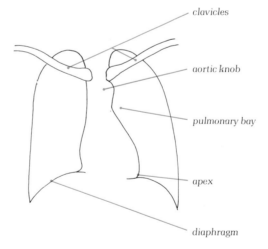

clavicles

aortic knob

pulmonary bay

apex

diaphragm

Fig. 1.16   A typical chest radiograph from a
person of normal build, showing the position
of the cardiac silhouette.

identified since it articulates with the
sternum at the sternal angle (angle of
Louis, *fig. 1.15*). The body of the heart
extending to the apex is behind the
fourth and fifth interspaces and the
normal position of the apex is usually
taken to be the fifth intercostal space
in the midclavicular line. The lower
border of the silhouette is directly on
the diaphragm and is a horizontal line
in the area of the sixth rib, extending
across to the sixth costal cartilage at
the right border of the sternum. The
right border of the heart is then a
slightly curved line between the right
sixth and third cartilages which peeps
out behind the right border of the
sternum. These landmarks are best
appreciated by viewing a chest
radiograph *(fig. 1.16)*. Although the

1.11

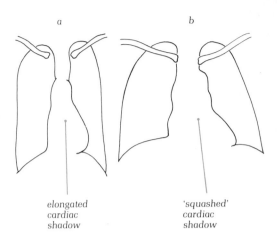

elongated cardiac shadow

'squashed' cardiac shadow

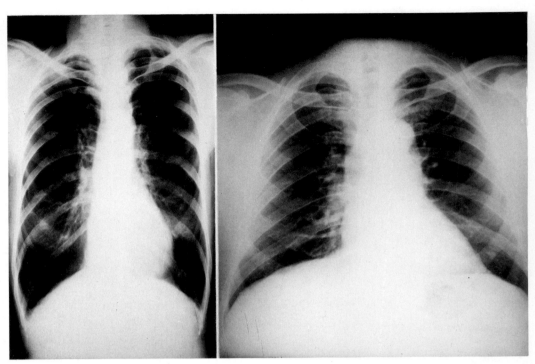

Fig. 1.17 Chest radiographs showing the effect of build on the cardiac silhouette, fig. 1.17a from a tall thin individual and fig. 1.17b from a thick-set individual.

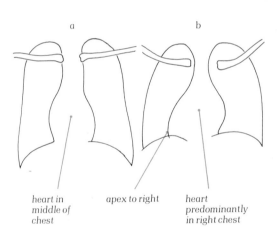

heart in middle of chest

apex to right

heart predominantly in right chest

Fig. 1.18 Chest radiographs showing alternative positions which may be occupied by the heart within the chest. Fig. 1.18a is a midline heart (mesocardial) and fig. 1.18b is a heart in the right chest (dextrocardial).

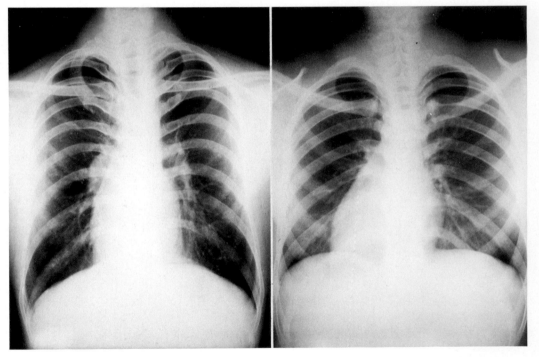

above configuration is described as 'normal', many normal persons have different cardiac silhouettes. Shape has a considerable effect. Tall thin individuals tend to have elongated cardiac silhouettes while thick-set people have squat silhouettes (compare figs. 1.17a & 1.17b). These factors must be taken into consideration when evaluating the shape of the heart as regards normality. Similarly, the position of the heart may vary from one individual to another. Although the cardiac silhouette usually has two-thirds of its bulk to the left of the midline of the chest (so-called laevocardia, fig. 1.16), the silhouette may be placed more directly in the middle of the thorax (mesocardia, fig. 1.18a) or it may be situated with its greater part in the right chest (dextrocardia, fig. 1.18b). Because the position of the heart conveys no information regarding its internal architecture, our preference is to reserve the terms laevocardia, mesocardia and dextrocardia to describe only the position of the heart within the chest, irrespective of the

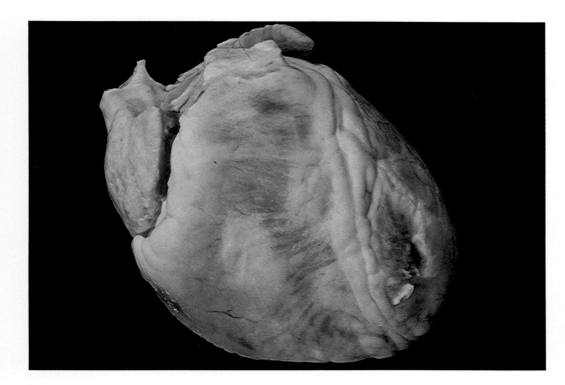

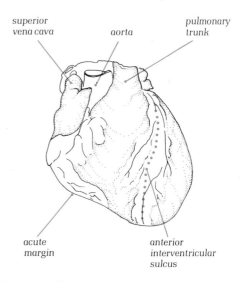

Fig. 1.19 The heart in its in situ position showing the position of the superior vena cava and pulmonary artery and the anterior interventricular sulcus.

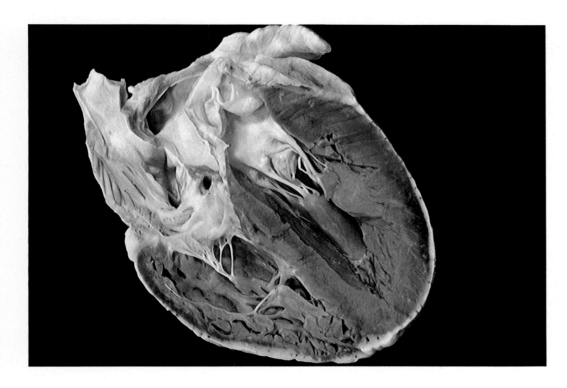

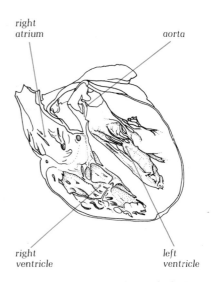

Fig. 1.20 Sagittal section through the heart in its in situ position showing that the right ventricle is inferior to as well as to the right of the left ventricle.

Cardiac Chambers Relative to the Silhouette

Having established the 'normal' position of the heart relative to the frontal view of the chest, it is then necessary to locate chamber position within the silhouette. Examination of an isolated heart orientated in its *in situ* position shows that the superior vena cava enters the upper border of the right margin of the base while the pulmonary artery exits from the left upper border (fig. 1.19). Furthermore, the anterior interventricular sulcus descends to the apex almost parallel to and close to the left cardiac margin. As the heart lies *in situ* then, the so-called 'right-sided' chambers are anterior to their 'left-sided' counterparts. The right ventricular trabecular zone lies in part inferior to its left-sided companion (fig. 1.20). The anterior

direction of the apex or its chamber connexions. However, there is no consensus regarding the use of these terms, and some authors base complex systematizations of congenital malformations on the use of laevocardia, dextrocardia and mesocardia (*Lev et al., 1968; Lev et al., 1971; Liberthson et al., 1973*).

1.13

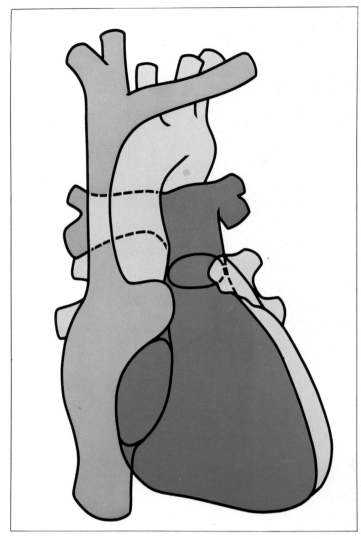

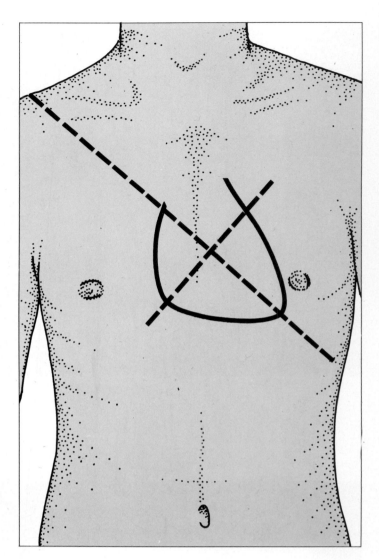

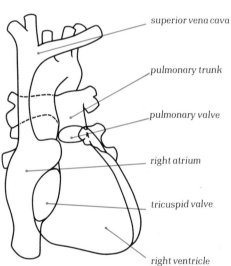

superior vena cava

pulmonary trunk

pulmonary valve

right atrium

tricuspid valve

right ventricle

Fig. 1.21   The positions of the right heart chambers relative to the cardiac silhouette.

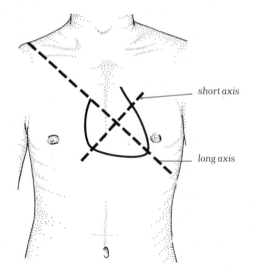

short axis

long axis

Fig. 1.22   The orientation of the long axis of the heart and atrioventricular junction relative to the vertical and horizontal planes.

projection of the cardiac silhouette is therefore composed for the most part of the right atrium and the right ventricle *(fig. 1.21)*. The right atrium forms the entire right border of the silhouette, the entrance of the superior vena cava forming its top and the entrance of the inferior vena cava its bottom. The right lower

border of the silhouette marks the inferior point of the atrioventricular sulcus and is where the right atrium joins the right ventricle *(figs. 1.16 & 1.19)*. The right ventricle forms the horizontal inferior border of the silhouette to the apex, where the left ventricular apex protrudes beyond it. The left border is the only part where

left-sided structures contribute, these being the left margin of the left ventricle and the left atrial appendage *(fig. 1.19)*. However, above the appendage a 'right-sided' structure again forms the left border of the heart, namely, the pulmonary artery. Thus, although the aorta arises from the left ventricle, it is to the right of

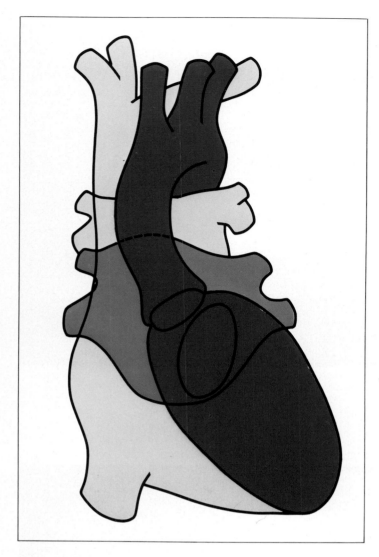

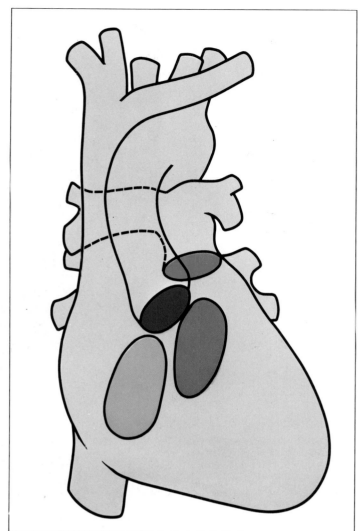

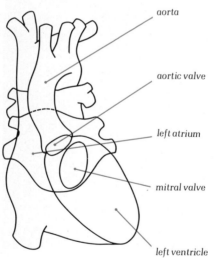

aorta

aortic valve

left atrium

mitral valve

left ventricle

Fig. 1.23 The positions of the left heart chambers relative to the cardiac silhouette.

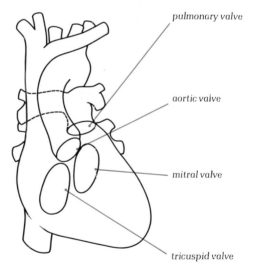

pulmonary valve

aortic valve

mitral valve

tricuspid valve

Fig. 1.24 The position of the cardiac valves relative to the cardiac silhouette.

the pulmonary artery at their ventricular origins. The long axis of the heart extends from the left hypochondrium towards the right shoulder, and because of this, the atrioventricular junction is closer to the vertical than the horizontal plane (figs. 1.19 & 1.22). From these facts, we can enunciate two basic 'rules' of normal cardiac anatomy: firstly, that right-sided structures (morphologically right atrium and ventricle) lie mostly anterior to their left-sided counterparts; and secondly, that atrial chambers are for the most part to the right of their corresponding ventricles. In terms of the cardiac silhouette, and hence their position, the left-sided chambers are posterior. The left atrium is the most posterior structure of the heart, lying directly adjacent to the oesophagus in the bifurcation of the trachea. It is overlaid anteriorly by part of the right atrium, the ascending aorta and the pulmonary trunk (fig. 1.23). Only its atrial appendage pokes round the

1.15

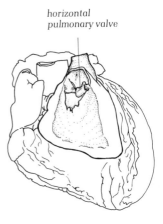

horizontal
pulmonary valve

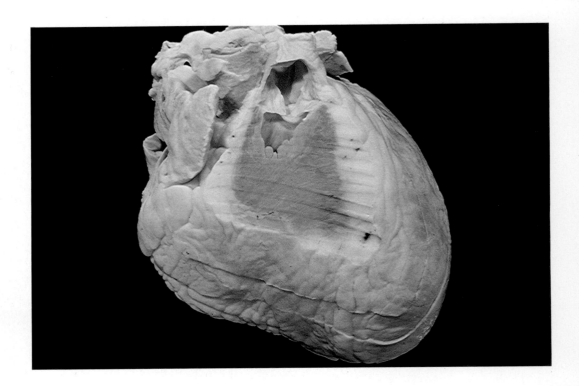

Fig. 1.25   Sagittal section through the heart
in its in situ position showing the horizontal
position of the pulmonary valve.

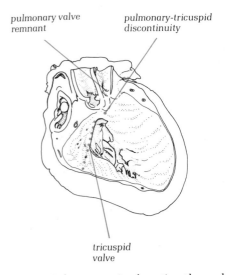

pulmonary valve
remnant

pulmonary-tricuspid
discontinuity

tricuspid
valve

Fig. 1.26   A deeper sagittal section through
the same heart as in fig. 1.25 showing the
position of the tricuspid valve.

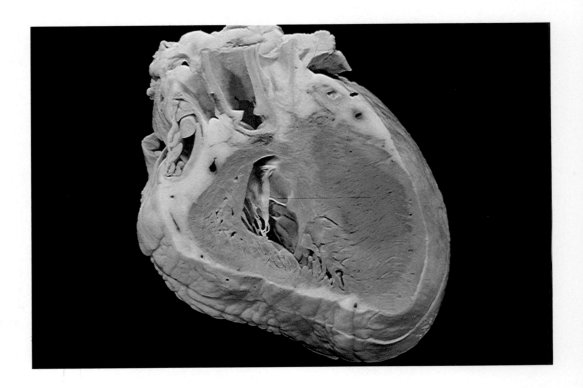

pulmonary trunk to form part of the
silhouette (fig. 1.19). The left ventricle
is behind the outflow tract of the
right ventricle but does reach the left
edge of the cardiac silhouette
(fig. 1.23). The aorta is very much a
deep structure, springing from

between the right atrium and the
pulmonary trunk and only becoming
part of the silhouette as its arch
reaches upwards and backwards
(fig. 1.16).
    A further important consideration
in elucidating cardiac anatomy is to

place the positions of the four cardiac
valves within the cardiac silhouette.
Since the atrioventricular junction is
oblique, with its axis veering towards
the vertical (fig. 1.22), the valves will
occupy a similar orientation. The most
superior valve is the pulmonary valve

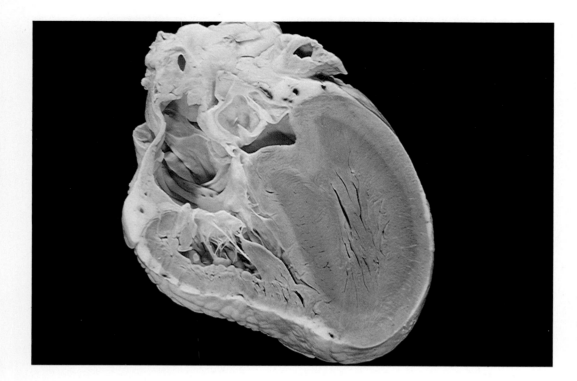

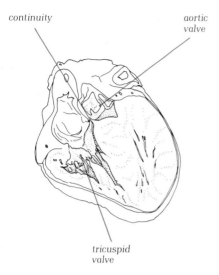

Fig. 1.27   *Further sagittal section through the same heart as in figs. 1.25 and 1.26 showing the relationship of the aortic, tricuspid and pulmonary valves.*

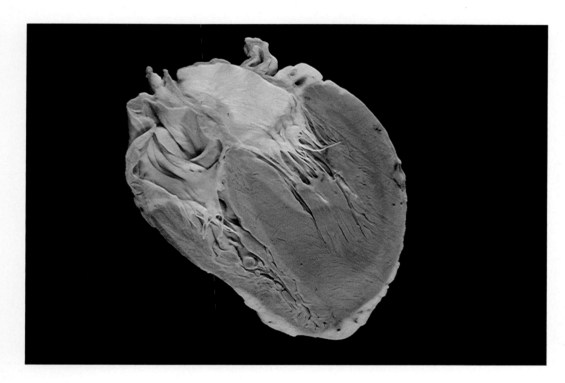

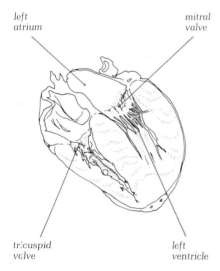

Fig. 1.28   *Further sagittal section of the heart shown in figs. 1.25 through 1.27 showing that the mitral valve is the most posterior of the four cardiac valves.*

which is a horizontal structure lying behind the third costal cartilage (*figs. 1.24 & 1.25*). Posterior to the pulmonary valve and falling downwards and away from it is the aortic valve, which lies above the tricuspid valve, the latter continuing the downward arc from obtuse to acute margins of the silhoutte (*figs. 1.26 & 1.27*). The mitral valve is more posterior and lies behind the aortic valve, overlapping the tricuspid valve (*fig. 1.28*). Understanding the precise position of the aortic valve is of particular importance. It is posterior to the right ventricle, occupying a position more or less in the middle of the heart. This is best appreciated by viewing a section of the atrioventricular junction from the right shoulder (*fig. 1.29*). This illustrates the 'wedge position' of the aorta, the key to full knowledge of cardiac anatomy.

1.17

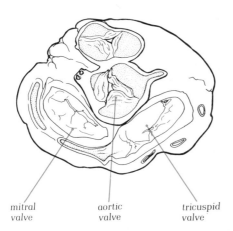

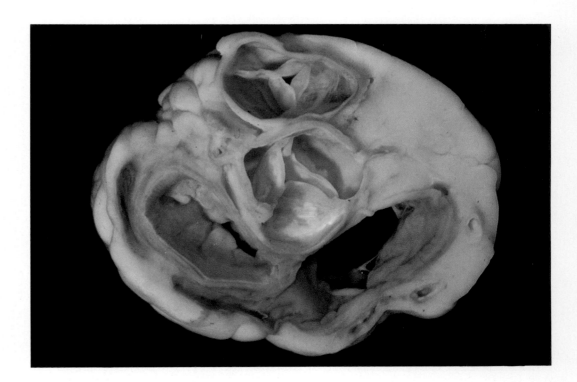

mitral
valve

aortic
valve

tricuspid
valve

Fig. 1.29   Dissection of the atrioventricular
junction viewed from the atrial aspect
showing that the aortic valve occupies a
position in the centre of the heart wedged
between the mitral and tricuspid valves.

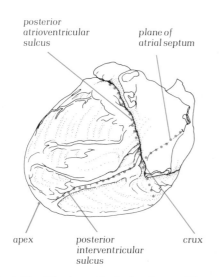

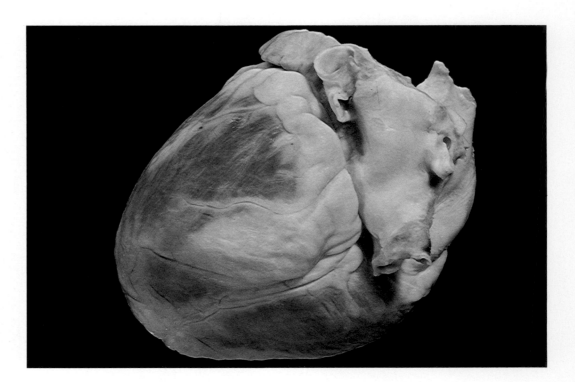

posterior
atrioventricular
sulcus

plane of
atrial septum

apex

posterior
interventricular
sulcus

crux

Fig. 1.30   The heart in its in situ position
viewed from behind showing the orientation
of the posterior atrioventricular and
interventricular sulci and the crux of the
heart.

Having considered the position of the heart *in situ*, we can now re-emphasize its own landmarks in this orientation. The anterior atrioventricular sulcus as described (fig. 1.19) runs from the right inferior to the left superior margins of the cardiac silhouette, and is closer to the vertical than the horizontal plane. Extending down from just beneath the superior margin of the

atrioventricular sulcus is the anterior interventricular sulcus which runs obliquely along the obtuse margin of the heart to the apex (fig. 1.19). The posterior interventricular sulcus is seen on the diaphragmatic surface of the heart, and requires a posterior approach to appreciate its *in situ* position (fig. 1.30). It runs from the midpoint of the posterior

atrioventricular sulcus as viewed from behind and again extends outwards and leftwards to the cardiac apex. The point at which the posterior interventricular sulcus leaves the atrioventricular sulcus is also the point at which the line of the atrial septum crosses the atrioventricular sulcus. This crossing point is termed the crux of the heart (fig. 1.30).

2 The Atria

The Morphologically Right Atrium
The Morphologically Left Atrium
The Interatrial Septum

The Morphologically Right Atrium

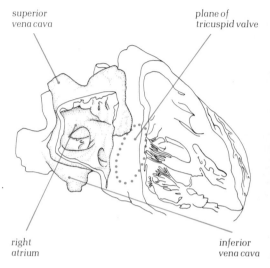

Fig. 2.1   *The heart in its in situ position dissected to show the position of the right atrium and the right ventricle.*

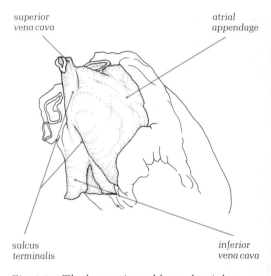

Fig. 2.2   *The heart viewed from the right showing how the great veins open into the posterior part of the right atrial chamber. The anterior part, the atrial appendage, is seen extending round the aorta.*

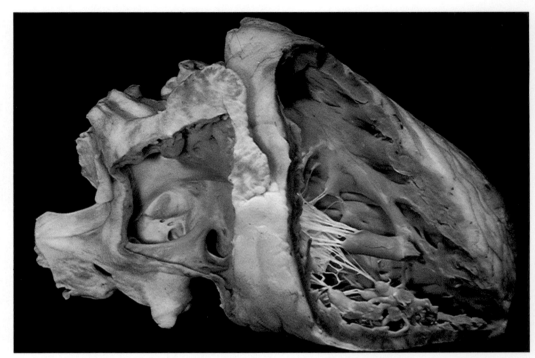

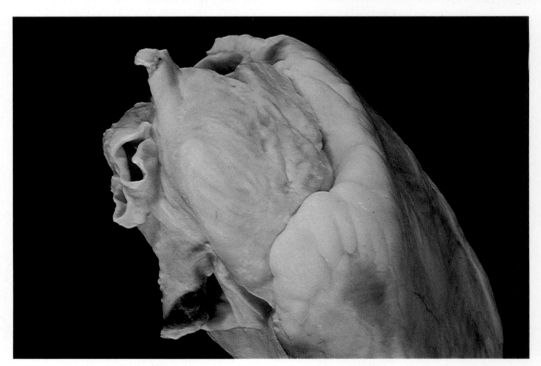

In the normal heart, this structure forms the rightward and anterior part of the cardiac mass, overlapping the right hand margin of the left atrium and communicating with the right ventricle to its right side (fig. 2.1). Externally, the chamber consists of a posterior part which receives the superior and inferior venae cavae, termed the sinus venarum (fig. 2.2) and an anterior part which extends forwards in pouch-like fashion to encircle the right border of the aorta, the right atrial appendage* (fig. 2.3). The border between the two is marked by a groove, the sulcus terminalis (fig. 2.2) which is variably developed and in some hearts may be

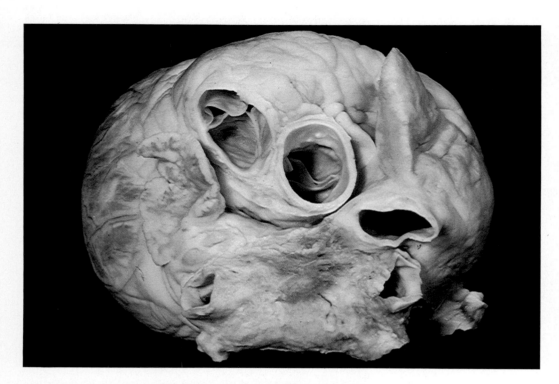

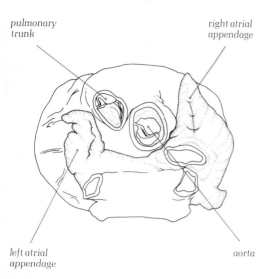

pulmonary
trunk

right atrial
appendage

left atrial
appendage

aorta

Fig. 2.3   The heart viewed from above
showing how the atrial appendages encircle
the roots of the great arteries.

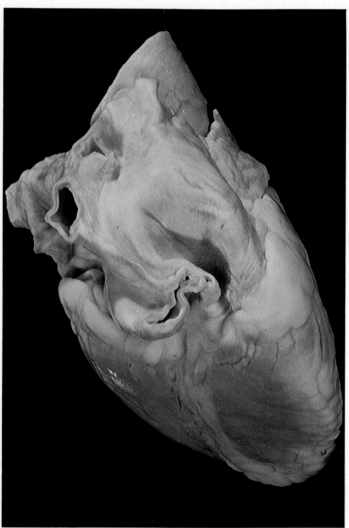

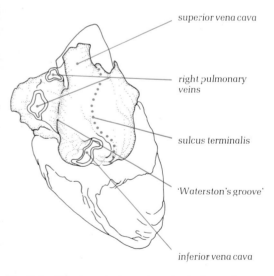

superior vena cava

right pulmonary
veins

sulcus terminalis

'Waterston's groove'

inferior vena cava

Fig. 2.4   The heart viewed posteriorly and
from the right showing the groove between
the pulmonary veins and right atrium.

inconspicuous. The left hand margin
of the right atrium is marked
posteriorly by the groove between the
superior vena cava and the right
pulmonary veins (fig. 2.4). Beneath the
groove, the left border of the inferior
vena cava is in the same plane as the
atrial septum, running inferiorly to
the crux cordis. Superiorly, the roof of
the atrium curves posteriorly behind
the aorta, a small groove sometimes
being seen at the site of the septum, to
become continuous with the left
atrial wall (fig. 2.3).

*Although the Nomina Anatomica terms this part of the
chamber simply the 'auricle', the term 'atrial appendage' is
in widespread clinical use and is preferred for this reason.

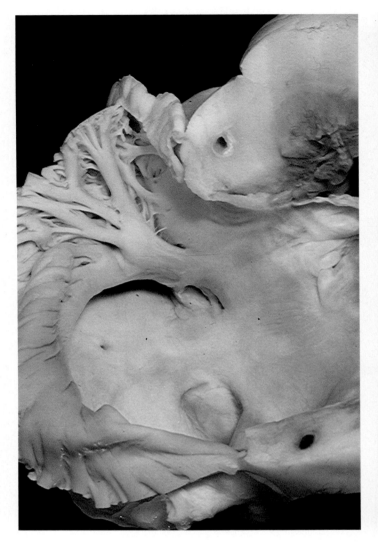

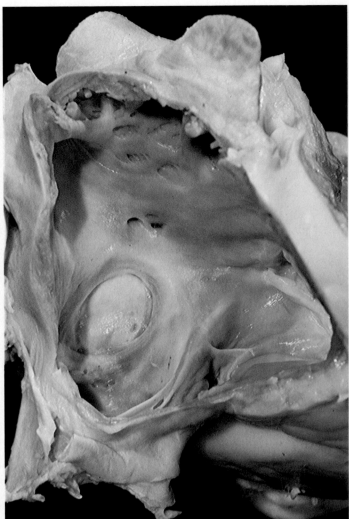

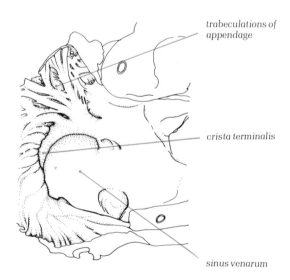

trabeculations of
appendage

crista terminalis

sinus venarum

Fig. 2.5   Dissection of the right atrium
viewed from the front showing the crista
terminalis separating the posterior smooth-
walled sinus venarum and the trabeculated
atrial appendage.

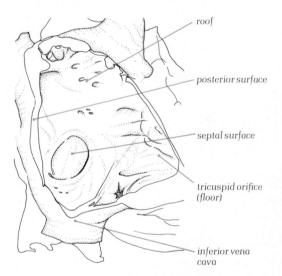

roof

posterior surface

septal surface

tricuspid orifice
(floor)

inferior vena
cava

Fig. 2.6   The right atrium viewed from the
right following removal of the parietal wall
and showing its surfaces.

When the atrium is opened, the
distinction between the posterior
smooth-walled sinus venarum and the
anterior trabeculated appendage is
much more readily apparent (fig. 2.5).
The junction between the two is
marked by a well-formed muscle
bundle, the crista terminalis (fig. 2.5).
The trabeculae tend to run at right
angles to the crista. The inside of the
right atrial chamber presents a
posterior surface, a septal surface, a

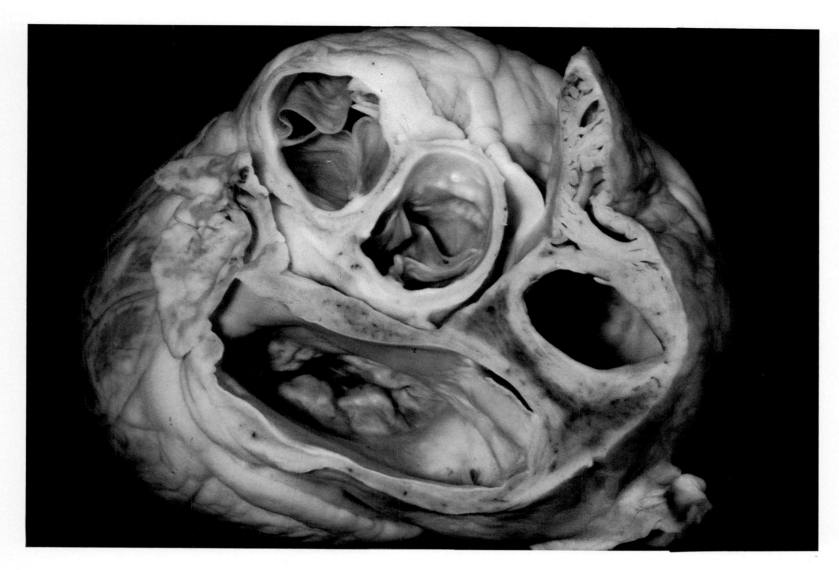

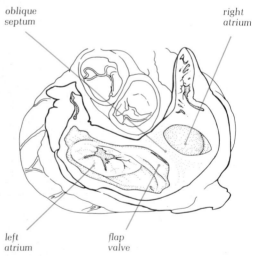

Fig. 2.7　Section through the short axis of the
atrial chambers showing oblique orientation
of the atrial septum.

roof and an anterior surface. The floor
of the chamber can be considered as
the tricuspid valve orifice orientated
obliquely to the right (fig. 2.6)
although the inferior vena cava opens
into the junction of the posterior wall
and the floor. The superior vena cava
orifice is in the roof of the chamber,
and the septal surface is obliquely
orientated, running from a right
posterior to left anterior position
(fig 2.7). The crista terminalis runs

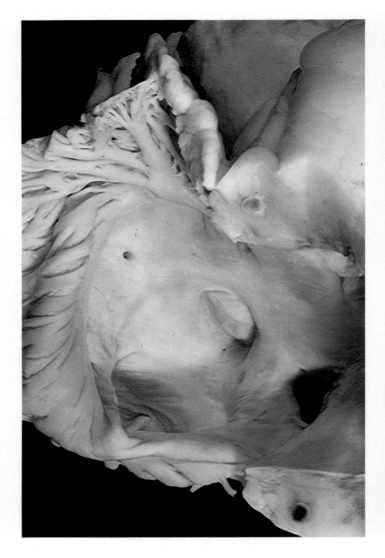

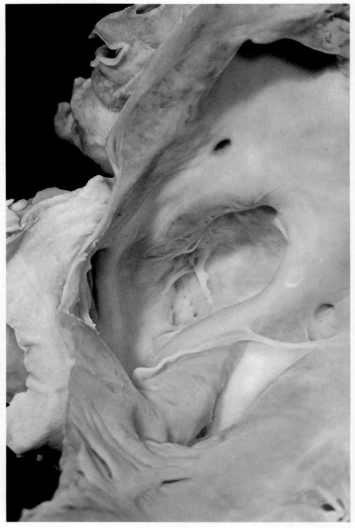

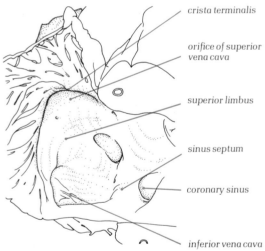

Fig. 2.8   Dissection showing how the
superior vena cava enters the right atrium
between the crista terminalis and the superior
limbus of the fossa ovalis.

crista terminalis

orifice of superior
vena cava

superior limbus

sinus septum

coronary sinus

inferior vena cava

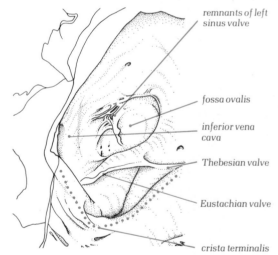

Fig. 2.9   Dissection of the lateral wall of the
right atrium showing the relationship of the
crista terminalis to the inferior vena cava, the
fossa ovalis and the coronary sinus.

remnants of left
sinus valve

fossa ovalis

inferior vena
cava

Thebesian valve

Eustachian valve

crista terminalis

from the anterior part of the septal
surface and swings in front of the
orifice of the superior vena cava
which enters the right atrium between
the crista and the superior limbus of
the fossa ovalis (fig. 2.8). Having
skirted the superior caval orifice, the
crista turns down the right side of the

inferior vena cava and curves in
towards the tricuspid orifice, passing
beneath the ostium of the coronary
sinus (fig. 2.9). The margin of the
crista terminalis is reinforced in fetal
life by sheet-like structures which
separate the orifices of the inferior
vena cava and coronary sinus from

the atrial appendage. These become
the valves of the inferior vena cava
(Eustachian valve) and coronary
sinus (Thebesian valve) and may be
seen to variable extent in adult hearts.
The Thebesian valve is usually
reasonably formed, but the
Eustachian valve is less well formed

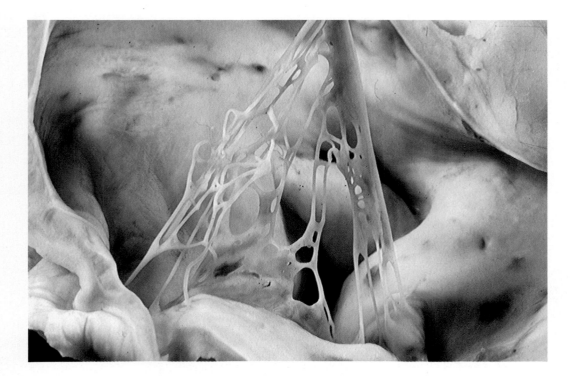

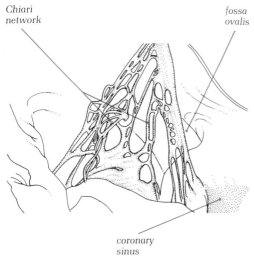

Fig. 2.10   Remnants of the extensive right valve of the sinus venosus termed a Chiari network.

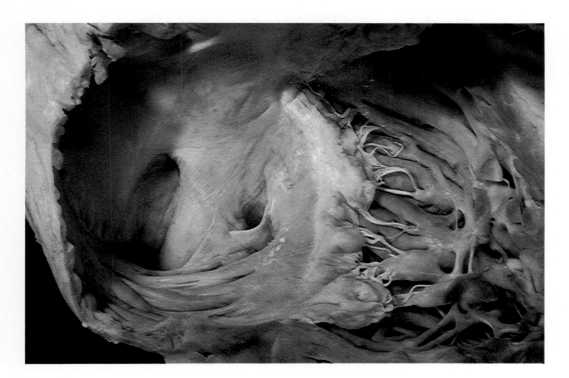

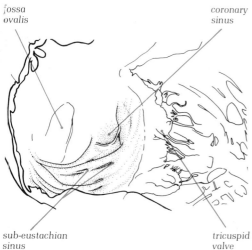

fossa ovalis

coronary sinus

sub-eustachian sinus

tricuspid valve

Fig. 2.11   Opened right atrium showing the extensive trabecular pouch found beneath the orifice of the inferior vena cava (the so-called sub-eustachian sinus).

(fig. 2.9). Fibrous strands may exist between the various parts of the crista which extend across the cavity of the right atrium. They, like the valves, are remnants of the extensive right valves of the sinus venosus seen during development (see *Chapter 10*) and are termed Chiari networks (fig. 2.10). Similar remnants may be seen across the fossa ovalis. They are remnants of the left sinus venosus valve (fig. 2.9). The atrial appendage usually shows a considerable pouch at its junction with the atrium anterior and inferior to the orifice of the inferior vena cava, the so-called sub-eustachian sinus (fig. 2.11). The crista itself runs forwards onto the posterior margin of the tricuspid orifice as a muscular sheet which inserts into the inferior and septal leaflets of the tricuspid valve (fig. 2.11).

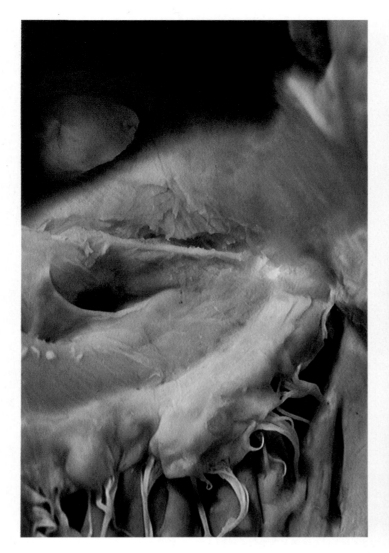

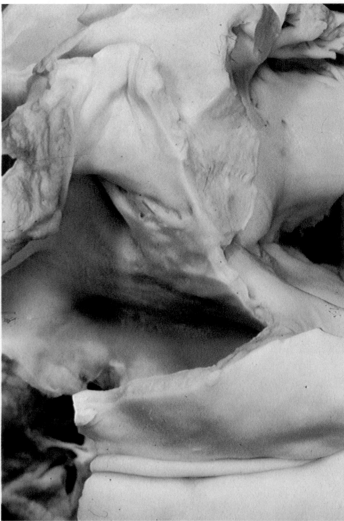

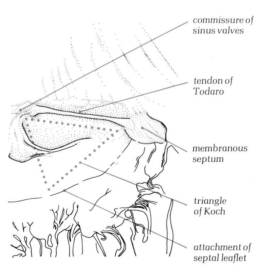

commissure of
sinus valves

tendon of
Todaro

membranous
septum

triangle
of Koch

attachment of
septal leaflet

Fig. 2.12   Dissection of the sinus septum
showing the tendon of Todaro. The heart
has been transilluminated from the left
ventricle to show the position of the
membranous septum.

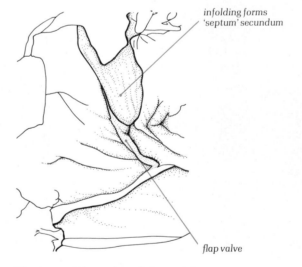

infolding forms
'septum' secundum

flap valve

Fig. 2.13   Dissection of the atrial septum
from behind showing that the limbus of the
fossa ovalis is an infolding of the atrial roof
and showing the position of the flap valve.

The posteroseptal surface of the chamber is, at first sight, extensive and is characterized by the fossa ovalis and the orifice of the coronary sinus, the third of the systemic venous channels which drain to the right atrium (fig. 2.12). The fossa ovalis is the depression at the site of the fetal interatrial communication termed the foramen ovale. In fetal life, this hole permits richly oxygenated inferior cava blood (coming from the placenta) to reach the left atrium and has a well-marked rim or limbus.

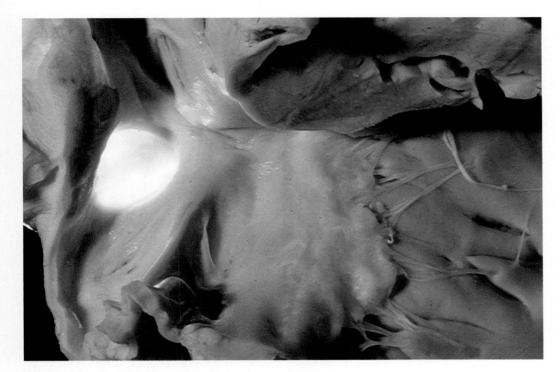

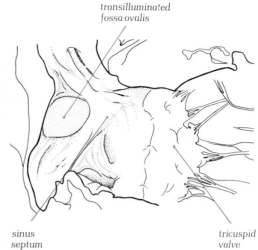

sinus
septum

tricuspid
valve

Fig. 2.14   Transillumination of the atrial
septum showing the position of the fossa
ovalis.

Superiorly, the limbus forms the
'septum secundum' between the
superior vena cava and the pulmonary
veins (fig. 2.9). Anteriorly, the limbus
is the interatrial groove running
behind the aorta. Inferiorly, the
limbus overlies the central fibrous
body and continues backwards as the
structure separating the orifice of the
coronary sinus from that of the
inferior vena cava. This structure is
termed the sinus septum (fig. 2.9). The
degree of accentuation of the limbic
structures (compare figs. 2.8 & 2.9)
depends on the amount of fat in the
interatrial grooves. A tendinous
structure extends through the sinus
septum in most hearts, being a
continuation of the commissure
between the Eustachian and
Thebesian valves. It runs
intramyocardially to insert into the
central fibrous body but can be easily
demonstrated by superficial
dissection (fig. 2.12). It is termed the
tendon of Todaro and is a vital
structure in demarcating the position
of the atrioventricular node (see
Chapter 6). The posterior limbus of
the fossa ovalis is very variable in its
formation. In some hearts, a well-
formed posterior lip is seen (fig. 2.6);
in others, the posterior wall of the
fossa is directly continuous with the
left wall of the inferior vena cava
(fig. 2.9). The floor of the fossa ovalis
is a thin fibromuscular partition – the
flap valve (fig. 2.13). It can be easily
transilluminated (fig. 2.14). In normal
hearts, the flap valve is of sufficiently
large size to close completely the fossa
ovalis. However, it is not always
adherent at its superior margin, and
in approximately 25% of normal
hearts, a probe can be passed through

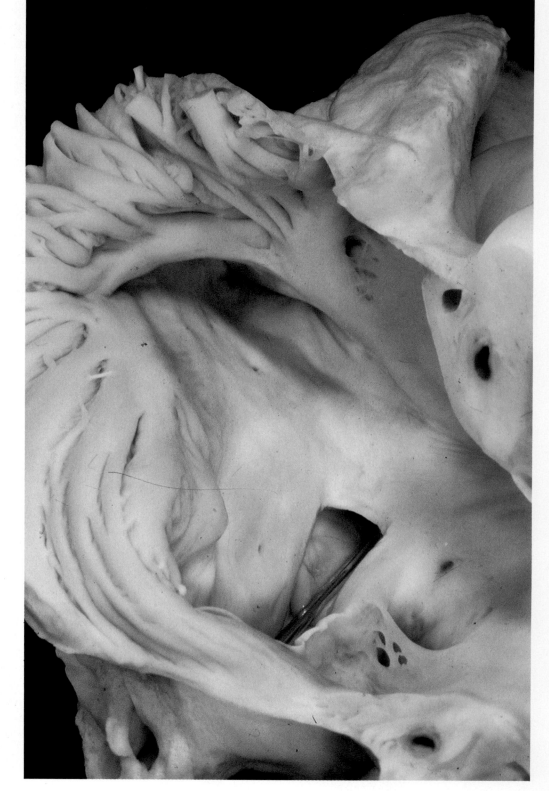

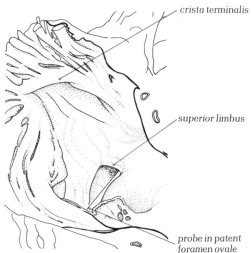

crista terminalis

superior limbus

probe in patent foramen ovale

Fig. 2.15 The heart with a probe-patent foramen ovale. The probe has been passed through the gap between the flap valve and the superior limbus (compare with fig. 2.27).

this site from right to left atrium producing a so-called probe-patent foramen ovale (fig. 2.15). However, because of this valve-like architecture, such a probe-patent foramen ovale does not permit an interatrial shunt as long as the left atrial pressure is higher than that of the right atrium.

The size of the opening of the coronary sinus is variable, but it is always placed between the sinus septum and the inferior extension of the crista terminalis (fig. 2.16). An extensive band of atrial muscle is present inferior to the orifice which extends into the leaflets of the tricuspid valve. Although this is the

wall of the right atrium, it also overlies the ventricular musculature due to the low attachment of the tricuspid valve leaflets. The area is not part of the atrial septum. Anteriorly, this muscle band merges with the anterior limbus and sinus septum, forming the overlay fibres above the atrioventricular node (see

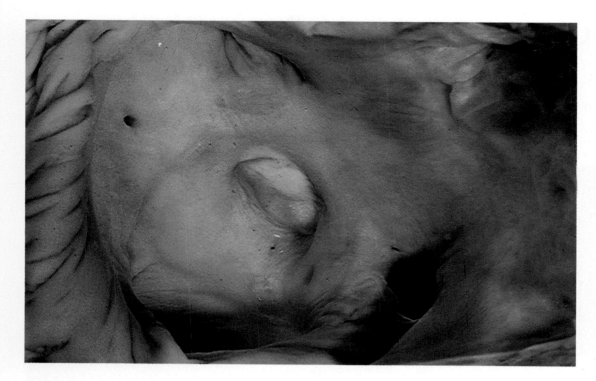

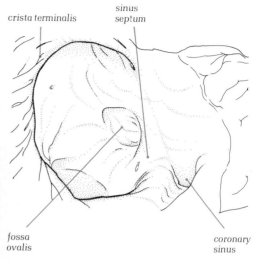

Fig. 2.16   The septal surface of the right
atrium showing the relationship of the
fossa ovalis and the ostium of the coronary sinus.

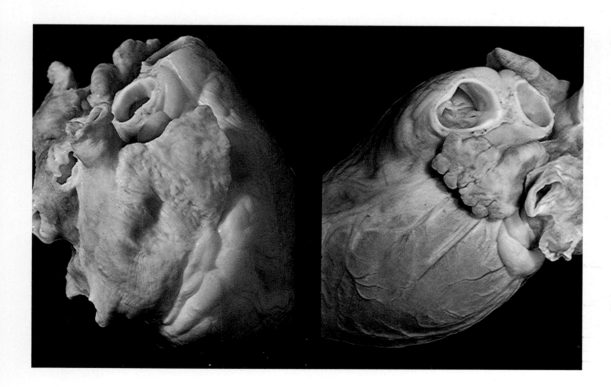

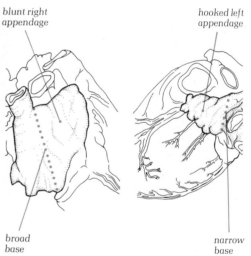

Fig. 2.17   The differing morphology of the
right and left atrial appendages.

Chapter 6). Frequently, small openings are present in this sheet from which venous channels extend into the conduction tissues of the atrioventricular junctional area. These, together with the tendon of Todaro, form better markers of the site of the atrioventricular node than the orifice of the coronary sinus.

The anterior wall of the right atrium is the atrial appendage. Seen externally, it has a characteristic blunt shape which serves to distinguish it from the left appendage (fig. 2.17). Internally, the appendage is lined by multiple trabeculae which extend at right angles to the crista terminalis all along its length,

continuing inferiorly into the sub-eustachian sinus (figs. 2.5, 2.11 & 2.15). In the roof of the atrium, one of the trabeculae is frequently prominent and is sometimes termed the septum spurium.

The morphology of the tricuspid orifice will be described in a separate section devoted to the tricuspid valve.

The Morphologically Left Atrium

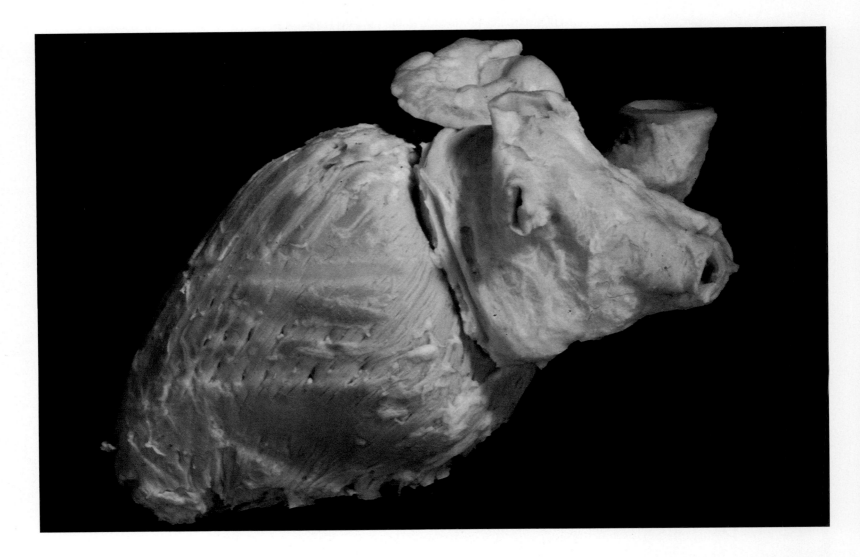

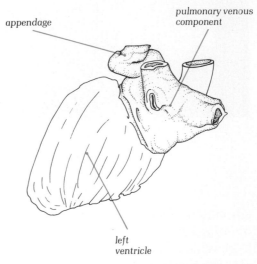

appendage

pulmonary venous component

left ventricle

Fig. 2.18   *Dissection viewed from behind showing the left-sided chambers. The left atrium is the most posterior and receives the four pulmonary veins at its four corners. The appendage passes forwards to hook round the great arteries.*

This is the most posterior chamber in the heart and, like the right atrium, has a smooth-walled portion which receives the venous drainage and an atrial appendage which hooks around the pulmonary artery *(fig. 2.18)*. The

atrial appendage is the only part of the left atrium to project directly on the cardiac silhouette *(fig. 1.19)*. The junction between smooth-walled atrium and appendage is much smaller than that of the right atrium

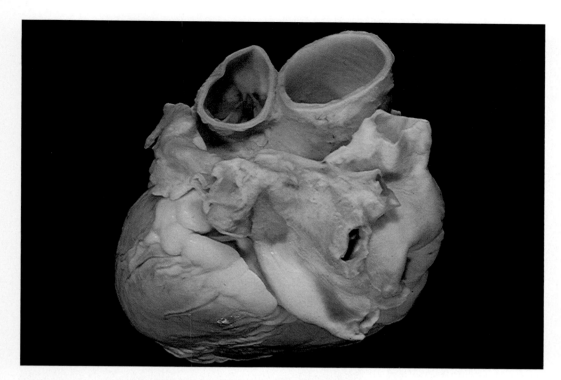

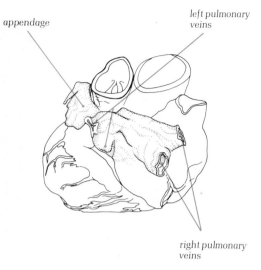

Fig. 2.19   The left atrium in an intact heart viewed from above and from the left. It shows the pulmonary veins entering the posterior aspect and the appendage hooking round the great arteries.

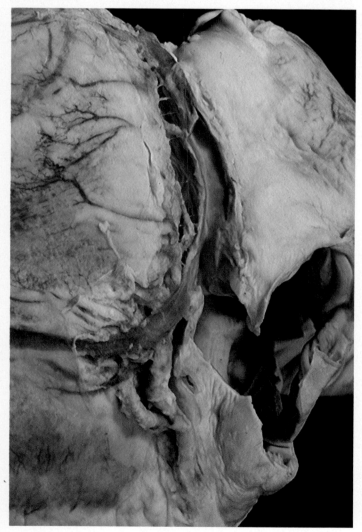

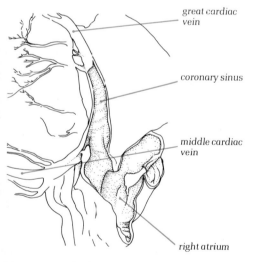

Fig. 2.20   The heart viewed from behind and orientated in its in situ position. The position of the coronary sinus is shown in the left atrioventricular groove between the left atrium and the left ventricle.

and is not marked by any specific sulcus. This is because the appendage is much narrower at its junction with the atrium (fig. 2.17). The appendage is hook-shaped and characteristically shows several constrictions along its length. The smooth-walled part of the atrium is considerably larger than the appendage (fig. 2.19) and superiorly receives the four pulmonary veins, two to each side (figs. 2.18 & 2.19).

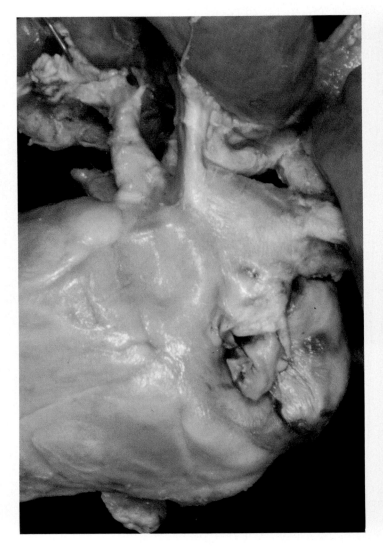

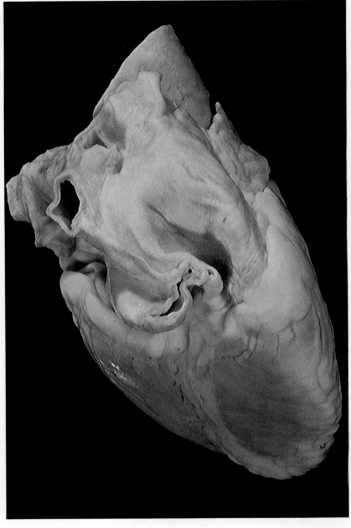

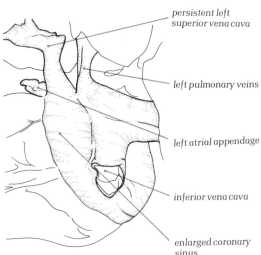

persistent left
superior vena cava

left pulmonary veins

left atrial appendage

inferior vena cava

enlarged coronary
sinus

Fig. 2.21   Posterior view of a heart with a
persistent left superior vena cava. The vein
runs down between the appendage and the
pulmonary venous portion to drain into the
right atrium via the coronary sinus.

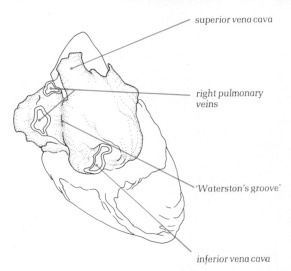

superior vena cava

right pulmonary
veins

'Waterston's groove'

inferior vena cava

Fig. 2.22   View of the heart from behind
showing the prominent groove (Waterston's
groove) between the right pulmonary veins
and the right atrium.

Inferiorly, the coronary sinus is
found along the posterior wall of the
left atrium occupying the left
atrioventricular sulcus (fig. 2.20). In
hearts with a persistent left superior
vena cava which drains to the
coronary sinus, the left-sided cava
forms a channel between the left

atrial appendage and the left
pulmonary veins (fig. 2.21). In some
hearts, a fibrous strand representing
the site of the left cava present during
development can be observed in a
similar position. The lower end of the
strand is frequently patent, forming
the oblique vein of the left atrium

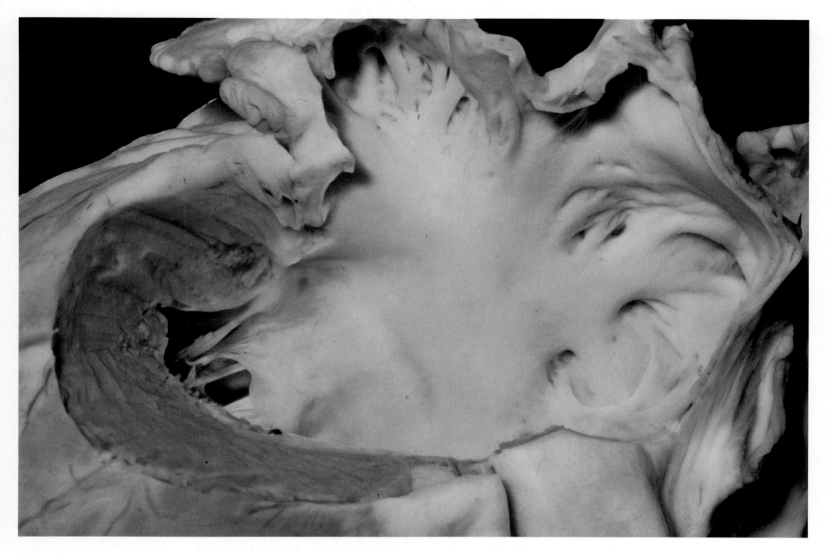

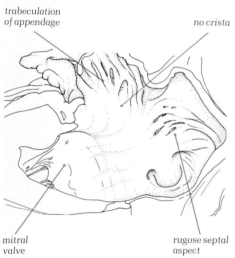

Fig. 2.23   *Cutaway view showing the
interior of the left atrium viewed from the left
and behind. The appendage is trabeculated
while the pulmonary venous component and
the septal surface are relatively smooth.*

which drains to the coronary sinus.
To the right, the right pulmonary
veins are separated from the right
atrium by the sulcus marking the
site of the superior limbus of the
fossa ovalis (fig. 2.22).

Internally, the appendage of the left
atrium is trabeculated as is the right
appendage; but the junction of
trabeculae and venous atrium on the
left is not marked by the presence of
any structure comparable to the
crista terminalis, and the trabeculae
are less pronounced (fig. 2.23). The
left atrium has a roof, a floor, a
posterior wall, an anterior wall and a

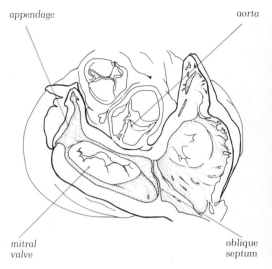

appendage   aorta

mitral   oblique
valve   septum

Fig. 2.24   Cross-section through the atria viewed as if it were from the right shoulder. Note the oblique orientation of the atrial septum.

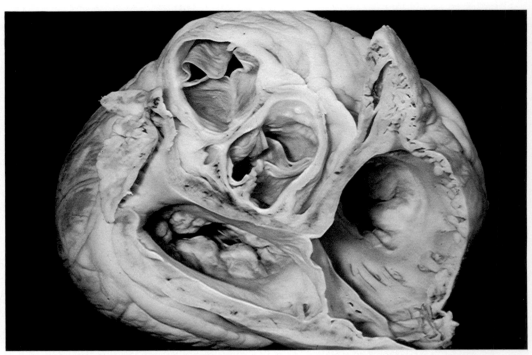

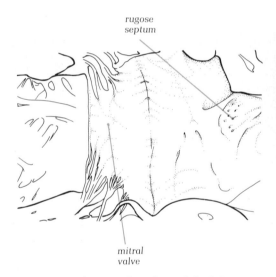

rugose
septum

mitral
valve

Fig. 2.25   The septal surface of the left atrium and the vestibule of the mitral valve. Note the roughened aspect of the septal surface which is the flap valve of the fossa ovalis.

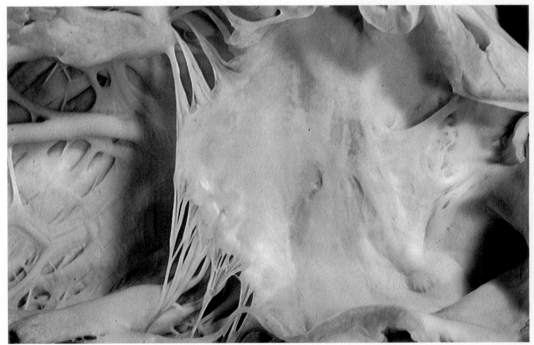

septal surface. The roof is formed by the tissue between the four pulmonary veins and this wall continues over into the posterior surface. The floor is the orifice of the mitral valve, considered along with the valve in its separate section. Anteriorly is the small ostium of the atrial appendage, abutting inferiorly on the mitral orifice. The left atrium also has an extensive anterior wall composed solely of roughened musculature which lies posterior to the aorta (fig. 2.24). The septal surface is oblique and consists of the left atrial surface of the fossa ovalis.

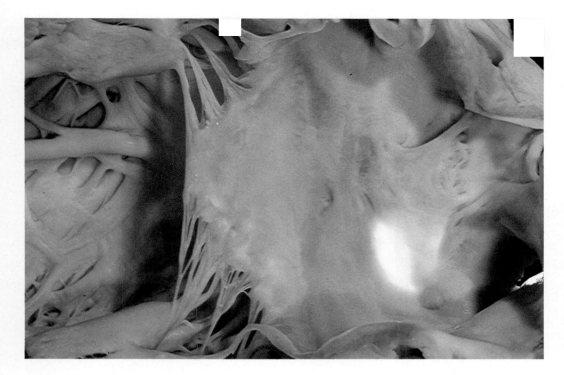

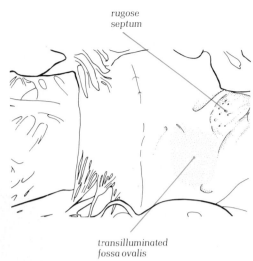

rugose
septum

transilluminated
fossa ovalis

Fig. 2.26   The same specimen as in fig. 2.25
transilluminated from the right side. The
fossa ovalis is well posterior and inferior to
the flap valve noted on the left septal surface.

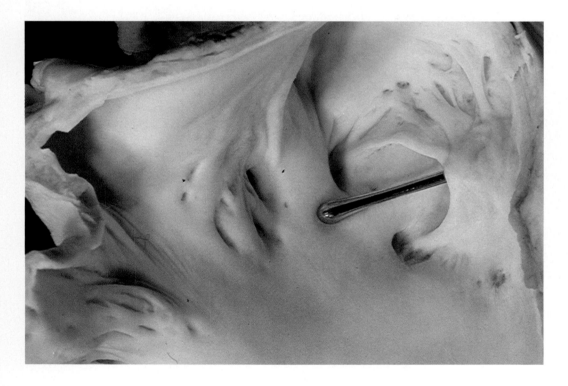

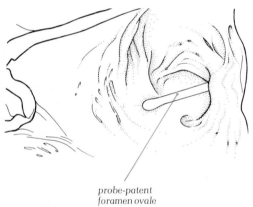

probe-patent
foramen ovale

Fig. 2 27   A probe-patent foramen ovale
with a probe inserted from the right atrium
between the limbus and the flap valve. The
right side of this heart is shown in fig. 2.15.

There is no rim to the fossa on the left atrial side; but anteriorly, the flap valve is usually plastered down onto the anterior wall, the junction being marked by a characteristic rough area (fig. 2.25). When the septum is transilluminated, it is found that the floor of the fossa ovalis visible in the right atrium is posterior to the rugose area of the left atrial wall (compare figs. 2.13, 2.14 , 2.25 & 2.26). When the anterior part of the flap valve is not adherent to the anterior atrial wall, then probe-patent foramen ovale results (fig. 2.27).

The Interatrial Septum

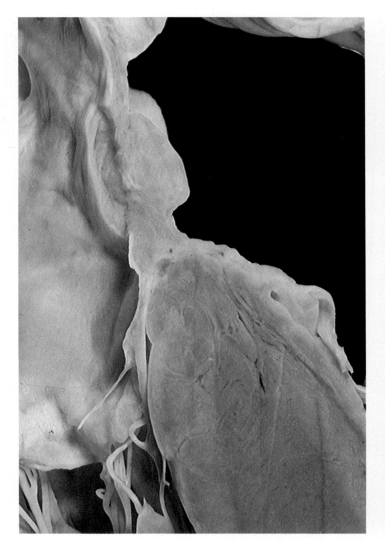

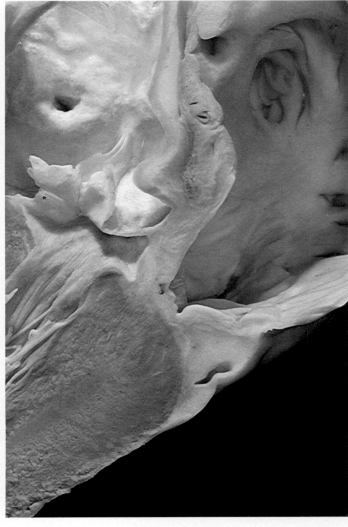

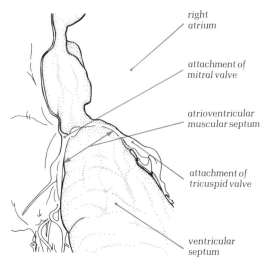

right
atrium

attachment of
mitral valve

atrioventricular
muscular septum

attachment of
tricuspid valve

ventricular
septum

Fig. 2.28   Section through the atrial and
ventricular septa viewed from behind.
Part of the inlet septum interposes between
the left ventricular inlet and the right atrium.

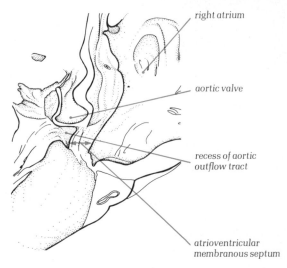

right atrium

aortic valve

recess of aortic
outflow tract

atrioventricular
membranous septum

Fig. 2.29   Oblique section through the aortic
outflow tract showing its relationship to the
right atrium. This area is the atrioventricular
membranous septum.

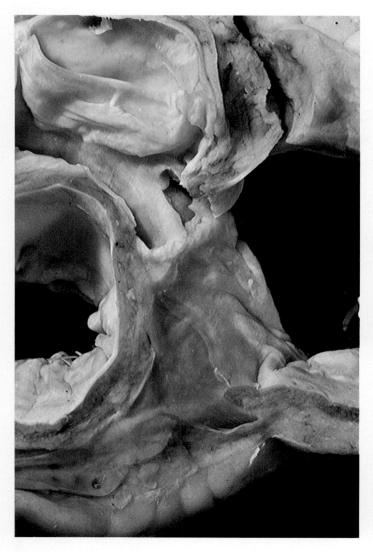

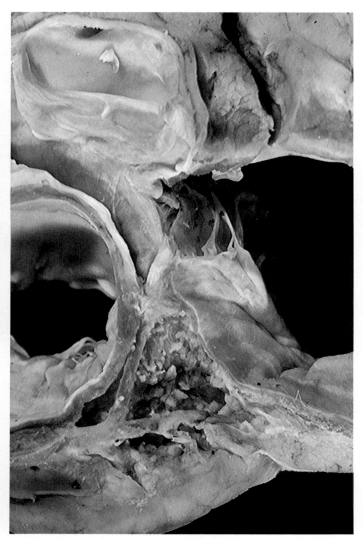

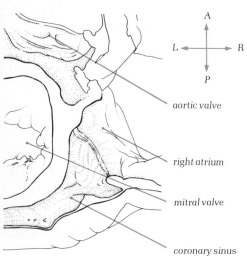

A
L ← → R
P

aortic valve

right atrium

mitral valve

coronary sinus

Fig. 2.30   Transverse section viewed
superiorly through the base of the atrium
showing the floor of the coronary sinus and
the aortic outflow tract.

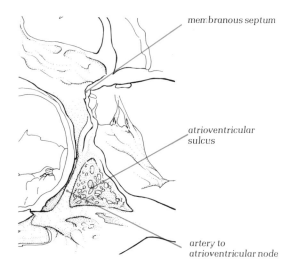

membranous septum

atrioventricular
sulcus

artery to
atrioventricular node

Fig. 2.31   The heart shown in fig. 2.30 after
removal of the floor of the coronary sinus.
This is not septum but the atrioventricular
sulcus.

By comparison of the transilluminated
figures (figs. 2.14 & 2.26) and
examination of the cross-sections
(figs. 2.7, 2.24 & 2.28), it can be seen
that the interatrial septum occupies
only a small part of the atrial walls
described as 'septal surface'. Much
of the superior limbus is simply the
infolded sulcus between the superior
vena cava and the right pulmonary
veins (fig. 2.13). The anterior limbus is
mostly the anterior atrial wall and in
this position is in direct relation to the
anterior root of the aorta, being
separated from it by the transverse
sinus of the pericardium (fig. 2.24).
The inferior limbus is in part true
atrial septum; but, owing to the origin
of the tricuspid valve from the septum
being much more towards the
ventricular apex than that of the
mitral valve (fig. 2.28), much of the
inferior limbus is positioned between
the right atrium and the inlet portion
of the left ventricle. Similarly, the
anterior part of the limbus overlying
the central fibrous body is

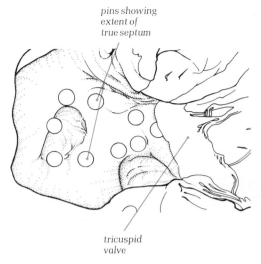

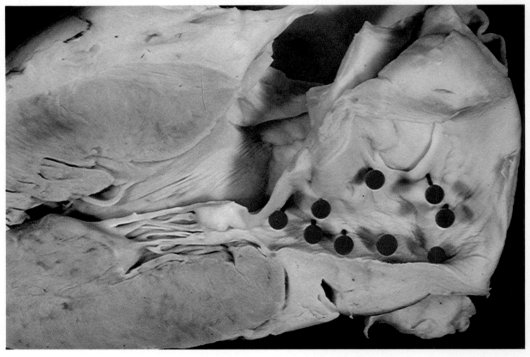

tricuspid
valve

Fig. 2.32 *The right aspect of the atrial 'septum'. Pins have been inserted to show the true confines of the interatrial septal surface. This is considerably smaller than may be anticipated.*

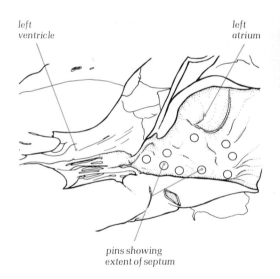

left
ventricle

left
atrium

pins showing
extent of septum

Fig. 2.33 *Left atrial view of the septum shown in fig. 2.32.*

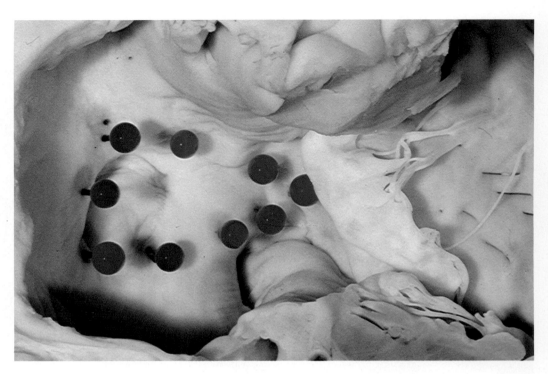

continuous with the atrioventricular component of the membranous septum and is located between the right atrium and the aortic outflow tract (fig. 2.29). The area around the coronary sinus is related directly to atrioventricular sulcus tissue. Consequently, it is not part of the septum (figs. 2.30 & 2.31). Finally, the area of the posterior limbus is directly continuous with the wall of the inferior vena cava and only a small part is true atrial septum. The small area of the true septum can be illustrated by inserting markers at its margins (figs. 2.32 & 2.33) and by removing the septum (figs. 2.34 & 2.35). The importance of this is largely surgical, since incisions placed outside the area of the septum will carry the surgeon outside the heart. Similarly, 'septal' puncture

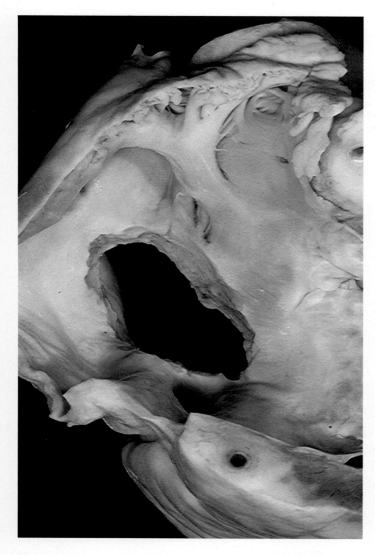

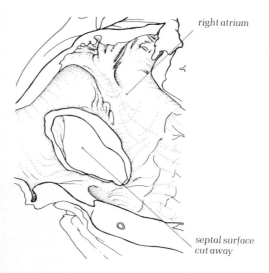

right atrium

septal surface
cut away

Fig. 2.34   Further view of the right side of the
atrial 'septum'. The true interatrial surface
has been removed to show the extent of the
septum.

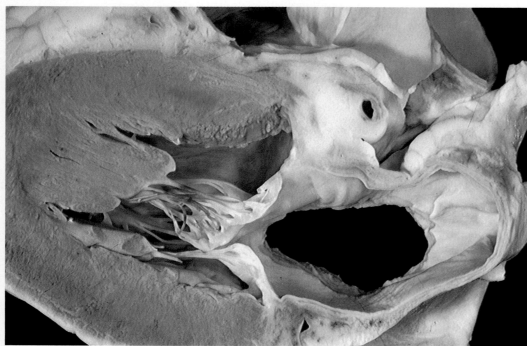

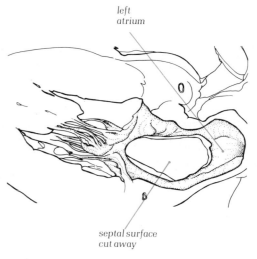

left
atrium

septal surface
cut away

Fig. 2.35   Left atrial view of the septum
shown in fig. 2.34.

performed at catheterization in a
position anterior to the area of the
fossa ovalis where there is frequently
a recess in the anterior wall of the
right atrium (fig. 2.36) will produce
cardiac rupture. A catheter lodged in
this recess can easily simulate a
position in the fossa ovalis. If pushed
through the recess, the catheter will
pass through the transverse sinus
and into the aorta or pulmonary
artery.

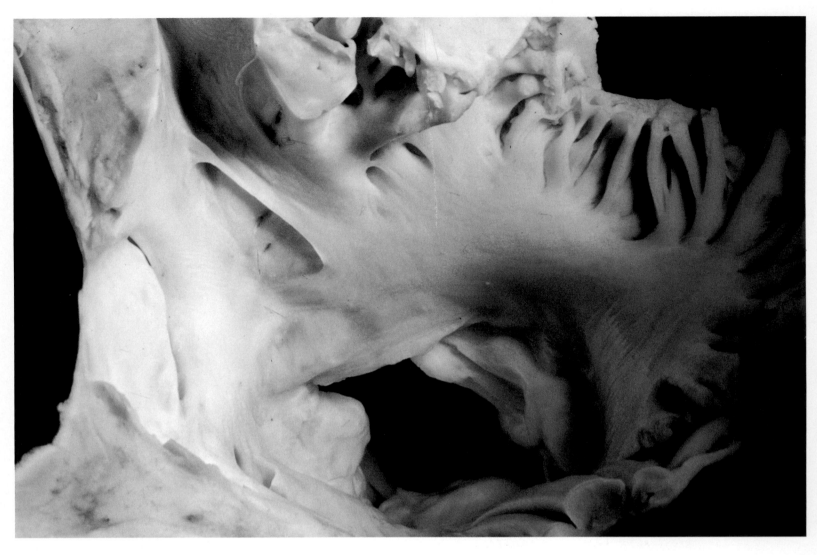

Differences between Morphologically Right and Left Atria

It is important for the paediatric cardiologist to be able to distinguish a morphologically right atrium from a morphologically left atrium. In most instances, this may be achieved easily because the morphologically right atrium receives the systemic venous return and the left atrium the pulmonary venous return. However, the fact that anomalous venous return can occur, particularly in situations where it is most important to identify atrial morphology, makes it necessary to be aware of the morphological differences which permit atrial distinction. The morphologically right atrium has a crista terminalis, a limbus to the fossa ovalis and frequently possesses remnants of the venous valves. The morphologically left atrium has no crista, possesses the rugose aspect of the flap valve of the fossa ovalis and has no venous valve remnants. All these features make differentiation easy for the morphologist but are of little value to the clinician who is dependent upon features which may be shown angiographically, namely, the shape of the atrial appendages. Thus, the single most important feature permitting atrial distinction is the blunt shape of the morphologically right atrial appendage compared with the hooked and narrow shape of the morphologically left appendage (fig. 2.17).

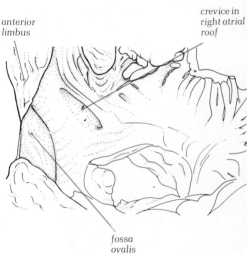

Fig. 2.36 *Transverse section superiorly viewed through the fossa ovalis. In front of the anterior limbus of the fossa there is a fold of endocardium producing a crevice in the anterior atrial wall.*

3 The Ventricles I

Introduction
The Morphologically Right Ventricle

Introduction

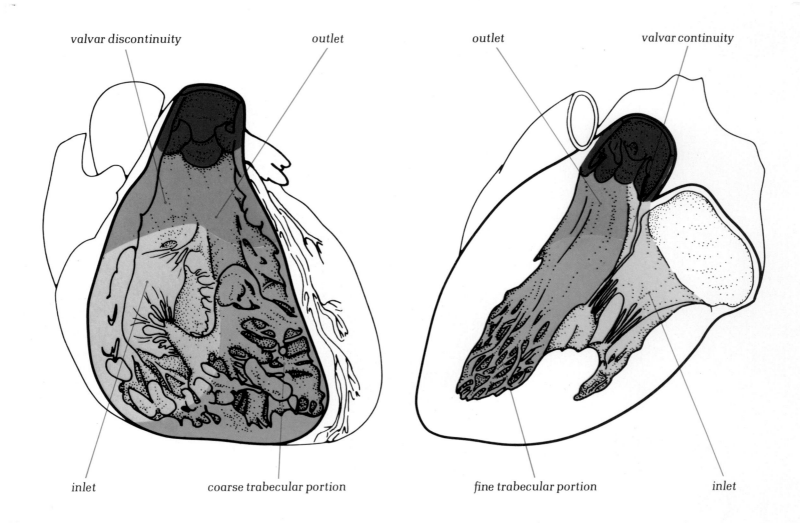

valvar discontinuity outlet   outlet valvar continuity

inlet coarse trabecular portion   fine trabecular portion inlet

Diagrammatic representation of the three basic components of the right and left ventricle. Each has an inlet component containing atrioventricular valve; an apical trabecular zone; and an outlet component supporting an arterial valve. See also figs. 3.16 & 4.3.

Each ventricle has basically the same pattern, composed of an inlet atrioventricular valve and its tension apparatus, a body and an outlet arterial valve. As with the atria, there are important morphological differences between the ventricles which permit their clinical distinction. We will, therefore, describe each ventricle, concentrating upon its inlet and outlet valves, and then describe the interventricular septum. Before that, however, some introductory remarks are necessary. It has been customary in the past to consider ventricles as possessing inflow and outflow tracts, or sinus and conus (infundibulum). This, to our minds, is a restrictive influence in terms of both development of the ventricles and their morphology. In this chapter, we prefer to describe ventricles in terms of three parts: an inlet, containing an atrioventricular valve and its tension apparatus; a trabecular body; and an outlet supporting an arterial valve. In similar fashion, we are then able to describe the muscular ventricular septum as composed of inlet (separating the atrioventricular valves); trabecular (between the trabecular zones); and outlet (between

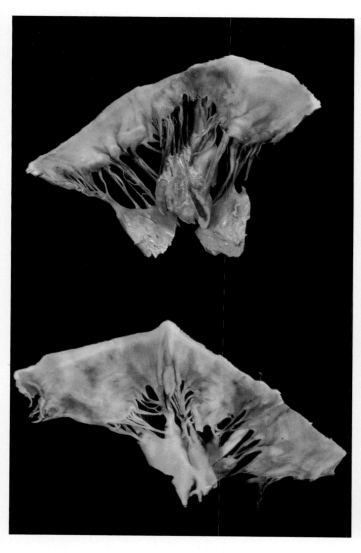

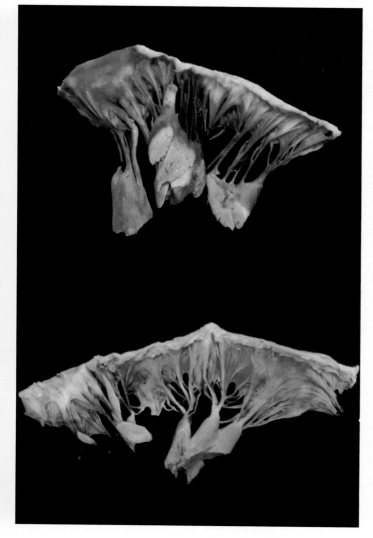

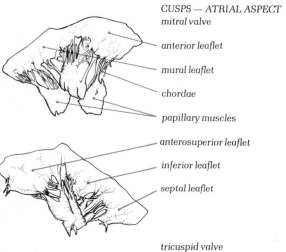

CUSPS — ATRIAL ASPECT
mitral valve

anterior leaflet

mural leaflet

chordae

papillary muscles

anterosuperior leaflet

inferior leaflet

septal leaflet

tricuspid valve

Fig. 3.1   The removed mitral (upper) and tricuspid (lower) valves viewed from their atrial aspect.

CUSPS — VENTRICULAR ASPECT
mitral valve

attachment (annulus)

anterior leaflet

mural leaflet

chordae

papillary muscles

septal leaflet

inferior leaflet

anterosuperior leaflet

tricuspid valve

Fig. 3.2   The removed mitral (upper) and tricuspid (lower) valves viewed from their ventricular aspect.

the arterial valves) portions. This division is not meant to indicate that ventricular inlet and outlet portions lack trabeculations, although in many places they do have smooth walls. Rather it indicates that the apical trabecular zones are the most trabeculated and most distinctive from this standpoint in each ventricle. The morphology of the atrioventricular valves is similar in each ventricle (*figs. 3.1 & 3.2*) although distinctive differences exist and will be described in the sections devoted to the tricuspid and mitral valves. Basically, each valve is made up of a number of leaflets consisting of a fibrous tissue core, the major support of this being the atrioventricular annulus. The core is termed the fibrosa and is continuous distally with the chordae tendineae. The chordae tendineae, composed of dense collagen, are in turn attached to the ventricular myocardium, most coming from specialized papillary muscles but some chordae taking origin from the ventricular walls. The chordae and papillary muscles make up the valvar tension apparatus.

3.3

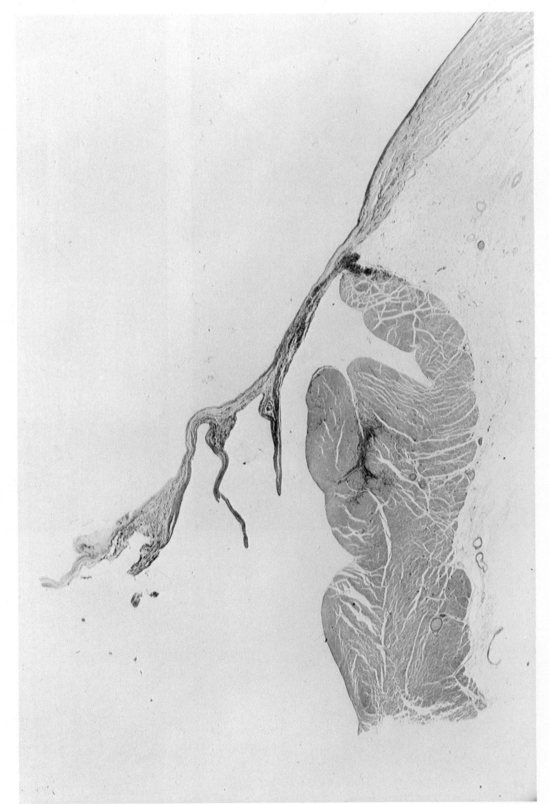

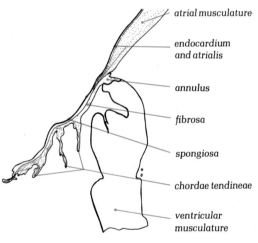

atrial musculature

endocardium
and atrialis

annulus

fibrosa

spongiosa

chordae tendineae

ventricular
musculature

Fig. 3.3   Histology of an atrioventricular
valve.

The fibrosa forms the ventricular
layer of the valve; on its atrial surface
is a superficial layer, the atrialis,
which is continuous with the atrial
endocardium and which is separated
from the fibrosa by a more loosely
textured layer of fibrous tissue termed

the spongiosa (fig. 3.3). The distal end
of the atrial myocardium may also
extend for a distance between the
atrialis and the fibrosa. Apart from
the blood vessels present in the atrial
musculature, the valve leaflets and
chordae are avascular structures.

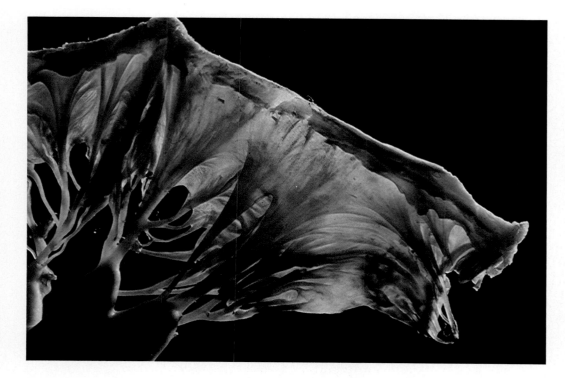

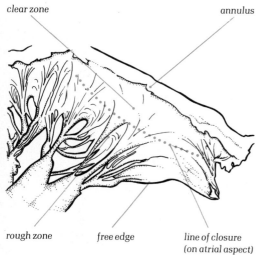

Fig. 3.4   Transilluminated mitral valve
showing the rough zone from the free edge to
the line of closure of the valve and the clear
zone between the line of closure and the
annulus.

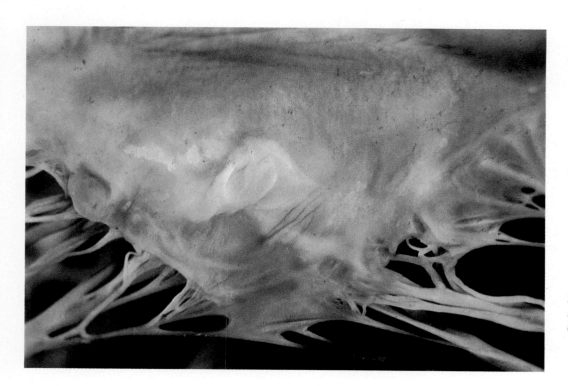

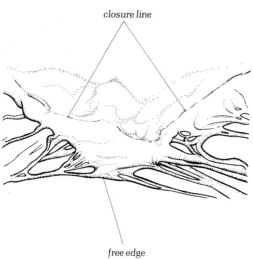

Fig. 3.5   The atrial surface of the mitral valve
showing how the line of closure is some
distance from the free edge of the valve.

The major chordae supporting a
leaflet insert either into its free edge,
or the area beyond the free edge on the
ventricular aspect up to the line of
closure of the leaflet. This area
between the free edge and the line of
closure is termed the rough zone in
contradistinction to the area between
the line of closure and the basal
attachment of the leaflet which is
easily transilluminated and is smooth
(fig. 3.4). It is important to remember
that the line of closure of a leaflet is
not its free edge (fig. 3.5).

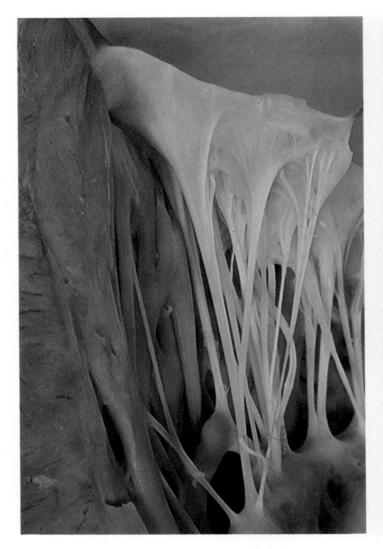

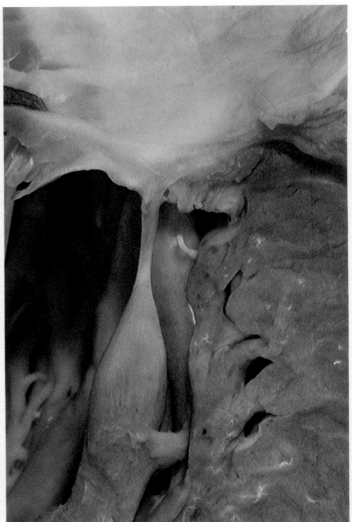

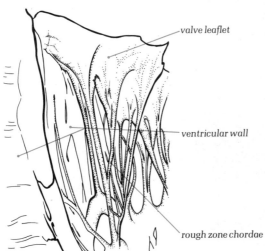

Fig. 3.6   The ventricular aspect of the mitral valve showing the attachment of rough zone chordae.

valve leaflet

ventricular wall

rough zone chordae

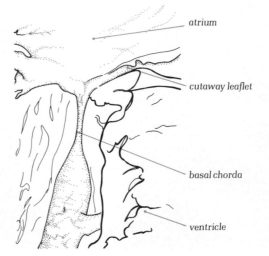

Fig. 3.7   Dissection of the mitral valve showing the morphology of a basal chorda.

atrium

cutaway leaflet

basal chorda

ventricle

The chordae inserting into the rough zone are called rough zone chordae (fig. 3.6). They are distinguished from basal chordae which pass from the ventricular myocardium to the ventricular aspect of the leaflet close to its attachment (fig. 3.7) and

commissural chordae which are the discrete fan-shaped chordae inserting into the free margin of the leaflet only and supporting two adjacent leaflets (figs. 3.8 & 3.9).

The atrioventricular valves are, therefore, intricate and complicated

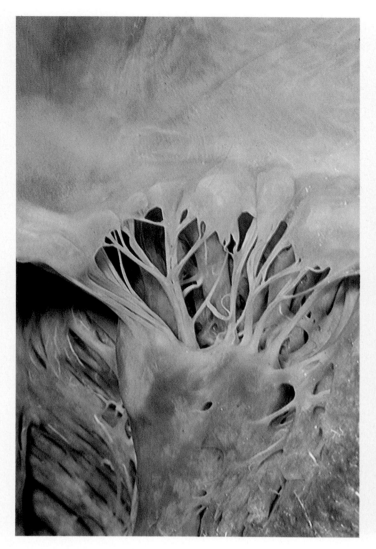

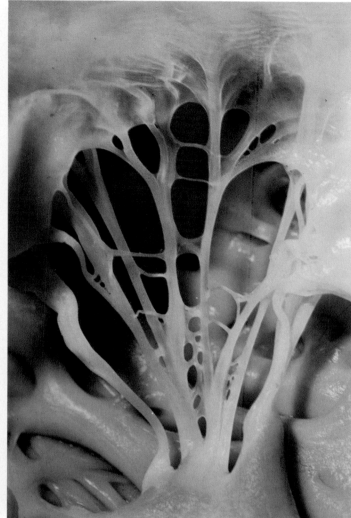

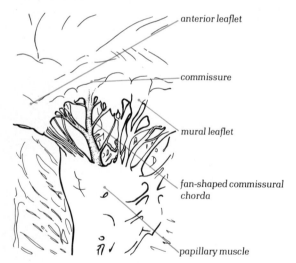

anterior leaflet

commissure

mural leaflet

fan-shaped commissural
chorda

papillary muscle

Fig. 3.8   Commissural chordae of the mitral
valve.

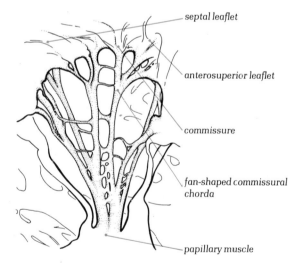

septal leaflet

anterosuperior leaflet

commissure

fan-shaped commissural
chorda

papillary muscle

Fig. 3.9   Commissural chordae of the
tricuspid valve.

structures, having several components. Each of these components must function correctly and in a coordinated fashion if the valve itself is to be competent. From a functional standpoint, the atrioventricular valves should not be considered solely in terms of the leaflets and chordae. For this reason, the term 'atrioventricular valve apparatus' is more apt (*Perloff & Roberts, 1972*).

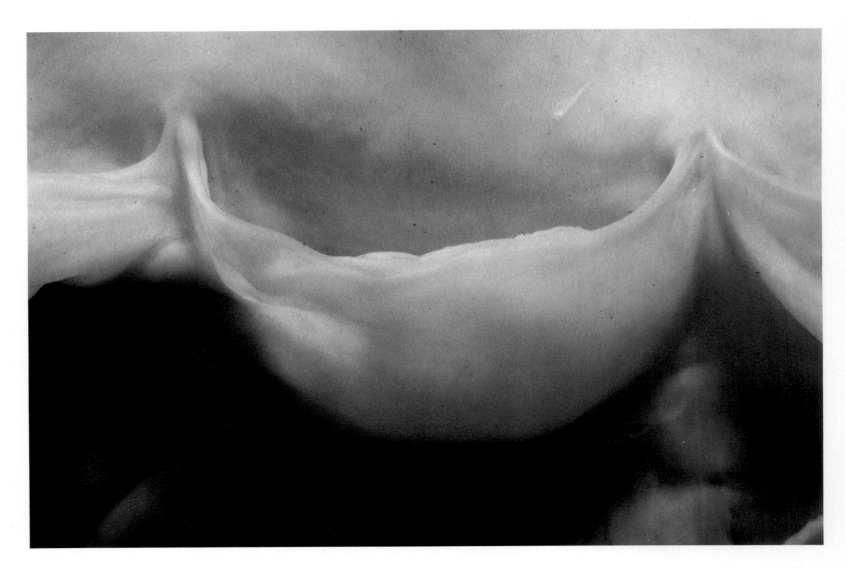

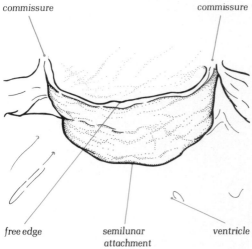

commissure   commissure

free edge   semilunar   ventricle
           attachment

Fig. 3.10   *The morphology of an arterial cusp.*

The arterial valves are considerably
simpler in pattern than the
atrioventricular valves. They are
composed of three cusps or leaflets
called the semilunar cusps. They have
a semilunar attachment to the junction
of the ventricular outlet with its great
artery (*fig. 3.10*). The distal ends of the
semilunar attachments meet, the site
of fusion of adjacent cusps being the

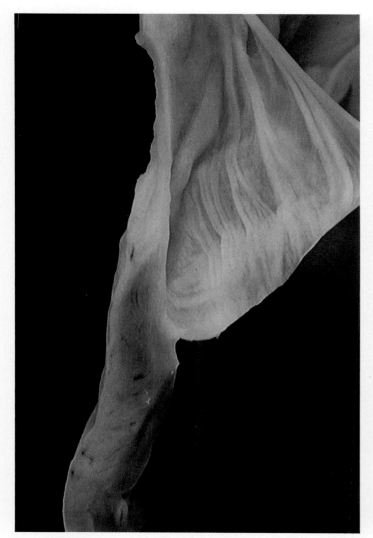

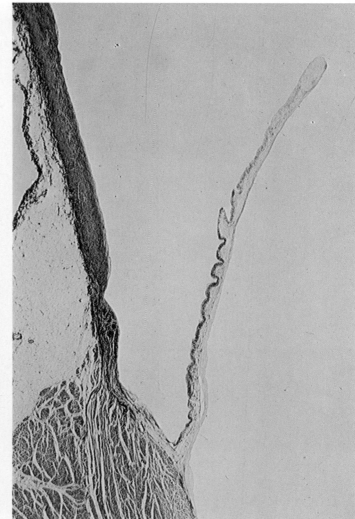

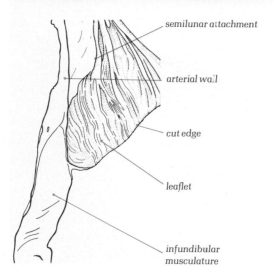

semilunar attachment

arterial wall

cut edge

leaflet

infundibular musculature

Fig. 3.11   *Bisection of one cusp of the pulmonary valve showing its attachment to its arterial muscular junction.*

arterial wall

arterialis

ventricularis

fibrosa

musculature

Fig. 3.12   *Histology of the valve shown in fig. 3.11.*

commissure. Histologically, each arterial cusp shows a main core of fibrous tissue, again termed the fibrosa (figs. 3.11 & 3.12). The cusp has endocardial linings on each surface, termed the ventricularis and arterialis respectively. The fibrosa is thickened at the midpoint of the free edge of each cusp to form the nodule.

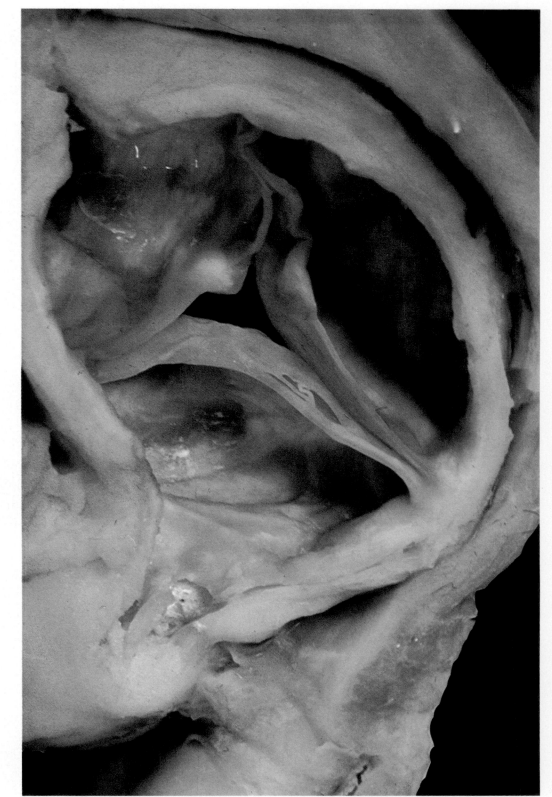

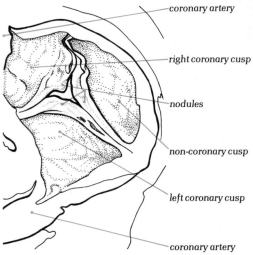

coronary artery

right coronary cusp

nodules

non-coronary cusp

left coronary cusp

coronary artery

Fig. 3.13   The aortic valve viewed from the aortic aspect showing how the nodules of the semilunar cusps meet together when it is in the closed position.

The nodules of the valve meet together when it is in the closed position (fig. 3.13), and become increasingly well developed with increasing age (fig. 3.14).

As with the atrioventricular valves, the line of closure is proximal to the free edge. Between the free edge and the line of closure the leaflet is extremely thin and can, on occasion, be fenestrated (fig. 3.15). This is not necessarily a pathological condition.

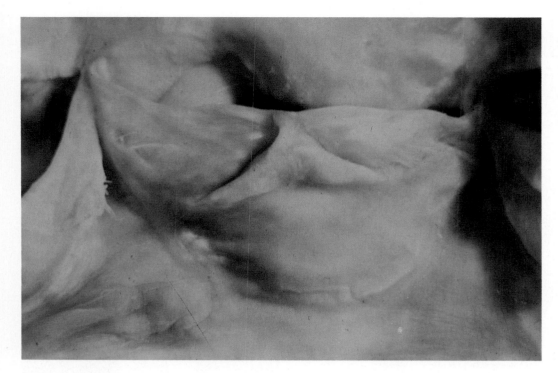

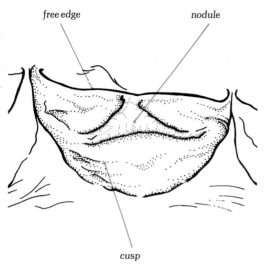

Fig. 3.14   Detail of a single arterial valve cusp from an old person showing the well developed nodule.

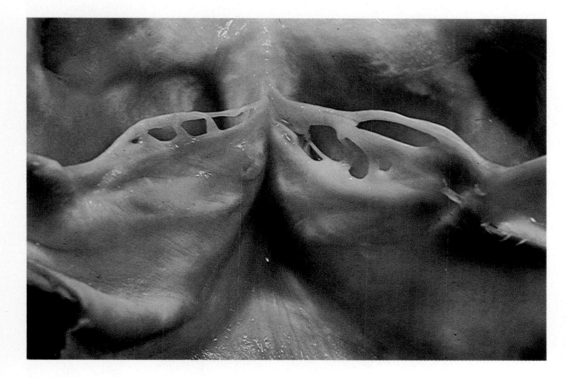

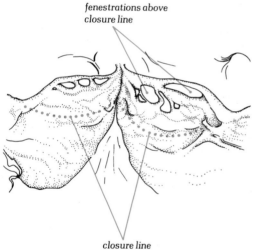

Fig. 3.15   As with the atrioventricular valve, arterial valves close some distance away from their free edge. The area between the line of closure and free edge can be fenestrated as shown here. This is a normal finding.

The three arterial valve cusps are not the same size in any given valve, and cusps vary in both height and width (*Vollebergh & Becker, 1977*).

With ageing, important changes may occur both in atrioventricular and arterial valves which affect the fibrosa and the valve annulus. Disruption may occur, and pooling of mucopolysaccharides may accompany this disruption. This change is in itself not necessarily a disease process.

The Morphologically Right Ventricle

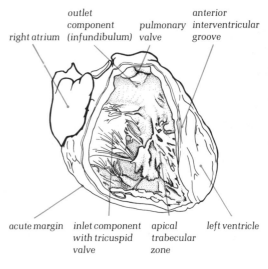

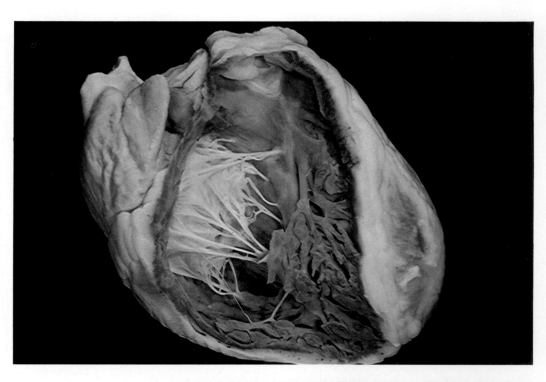

Fig. 3.16   The heart positioned in its in situ position with the anterior wall removed to show the extent of the morphologically right ventricle.

Labels (Fig. 3.16):
right atrium, *outlet component (infundibulum)*, *pulmonary valve*, *anterior interventricular groove*, *acute margin*, *inlet component with tricuspid valve*, *apical trabecular zone*, *left ventricle*

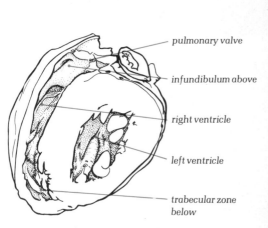

Fig. 3.17   Oblique section through the ventricular mass showing how the right ventricle sweeps from below to above the left ventricle.

Labels (Fig. 3.17):
pulmonary valve, *infundibulum above*, *right ventricle*, *left ventricle*, *trabecular zone below*

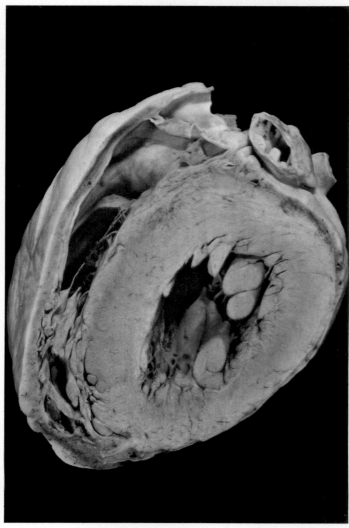

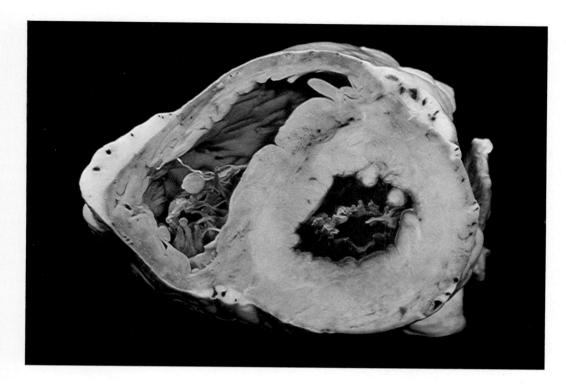

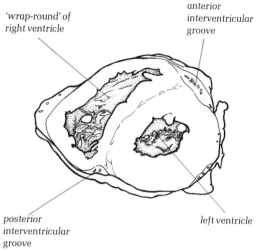

Fig. 3.18   Short axis section through the ventricular mass showing how the right ventricle wraps itself around the left ventricle.

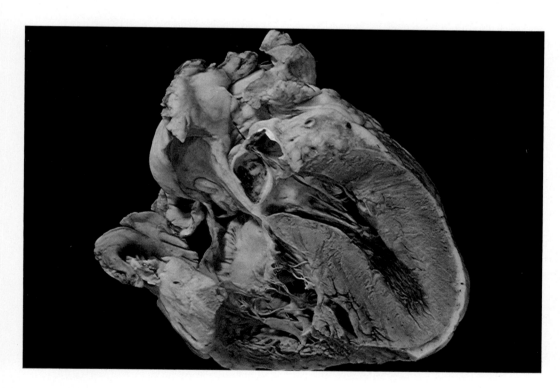

Fig. 3.19   Frontal section through the heart showing the junction between the inlet and trabecular portions of the right ventricle, with the inlet septum extending to the position of the crux (posterior junction of arterial and ventricular septa).

As described in the introductory section, the right and left ventricles have discrete morphological features. In congenitally malformed heart, these ventricles do not always occupy right-sided and left-sided positions. Indeed, as will be seen, in the normal heart the right ventricle is an anterior as well as a right-sided structure. For these reasons, the ventricles are distinguished in terms of their morphology, rather than their position, as the morphologically right

and morphologically left ventricles.

Thus the morphologically right ventricle occupies most of the anterior part of the frontal projection of the cardiac silhouette (fig. 3.16). It swings in front of the left ventricle from right (tricuspid valve) to left (pulmonary valve) in the anteroposterior projection (fig. 3.16) and from beneath to above the left ventricle in the lateral projection (fig. 3.17). In shape it is like an additional slice of tissue wrapped around the circular left

ventricle, particularly when viewed in a section across the short axis of the ventricular mass (fig. 3.18). Its right-sided inlet portion contains the tricuspid valve and extends posteriorly to the crux cordis, being separated from the left ventricle in this projection by the posterior or inlet interventricular sulcus running from the crux towards the apex (fig. 3.19).

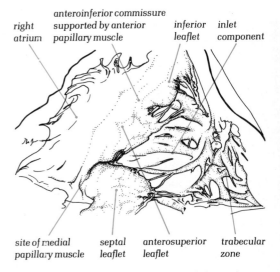

right atrium — anteroinferior commissure supported by anterior papillary muscle — inferior leaflet — inlet component

site of medial papillary muscle — septal leaflet — anterosuperior leaflet — trabecular zone

Fig. 3.20   The inlet component of the right ventricle viewed from behind showing the transition into the trabecular zone. Note also the leaflets of the valve separated by the commissures.

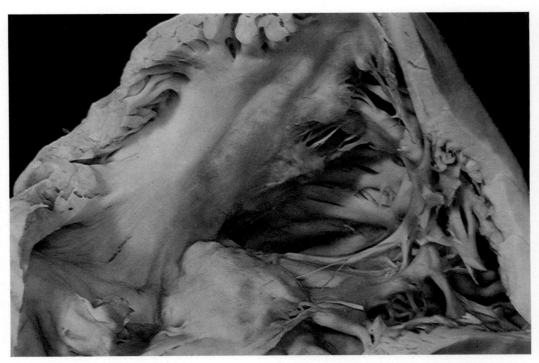

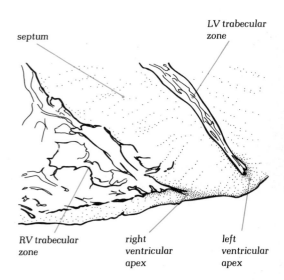

septum — LV trabecular zone

RV trabecular zone — right ventricular apex — left ventricular apex

Fig. 3.21   Section through the ventricular apex showing how thin both the right and left ventricular myocardia are at this point.

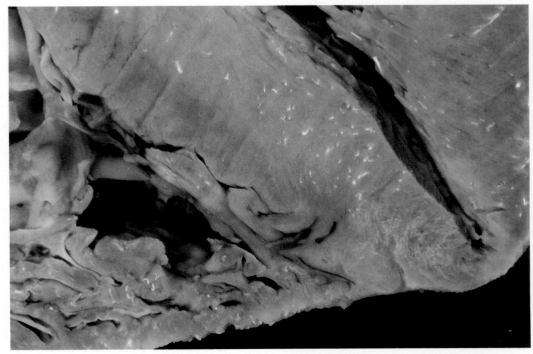

The limit of the inlet zone is the attachment of the papillary muscles, but a distinct line between inlet and trabecular portions is not seen (fig. 3.20). The apical trabecular zone extends inferiorly and more horizontally beyond the attachments of the papillary muscle towards the ventricular apex. The wall of the apex is frequently thinner compared to the

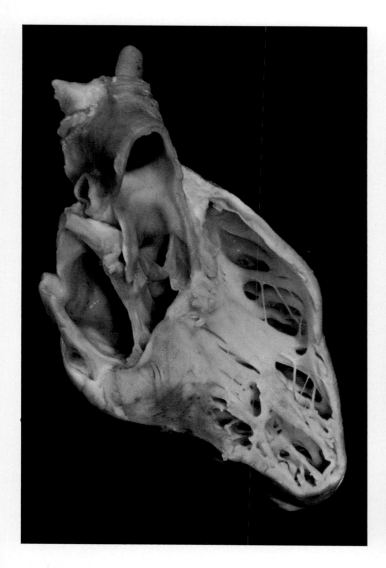

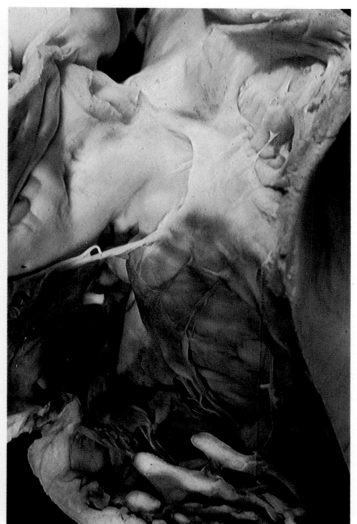

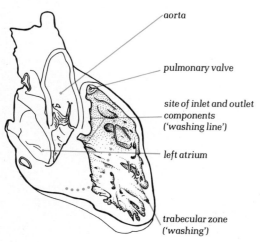

aorta

pulmonary valve

site of inlet and outlet
components
('washing line')

left atrium

trabecular zone
('washing')

Fig. 3.22   The ventricular mass of the heart
viewed from its right side after removal of the
inlet and part of the outlet components of the
right ventricle. It shows how the trabecular
zone is suspended like a piece of washing
from the washing line made up of the inlet
and outlet components.

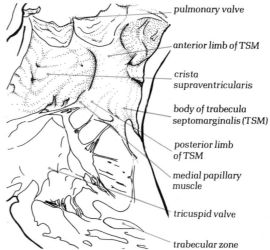

pulmonary valve

anterior limb of TSM

crista
supraventricularis

body of trabecula
septomarginalis (TSM)

posterior limb
of TSM

medial papillary
muscle

tricuspid valve

trabecular zone

Fig. 3.23   The right ventricle viewed from the
front showing the structure of the
infundibulum.

remaining wall thickness (fig. 3.21).
The trabecular zone hangs rather like
a piece of washing from the
'mainstream' of inlet and outlet
portions, which represent the

'washing line' (fig. 3.22). The outlet
portion of the right ventricle, or
infundibulum, is a muscular tube
which supports the pulmonary valve
(fig. 3.23).

3.15

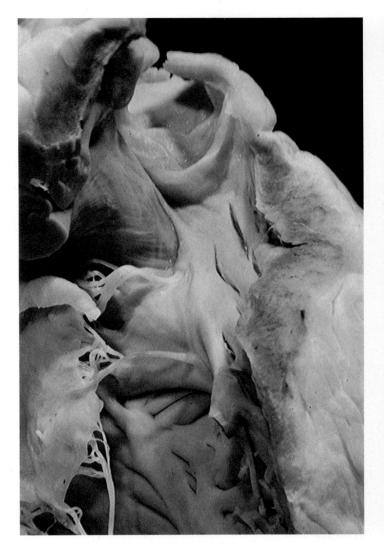

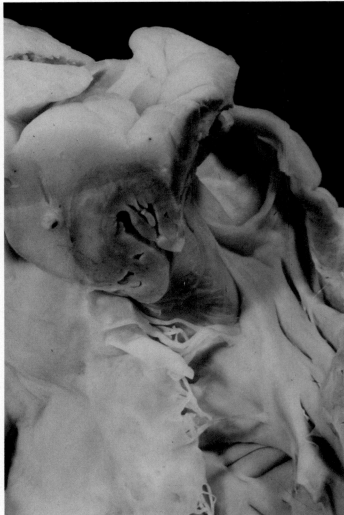

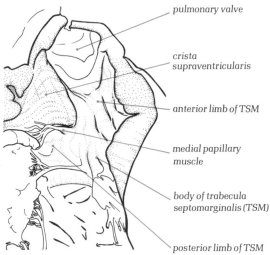

pulmonary valve

crista supraventricularis

anterior limb of TSM

medial papillary muscle

body of trabecula septomarginalis (TSM)

posterior limb of TSM

Fig. 3.24   Dissection of the outflow part of the right ventricle showing the difference between the crista supraventricularis (the supraventricular crest separating the tricuspid from the pulmonary valve) and the trabecula septomarginalis (TSM) which is an extensive septal trabeculation. Note the distinct raphe between the two structures.

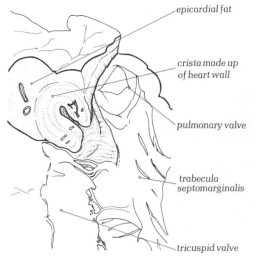

epicardial fat

crista made up of heart wall

pulmonary valve

trabecula septomarginalis

tricuspid valve

Fig. 3.25   Further dissection of the heart shown in fig. 3.24 demonstrates that most of the crista supraventricularis is made up of the heart wall rather than septal structures. Note its relationship to the epicardial fat and the coronary artery.

The inlet and outlet components are separated in the ventricular roof by a prominent muscular bar termed the crista supraventricularis (fig. 3.24).

In its parietal part, this bar is formed by the heart wall, specifically by the inner curvature of the wall or the ventriculo-infundibular fold (figs. 3.25 & 3.26). This fold extends towards the septal surface as it separates the pulmonary and tricuspid valves; but throughout this

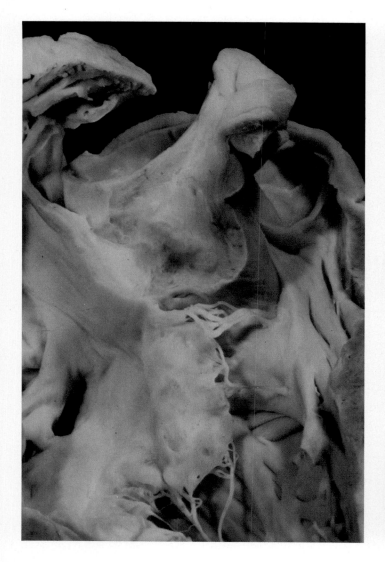

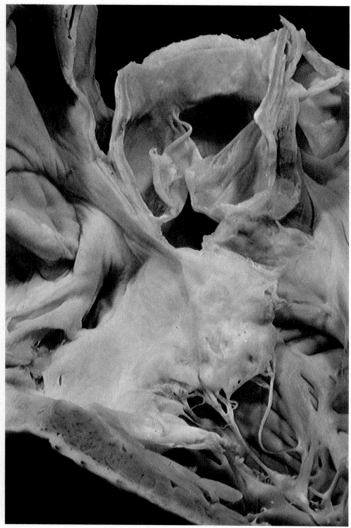

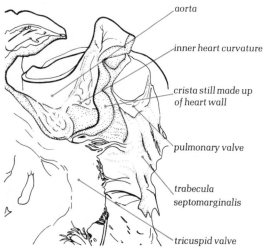

aorta

inner heart curvature

crista still made up
of heart wall

pulmonary valve

trabecula
septomarginalis

tricuspid valve

Fig. 3.26 Still further dissection confirms
that the crista is made up in its larger part of
the outer heart wall.

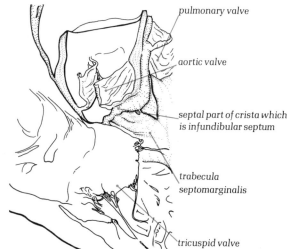

pulmonary valve

aortic valve

septal part of crista which
is infundibular septum

trabecula
septomarginalis

tricuspid valve

Fig. 3.27 Sectioning into the aorta in this
heart shows that only the extreme septal
insertion of the crista supraventricularis is
made up of infundibular septum.

extent, it is still external heart wall
(fig. 3.26). A raphe is usually seen at
the junction of fold with the septum,
and only the part of the crista at this
junction is made up of the infundibular
septum between pulmonary and
aortic valves (fig. 3.25). Medially,
therefore, the crista
supraventricularis merges with the
ventricular septum, inserting between
the limbs of the trabecula
septomarginalis (fig. 3.27).

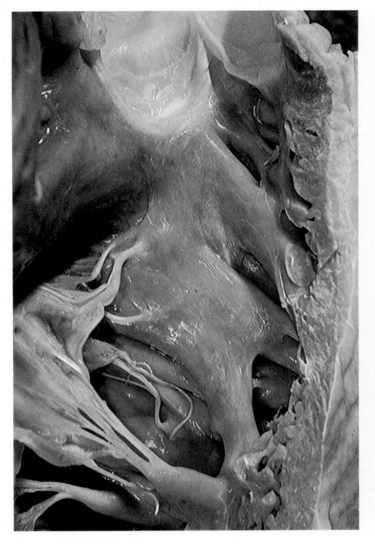

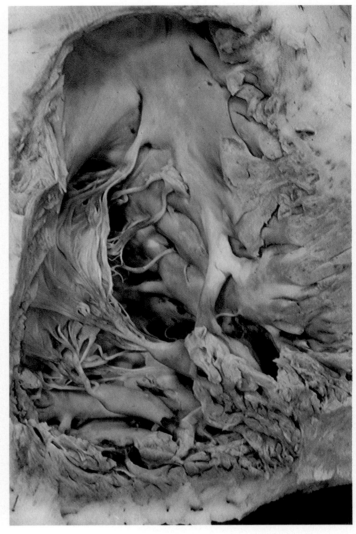

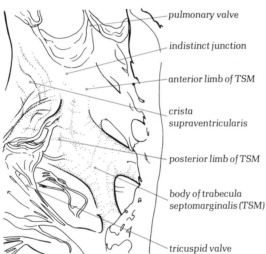

pulmonary valve

indistinct junction

anterior limb of TSM

crista supraventricularis

posterior limb of TSM

body of trabecula septomarginalis (TSM)

tricuspid valve

Fig. 3.28   The septal surface of the right ventricle. The raphe between trabecula septomarginalis and crista is less well seen in this heart than in the heart shown in fig. 3.24.

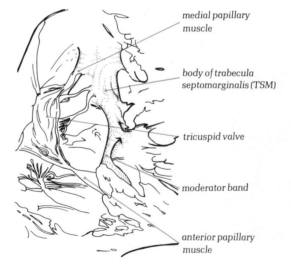

medial papillary muscle

body of trabecula septomarginalis (TSM)

tricuspid valve

moderator band

anterior papillary muscle

Fig. 3.29   The moderator band of the right ventricle. It is an extension from the apex of the trabecula septomarginalis.

The trabecula septomarginalis is a prominent trabecula plastered onto the right ventricular aspect of the septum. Usually, a distinct raphe is visible at the site of insertion of the crista (fig. 3.24); but in other hearts, the crista merges imperceptibly with the trabecula septomarginalis (fig. 3.28). As indicated, the trabecula septomarginalis itself bifurcates in the outlet component of the ventricle into two limbs which clasp the crista (fig. 3.27). The anterior limb ascends to support the pulmonary valve. The posterior limb runs onto and overlays the inlet septum, giving rise to the medial papillary muscle complex and other chordae to the septal leaflet of the tricuspid valve (fig. 3.28). When traced towards the apex, the body of the trabecula septomarginalis splits up to become continuous with the major papillary muscles supporting the anterosuperior and inferior

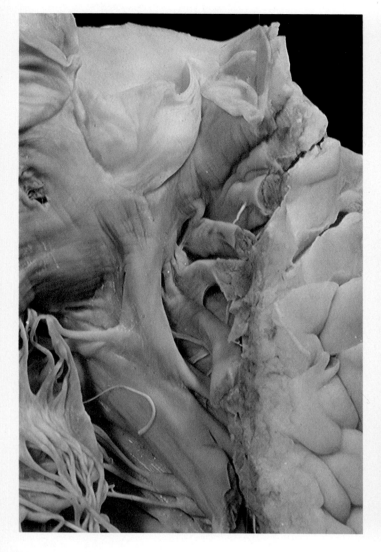

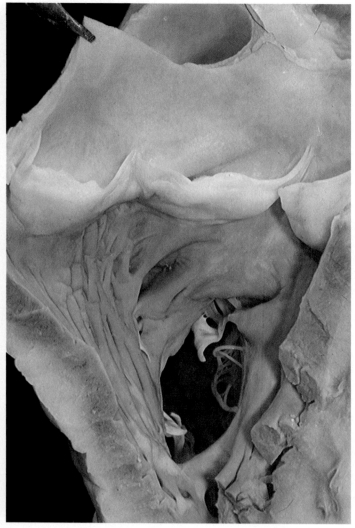

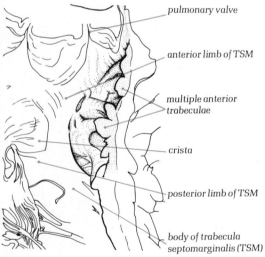

pulmonary valve

anterior limb of TSM

multiple anterior
trabeculae

crista

posterior limb of TSM

body of trabecula
septomarginalis (TSM)

Fig. 3.30   The multiple muscular bars which
line the anterior aspect of the infundibulum
of the right ventricle.

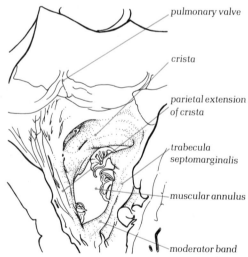

pulmonary valve

crista

parietal extension
of crista

trabecula
septomarginalis

muscular annulus

moderator band

Fig. 3.31   The infundibulum of the right
ventricle viewed from the front showing the
muscular annulus formed by the crista
supraventricularis and its parietal extension
and the trabecula septomarginalis together
with the moderator band.

tricuspid valve leaflets; and one band
passes prominently across the cavity
of the ventricle as the moderator band
(fig. 3.29). Usually the origin of the
moderator band is found well out
towards the apex, but early take-off is
not uncommon; while in other hearts

several prominent trabeculae can
cross the cavity of the ventricle
anterior to the edge of the trabecula
septomarginalis (fig. 3.30). In most
hearts, a muscle band on the
underside of the ventriculo-
infundibular fold is continued down

the parietal ventricular wall as a
prominent trabecula. Fusion of this
with the moderator band produces a
muscular annulus between the
ventricular inlet and the outlet and
trabecular components (fig. 3.31).

3.19

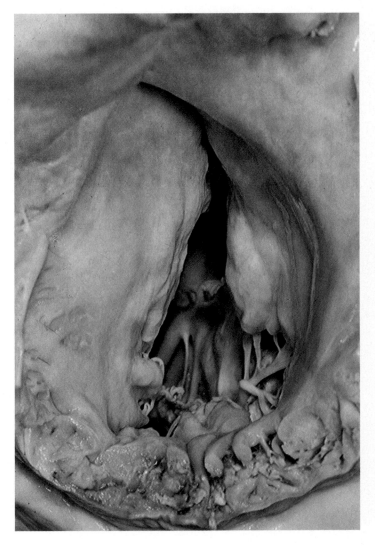

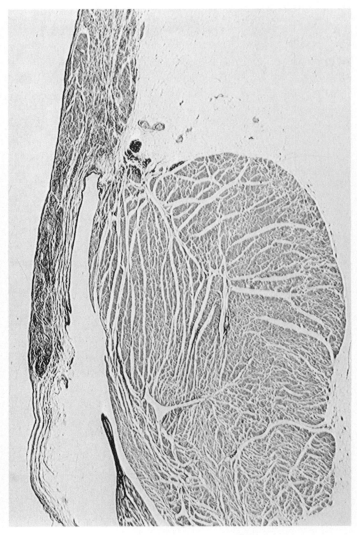

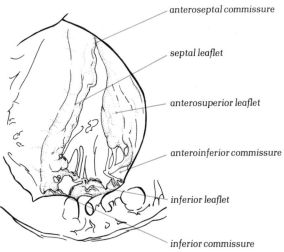

anteroseptal commissure

septal leaflet

anterosuperior leaflet

anteroinferior commissure

inferior leaflet

inferior commissure

Fig. 3.32   The tricuspid valve viewed from behind with the heart in its in situ position. The three leaflets occupy septal, anterosuperior and inferior positions.

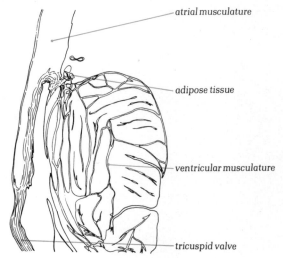

atrial musculature

adipose tissue

ventricular musculature

tricuspid valve

Fig. 3.33   Histology of the tricuspid ring. The leaflet does not spring from a strong well-formed annulus as in the mitral valve (compare with fig. 4.10).

The Tricuspid Valve

It is frequently difficult to identify three leaflets in this valve on superficial examination. However, if a search is made for commissural chordae springing from papillary muscles, then it is rare not to find three leaflets, frequently with the major leaflets themselves divided by clefts supported by cleft chordae as in the mitral valve. Considering the valve *in situ*, the three leaflets occupy septal, anterosuperior and inferior positions (fig. 3.32). Although the leaflets all spring from the atrioventricular junction, a distinct fibrous annulus such as seen in the mitral ring (see fig. 4.10) is not always identified. Instead, the fibrosa of the tricuspid valve tapers out in the adipose tissue of the atrioventricular sulcus (fig. 3.33). The commissures between the leaflets can be termed the anteroseptal, anteroinferior and inferior

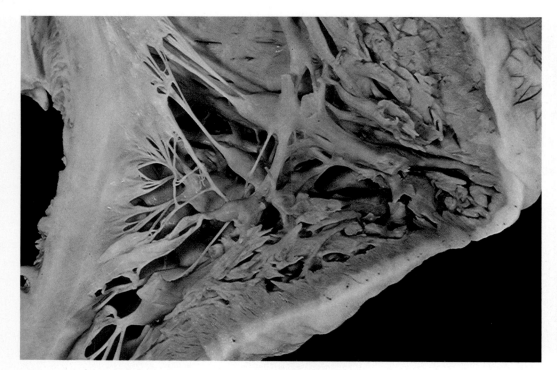

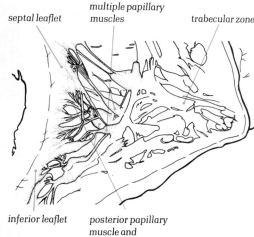

septal leaflet | multiple papillary muscles | trabecular zone

inferior leaflet | posterior papillary muscle and commissural chorda

Fig. 3.34   The inlet part of the right ventricle showing the multiple papillary muscles supporting the septal and inferior leaflets. However, only one, the posterior papillary muscle, gives rise to a commissural chord.

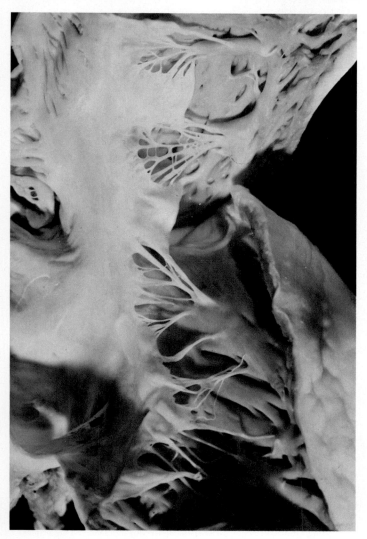

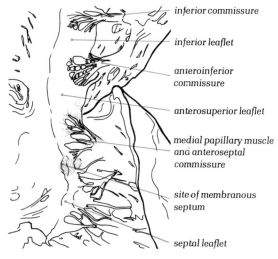

inferior commissure

inferior leaflet

anteroinferior commissure

anterosuperior leaflet

medial papillary muscle and anteroseptal commissure

site of membranous septum

septal leaflet

Fig. 3.35   The anteroseptal commissure of the tricuspid valve viewed from behind having opened the valve through the inferior commissure is supported by the medial commissure. Note that the anteroseptal papillary muscle is superior to and to the right of the membranous septum.

commissures (fig. 3.32). The papillary muscles supporting the valve leaflets spring mostly from the trabecula septomarginalis and its apical ramification; but, in the case of the septal and inferior leaflets, additional muscles or chordae take origin from the superficial trabeculations of the inlet septum (fig. 3.34).

The anteroseptal commissure is supported by the medial papillary muscle or papillary muscle complex, originating either singly or as a group of chordae from the posterior limb of the trabecula septomarginalis. The various chordae run to both the septal leaflet and the anterosuperior leaflet, but the commissural chord is found superior to and to the right of the membranous septum (fig. 3.35).

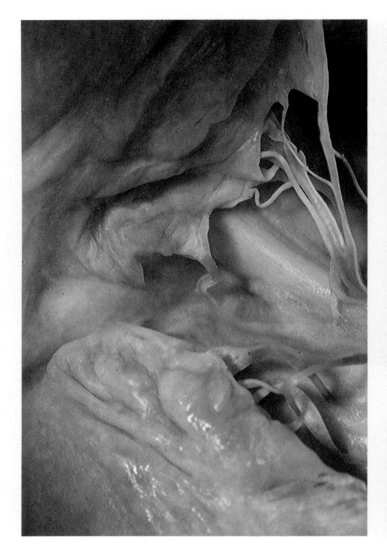

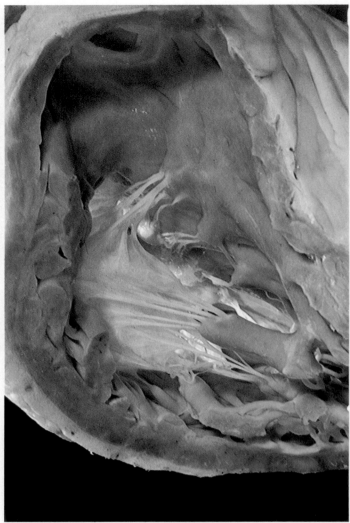

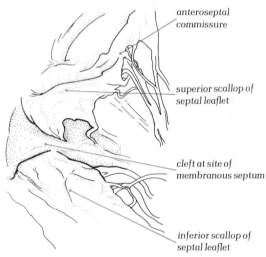

anteroseptal
commissure

superior scallop of
septal leaflet

cleft at site of
membranous septum

inferior scallop of
septal leaflet

Fig. 3.36   A heart with a cleft in the septal
leaflet of the tricuspid valve at the site of the
membranous septum.

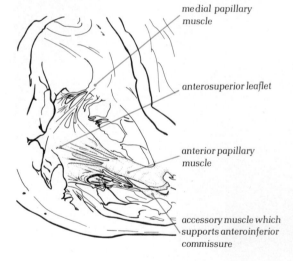

medial papillary
muscle

anterosuperior leaflet

anterior papillary
muscle

accessory muscle which
supports anteroinferior
commissure

Fig. 3.37   A frequent variant in tricuspid
valve morphology is for the large anterior
papillary muscle to support the midzone of
the anterosuperior leaflet. The anteroinferior
commissure in this heart is supported by an
accessory anterior papillary muscle.

This means that part of the septal
leaflet swings away from the septum
and membranous septal area,
frequently with a cleft between the
septal and free wall scallops of the
leaflet (fig. 3.36). Other investigators
have considered this cleft to be the
commissure; however, if the criterion

for a commissure is that it gives fan-
shaped chordae to the edges of
adjacent leaflets, then the more
superior structure is the commissure;
particularly since in many hearts the
cleft related to the membranous
septum has no chordal support
(fig. 3.36). The anterosuperior leaflet

(fig. 3.20) stretches from the medial
papillary muscle to the anteroinferior
commissure. Frequently, the major
anterior papillary muscle springing
from the trabecula septomarginalis
runs up to the midpoint of this leaflet,
and does not give rise to a commissural
chord. The commissure is usually

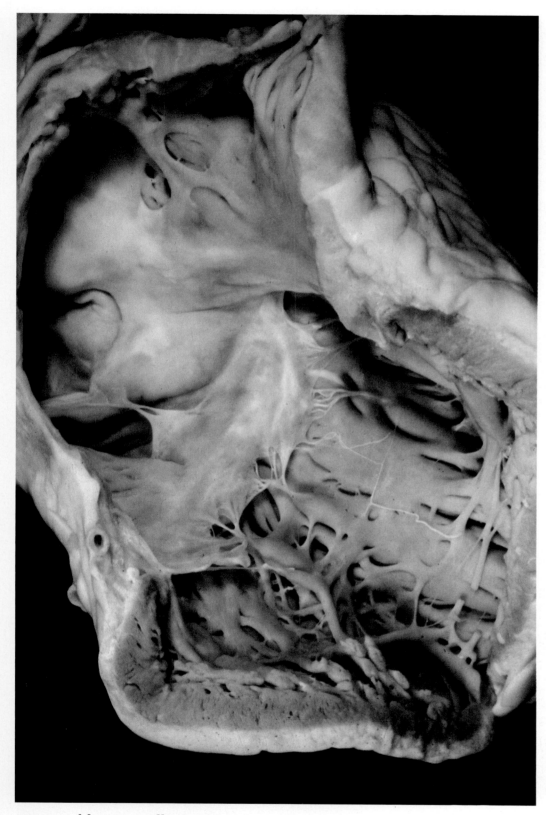

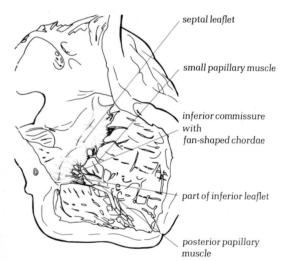

septal leaflet

small papillary muscle

inferior commissure
with
fan-shaped chordae

part of inferior leaflet

posterior papillary
muscle

Fig. 3.38   The opened inlet portion of the
right ventricle showing the inferior
commissure. Note that the other small
muscles do not give rise to commissural
chordae.

supported from a smaller anterior muscle arising from the same area (*fig. 3.37*). Many smaller muscles spring from the same area and support the inferior and septal leaflets; but only one of them gives rise to a commissural chord, this being the inferior commissure (*fig. 3.38*). The variation seen in tricuspid leaflet and papillary muscle pattern is considerable, but the above morphology can generally be recognized. At the point of insertion of the tricuspid papillary muscles and

chordae, the ventricular inlet portion merges with the trabecular portion of the right ventricle. The trabecular zone extends out to the apex, and has characteristic coarse trabeculae (*fig. 3.22*). At the apex, the myocardium is thinner than the remainder of the ventricle (*fig. 3.21*). Towards the base, the trabecular zone in turn merges with the outlet portion or infundibulum. The trabecular zone extends well up the left margin of the ventricle towards the base (*fig. 3.22*)

and its junction with the infundibulum is indistinct. The infundibulum generally has smoother walls. It is a muscular funnel which supports the pulmonary valve. It should be noted that the greater part of its posterior wall is the ventriculo-infundibular fold, being above the level of the aortic valve. It does not, therefore, constitute a true septum (*fig. 3.26*). This right lateral part of the infundibulum is the major part of the crista supraventricularis.

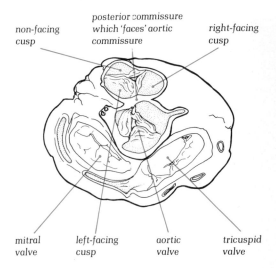

non-facing cusp — posterior commissure which 'faces' aortic commissure — right-facing cusp

mitral valve — left-facing cusp — aortic valve — tricuspid valve

Fig. 3.39 The atrioventricular junction viewed from its atrial aspect after removal of the atrial chambers and great arteries. It shows the relationships of the leaflets of the pulmonary and aortic valves. Two leaflets of these valves always face each other, permitting the nomination of right-facing and left-facing leaflets of the pulmonary valves.

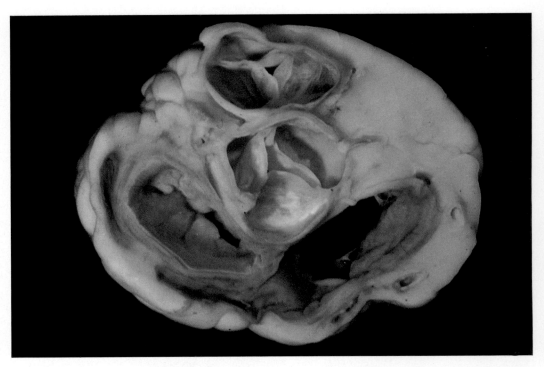

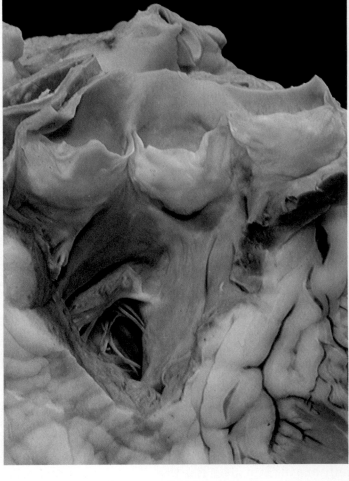

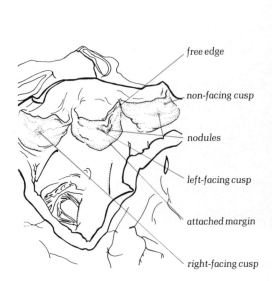

free edge

non-facing cusp

nodules

left-facing cusp

attached margin

right-facing cusp

Fig. 3.40 The infundibulum of the right ventricle opened from the front showing the morphology of the pulmonary valve.

The pulmonary valve is the trifoliate arterial valve of the right ventricle. The posterior commissure of the valve is positioned so as to face the commissure between the left and right aortic coronary cusps (fig. 3.39). This means that two of the pulmonary cusps 'face' the aortic coronary cusps, and can therefore be termed right-facing and left-facing pulmonary cusps. The third cusp is then the non-facing cusp (fig. 3.39). Each cusp is semilunar in shape and is attached to the infundibulum along its convex edge, flicking up into the pulmonary trunk in the open position (fig. 3.40). The central point of the free edge of each cusp is thickened to form the nodule, and the cusps close against each other at this point. The cusps are approximately equal in size. Hearts may be found with bicuspid or quadricuspid pulmonary valves, the findings being of no pathological significance.

4 The Ventricles II

The Morphologically Left Ventricle
The Interventricular Septum

The Morphologically Left Ventricle

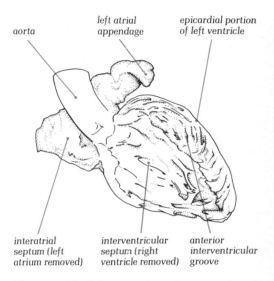

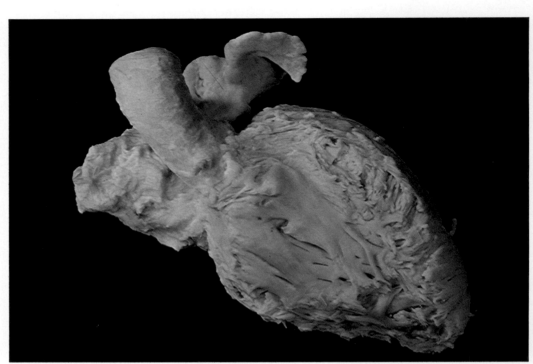

Fig. 4.1 The left ventricle and atrium after removal of the right-sided structures and viewed from the front.

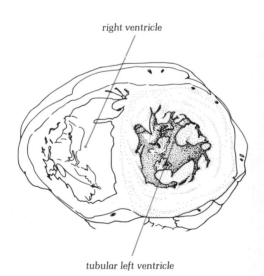

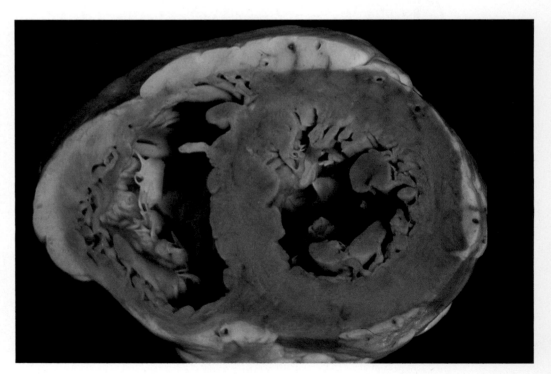

Fig. 4.2 Short axis section of the ventricular mass showing the tubular nature of the left ventricle.

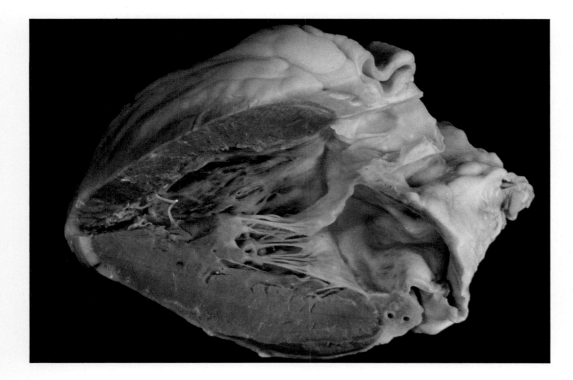

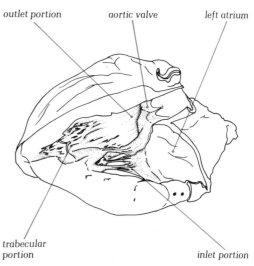

outlet portion · aortic valve · left atrium

trabecular portion · inlet portion

Fig. 4.3   The opened left ventricle showing inlet, trabecular and outlet portions.

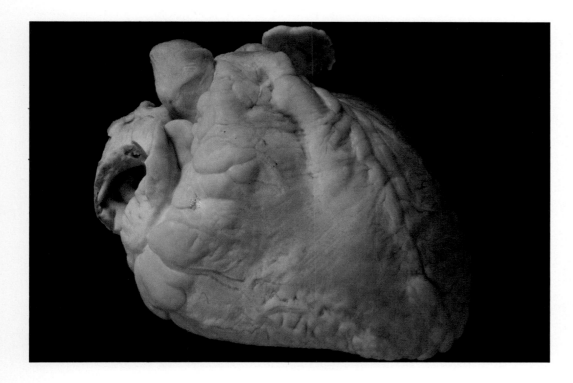

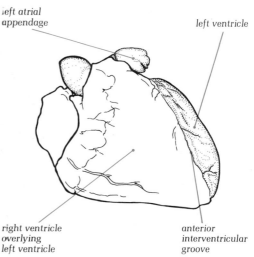

left atrial appendage · left ventricle

right ventricle overlying left ventricle · anterior interventricular groove

Fig. 4.4   A heart viewed from the front. Comparisons with fig. 4.1 will show how most of the left ventricle is overlaid by the right ventricle.

The left ventricle is a conical structure (fig. 4.1) with tubular walls (fig. 4.2) which narrow down to a rounded apex (fig. 4.1). It comprises an inlet portion, containing the mitral valve and its tension apparatus; an apical trabecular zone characterized by fine trabeculations and an outlet zone, supporting the aortic valve, which is incomplete posteriorly so that the aortic and mitral valves are in fibrous continuity (fig. 4.3). The left ventricle forms the greater part of the diaphragmatic surface of the heart but is overlaid anteriorly and superiorly by the trabecular zone and outlet of the right ventricle (fig. 4.4).

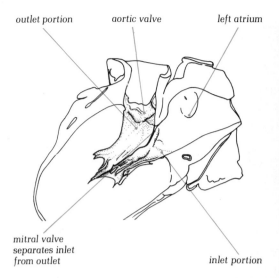

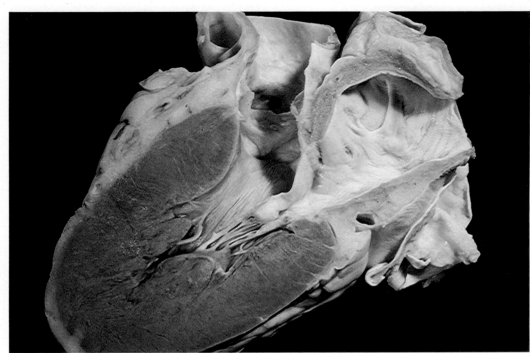

Fig. 4.5   Section through the left ventricle showing how the anterior mitral valve leaflet separates its inlet and outlet portions.

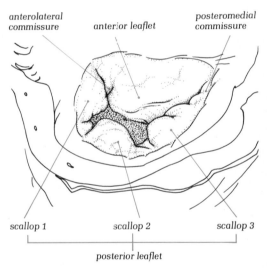

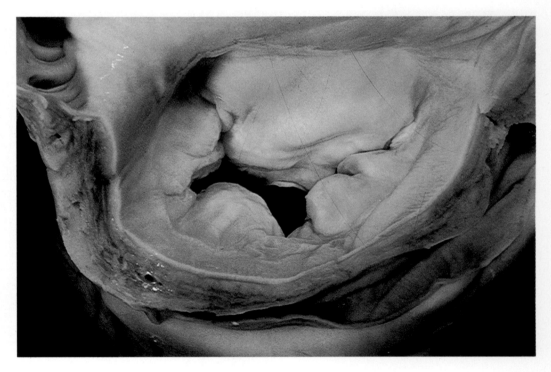

Fig. 4.6   Mitral valve viewed from above showing the anterior or septal leaflet and the posterior or mural leaflet with its three scallops.

In contrast to the right ventricle where there is a gentle curve between inlet and outlet portions, the left ventricle shows an acute angle between these portions, both extending down into the trabecular zone separated by the anterior leaflet of the mitral valve (fig. 4.5). Usually there is no structure comparable to the crista supraventricularis in the left ventricle owing to the fibrous continuity of the inlet and outlet valves, although in rare hearts, a muscular fold (ventriculo-infundibular fold) may interpose between the valves (*Becu, 1971; Rosenquist et al., 1977*). The septal surface of the left ventricle is smooth, so that there is no structure corresponding to the trabecula septomarginalis in the left ventricle (compare *figs. 4.5 & 3.29*).

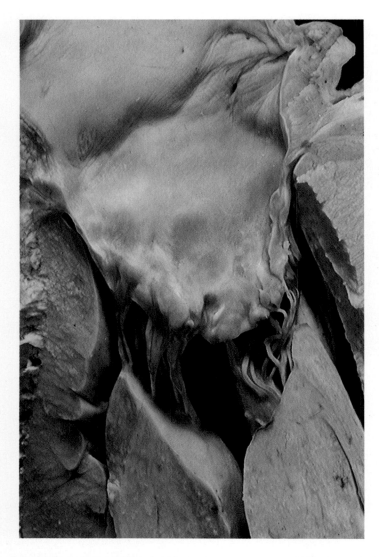

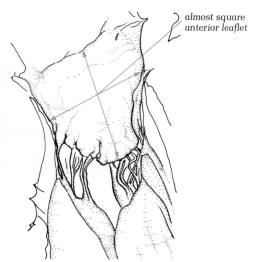

Fig. 4.7 The anterior or septal leaflet of the mitral valve viewed from behind after division of the valve through its commissure. The posterior or mural leaflet is shown in fig. 4.2. Note that the anterior leaflet is almost square.

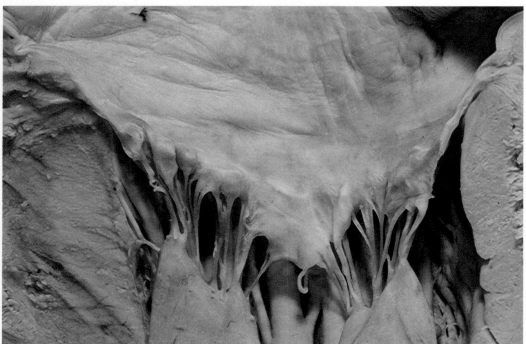

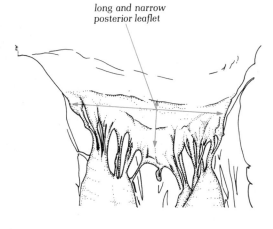

Fig. 4.8 The posterior or mural leaflet of the divided mitral valve shown in fig. 4.7 viewed from the front. Note that the posterior leaflet is long and narrow.

The Mitral Valve

The mitral valve is characteristically described as having two leaflets, the anterior or septal and posterior or mural leaflets. The leaflets are separated by the posteromedial and anterolateral commissures (fig. 4.6). The anterior leaflet is attached to less than half the circumference of the mitral annulus but has considerable height and consequently presents as a large leaflet (fig. 4.7). The posterior leaflet, in contrast, is attached to more than half the circumference (fig. 4.6) but is less tall (fig. 4.8), and occupies only about the same area as the anterior leaflet. Moreover, the posterior leaflet has a characteristic scalloped contour. In the usual case three scallops can be distinguished divided by clefts (fig. 4.6). These scallops are termed posteromedial, middle and anterolateral.

4.5

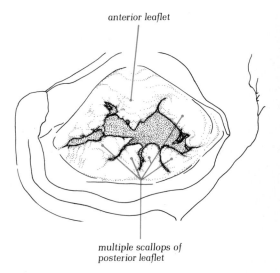

anterior leaflet

multiple scallops of
posterior leaflet

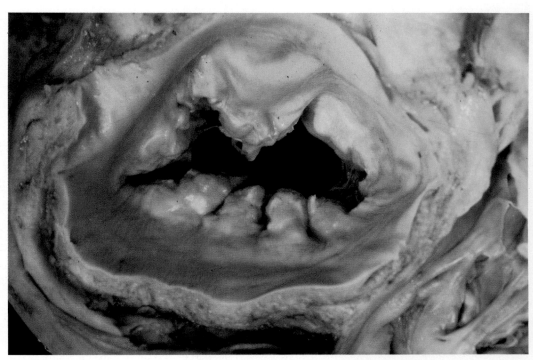

Fig. 4.9   Another normal mitral valve viewed
from above showing the variation which
exists in the number of scallops (compare
with fig. 4.6).

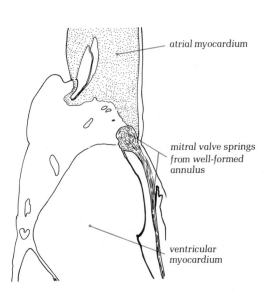

atrial myocardium

mitral valve springs
from well-formed
annulus

ventricular
myocardium

Fig. 4.10   Histological section through the
mitral valve ring. The leaflet takes origin from
a well-formed annulus (compare with fig. 3.34).

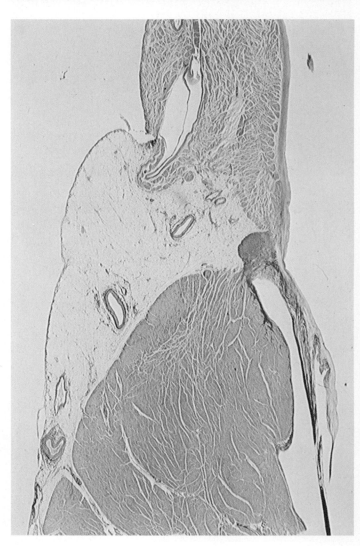

However, it is not at all unusual to
find aberrations from this pattern,
two, four, five or more scallops being
seen in otherwise normal valves
(fig. 4.9). The posterior leaflet
throughout its length is attached
to the mitral atrioventricular annulus

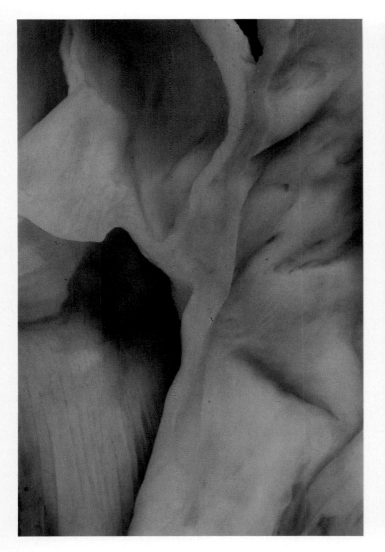

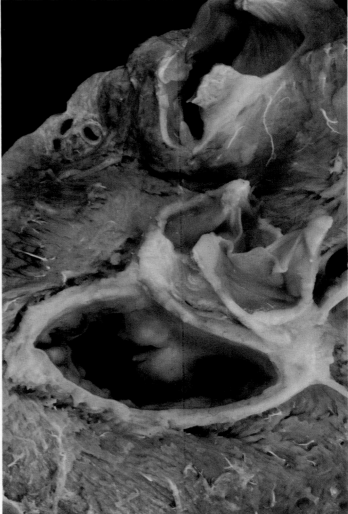

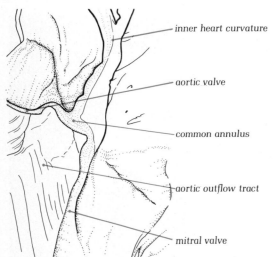

Fig. 4.11 *Section through the area of aortic-mitral fibrous continuity. The two valves have a common annulus.*

- inner heart curvature
- aortic valve
- common annulus
- aortic outflow tract
- mitral valve

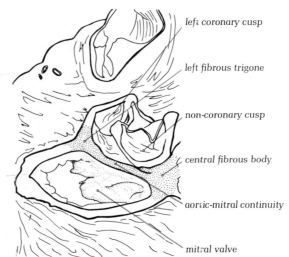

Fig. 4.12 *Dissection of the fibrous skeleton of the aortic and mitral valves viewed from above and behind showing the thickening at either end of the area of valvar continuity.*

- left coronary cusp
- left fibrous trigone
- non-coronary cusp
- central fibrous body
- aortic-mitral continuity
- mitral valve

(fig. 4.10). The anterior leaflet, in contrast, is in fibrous continuity with the aortic valve, the two valves having a common annulus (fig. 4.11) strengthened at each end by the right and left fibrous trigones (fig. 4.12).

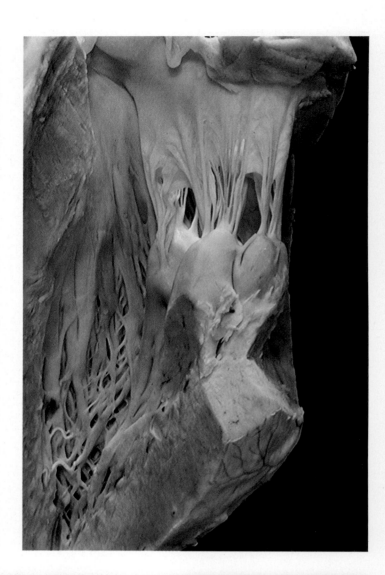

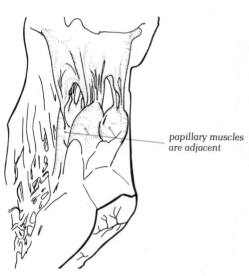

Fig. 4.13   Cutaway of the left ventricle showing the papillary muscle groups of the mitral valve. Note how they arise adjacent to each other when in their in situ position (compare with fig. 4.15).

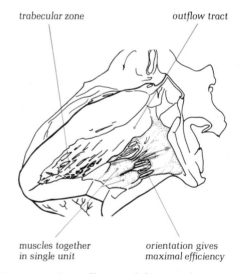

Fig. 4.14   Overall view of the mitral unit showing how the muscles act at maximum mechanical efficiency.

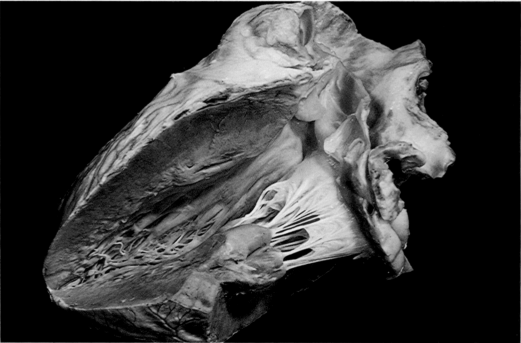

The mitral valve leaflets are supported by two papillary muscle groups situated underneath the commissural areas in posteromedial and anterolateral positions (fig. 4.13). Their position is such that the chordae between muscle and leaflet operate at the maximal mechanical efficiency (fig. 4.14). Each papillary muscle supports the adjacent part of both valve leaflets (fig. 4.15). There is considerable variation in

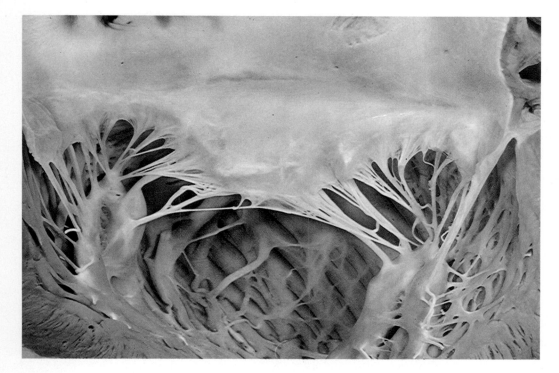

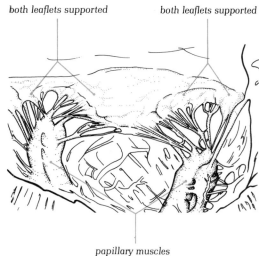

papillary muscles

Fig. 4.15 The opened mitral valve showing how each papillary muscle supports the adjacent part of both valve leaflets. The apparent separation of the papillary muscles is artefactual. See fig. 4.13 for the in situ position of the muscles.

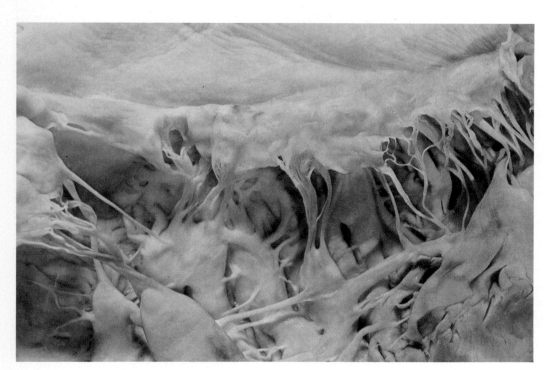

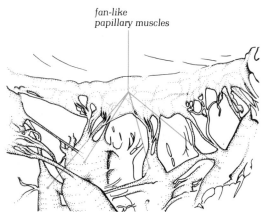

fan-like papillary muscles

Fig 4.16 With the considerable variation possible in papillary muscle, this group of fan-like muscles is in sharp contrast to the pillar-type muscles in fig. 4.15.

the morphology of the papillary muscles themselves, particularly the posteromedial muscle. They may be single pillar-like muscles or be composed of several heads of differing size (compare *figs. 4.15 & 4.16*).

The different papillary muscle architecture affects the chordal distribution (*vide infra*) and also affects the mode of arterial supply to the papillary muscle complex.

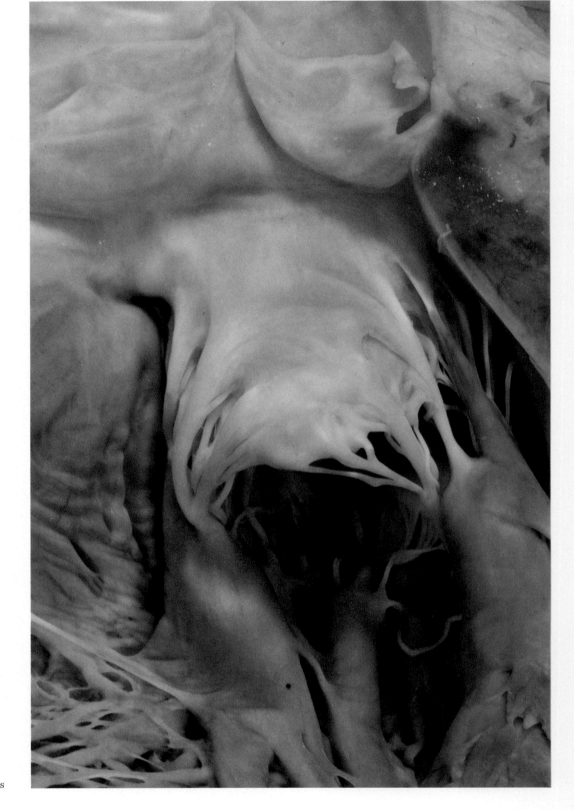

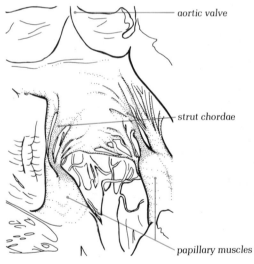

aortic valve

strut chordae

papillary muscles

Fig. 4.17 The anterior leaflet of the mitral valve viewed from the outflow tract showing the strut chordae.

Because of the different topography of the anterior and posterior leaflets, there are corresponding differences in the mode of chordal support which also show considerable individual variation.

These variations may leave part of the leaflet less well supported than would be anticipated. The anterior leaflet is supported only by rough zone chordae together with the two commissural chords (fig. 4.15). The rough zone

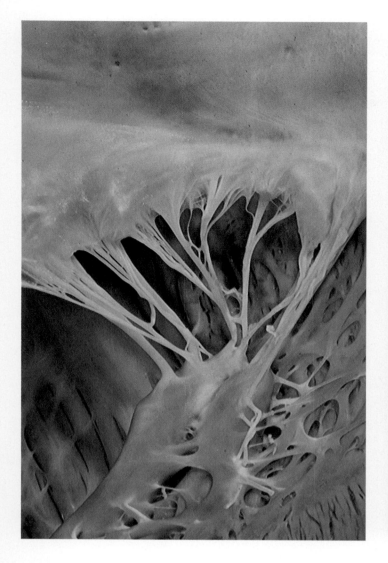

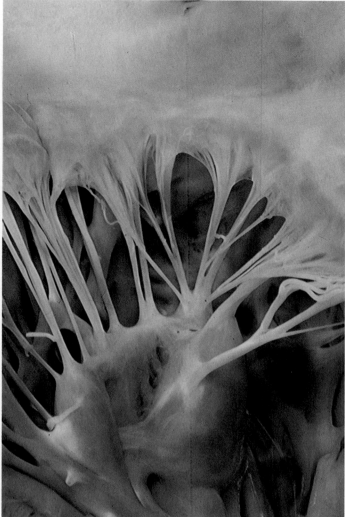

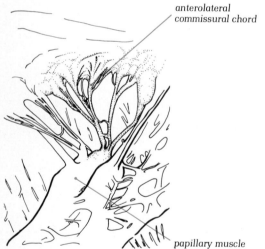

anterolateral
commissural chord

papillary muscle

Fig. 4.18   The posteromedial commissural
chordae of the mitral valve.

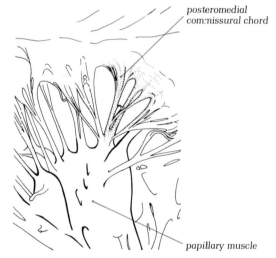

posteromedial
commissural chord

papillary muscle

Fig. 4.19   The anterolateral commissural
chordae of the mitral valve.

chords may be strengthened by
thicker tendinous structures, the
so-called strut chordae (fig. 4.17),
usually one for each half of the leaflet.
The commissural chords spring from
the tip of their papillary muscle
and fan out to attach to the free
margins of both leaflets. The
posteromedial commissural chord
usually fans out more than that of the
anterolateral commissure (compare
figs. 4.18 & 4.19)

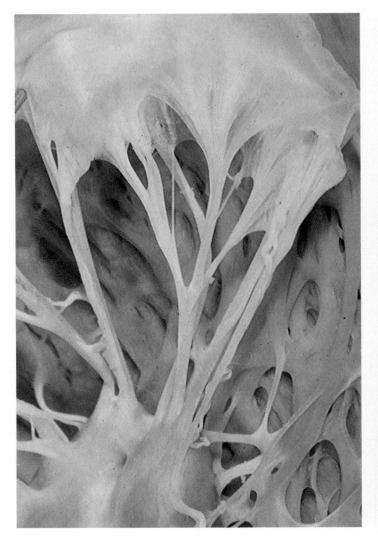

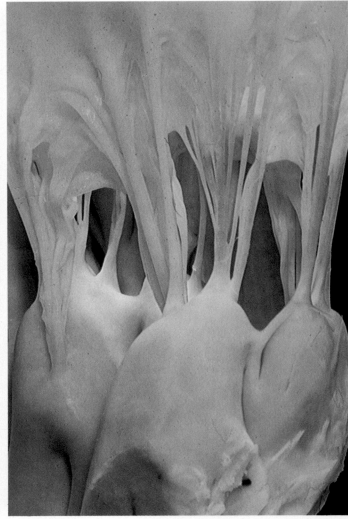

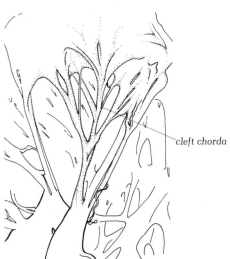

cleft chorda

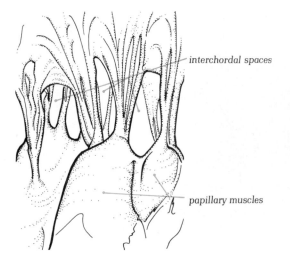

interchordal spaces

papillary muscles

Fig. 4.20 *Cleft chorda of the same valve as in figs. 4.18 & 4.19. Although supporting a cleft between 2 scallops, it is virtually indistinguishable from the commissural chords.*

Fig. 4.21 *Detail of the attachments of the chordae to the papillary muscles. The blood disperses into the left ventricle through the interchordal spaces.*

The scallops of the posterior leaflet, like the anterior leaflet, have their main support from rough zone and commissural chordae. In addition, the clefts between the scallops are supported by so-called cleft chordae which may be virtually indistinguishable from commissural chordae (*fig. 4.20*). The basal parts of the scallops of the posterior leaflet may show further support from basal chordae, although their number and distribution is variable. While the basic pattern described above for the mitral valve is usually apparent, the individual variability is considerable and such variations may well reflect the frequent variations from 'normality' observed in clinical practice (*Becker, 1979*).

On superficial examination it may appear that the mitral orifice consists solely of the area delineated by the leaflets. It must be remembered that the valve in its open state is a funnel from the annulus (point of attachment) down to the free margin

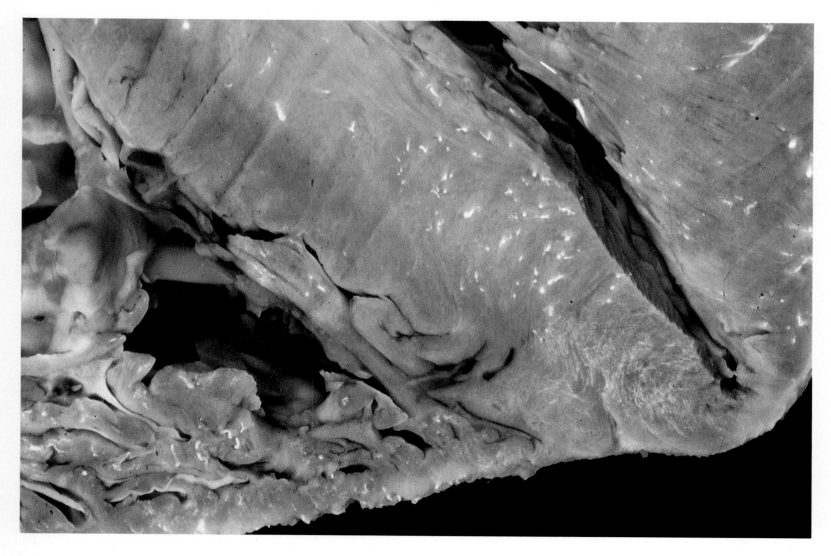

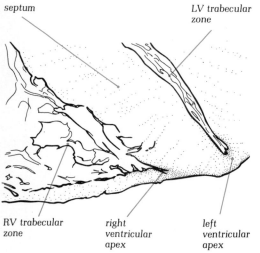

septum

LV trabecular zone

RV trabecular zone

right ventricular apex

left ventricular apex

Fig. 4.22   *Section of the ventricular apices showing how thin the myocardium is at this point.*

of the leaflets. This funnel leads into the inlet portion of the left ventricle which is surrounded by the chordae supporting the leaflets. From a functional standpoint, therefore, it is important that the interchordal spaces (fig. 4.21) do not obstruct dispersion of blood from the inlet to the remainder of the left ventricular cavity. The apparently wide gap between the papillary muscle groups and the two halves of the anterior leaflet (fig. 4.15) is artefactual. When the papillary muscles are *in situ* they and their chordae are in close apposition (figs. 4.13 & 4.14).

The trabecular portion of the left ventricle extends from the origin of the papillary muscles to the apex (fig. 4.3). It has the shape of a narrowing cone and its walls exhibit fine trabeculations. The thickness of the ventricular wall diminishes markedly towards the apex where it may be no more than 1–2mm thick (fig. 4.22).

4.13

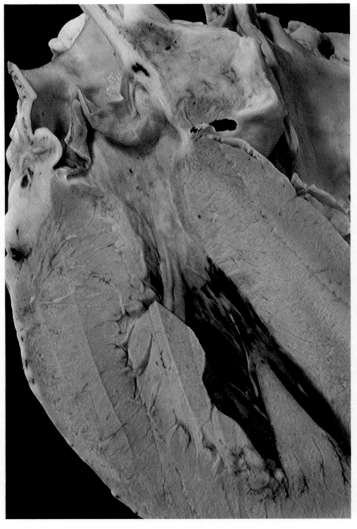

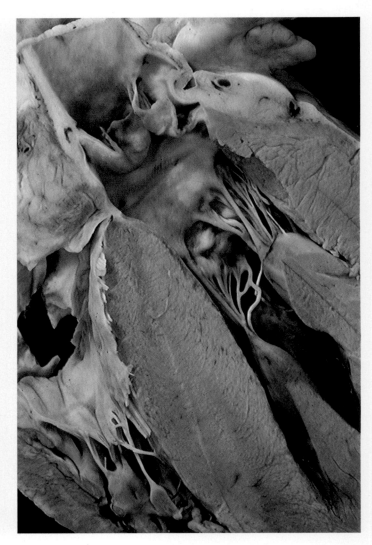

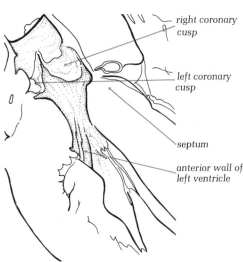

right coronary
cusp

left coronary
cusp

septum

anterior wall of
left ventricle

left coronary
cusp

non-coronary
cusp

aortic-mitral
continuity

septum

Fig. 4.23   The anterior half of the left
ventricular outflow tract viewed from behind.
The posterior part is shown in fig. 4.24.
Note that the anterior quadrants are muscular.

Fig. 4.24   The posterior half of the left
ventricular outflow tract shown in fig. 4.23.
Note the continuity between aortic and
mitral valves.

The outlet of the left ventricle
supports the aortic valve. The outlet
tract is a partly muscular and partly
fibrous structure (figs. 4.23 & 4.24).
The long axis of the outlet tract
subtends an angle to the long axis of
the inlet-trabecular portion of the
ventricle as viewed in both
anteroposterior (fig. 4.25) and lateral
(fig. 4.3) projection. The angulation

in anterolateral-posterior projection
approaches more of a right angle
with increasing age, and the septum
then has a sigmoid configuration
(fig. 4.26). The muscular part of the
outlet comprises the upper edge of
the smooth trabecular septum
medially, the infundibular septum
anteriorly and the left margin of the
ventriculo-infundibular fold laterally

(fig. 4.23). These structures merge
imperceptibly with the trabecular
zone towards the apex and support
the leaflets of the aortic valve at the
base (fig. 4.27). The fibrous part
consists of the area of aortic-mitral
continuity, the area of aortic wall
beneath the commissure of the non-
and left coronary cusps and the
recess beneath the central fibrous

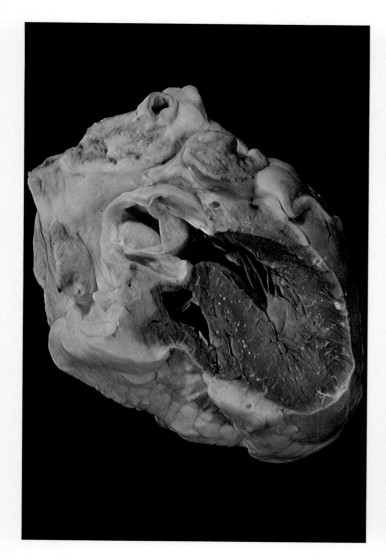

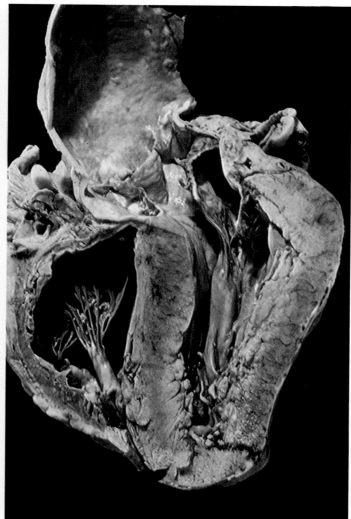

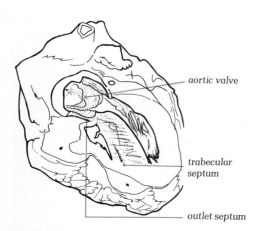

Fig. 4.25 Frontal section through a heart showing the considerable angle which exists between the trabecular and outlet parts of the left ventricle.

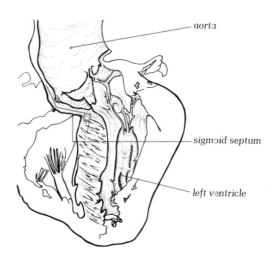

Fig. 4.26 Increase in the angle between trabecular and outlet portions leads to the sigmoid septum of old age (compare with fig. 4.25).

body walled on its right side by the compartments of the membranous septum (figs. 4.24 & 4.27) and the atrioventricular muscular septum. The extent of aortic-mitral continuity varies in individual hearts, as do the precise proportions of the cusps in continuity with the mitral leaflet. If a line is constructed to divide the anterior mitral leaflet into equal halves, it can intersect the aortic root anywhere between the midpoints of the non-coronary and left coronary cusps (fig. 4.27). It follows from this description that the left ventricular outlet has length in both its anterior and posterior walls, albeit less than the right ventricular outlet.

The major distinguishing feature between the ventricular outlets is that the posterior wall of the left ventricular outlet is a fibrous structure. Furthermore, although the outlet is very much in the middle of the heart, the intervalvar fibrous area forms the floor of the transverse sinus. In this area, therefore, the outlet is separated from the pericardial cavity only by this intervalvar fibrous tissue (fig. 4.11). The membranous ventricular septum

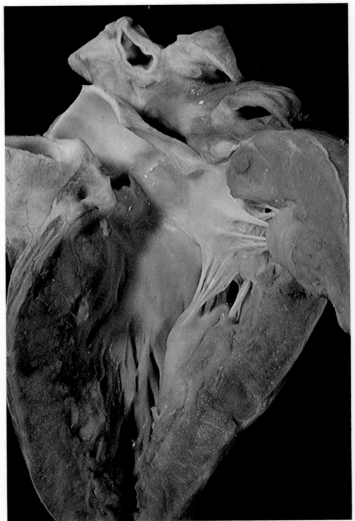

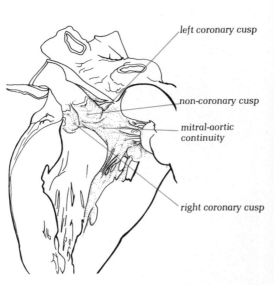

Fig. 4.27   The opened left ventricular outflow tract. The relationship of the aortic cusps to the mitral valve anterior leaflet is variable.

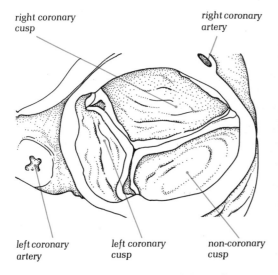

Fig. 4.28   Aortic leaflet viewed from above in the closed position. Note that the leaflets are not of the same size.

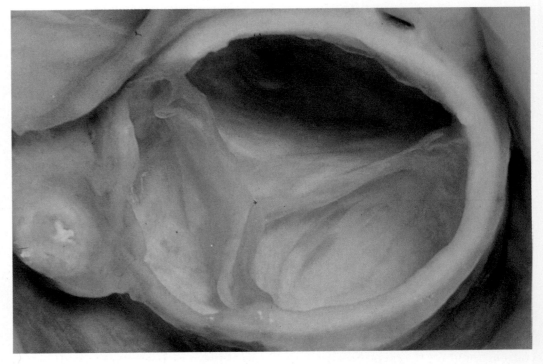

is an integral part of the left ventricular outlet but will be considered in the section devoted to the ventricular septum (see figs. 4.36 & 4.41).

The aortic valve is a trifoliate valve (fig. 4.28) having typical semilunar cusps (see fig. 3.10). There are various systems of naming the aortic cusps. Those using anterior and posterior in their titles give problems due to the oblique position of the aortic valve when the heart is in situ. This problem can be circumvented by taking account of the fact that cusps of the aortic valve always face two cusps of the pulmonary valve. As with the pulmonary valve (see fig. 3.39), the cusps could, therefore, be named right-facing, left-facing and non-facing. However, account is additionally taken of the feature that when two coronary arteries are present, they almost always arise from the sinuses related to the facing cusps. The cusps are therefore termed the right coronary, left

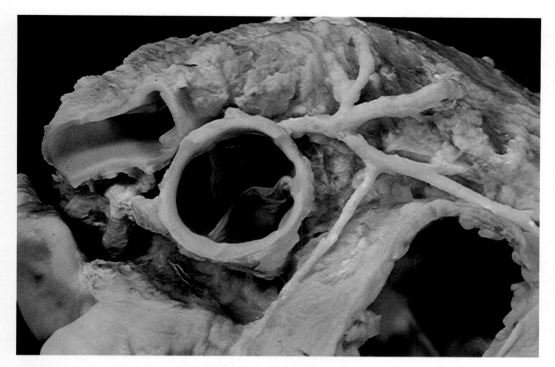

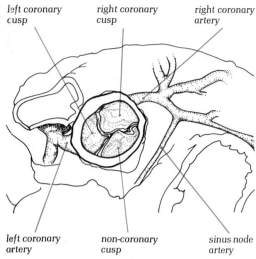

Fig. 4.29   The origin of the coronary arteries enables the leaflets of the aortic valve to be designated right coronary, left coronary and non-coronary leaflets.

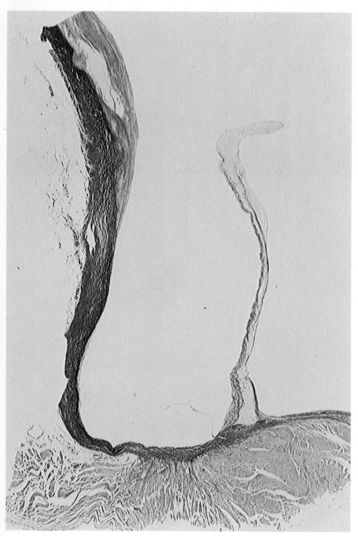

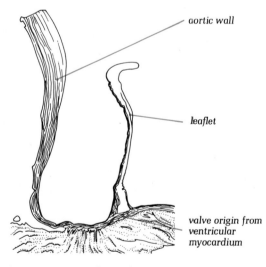

Fig. 4.30   Histological section showing the origin of the parietal part of an aortic leaflet from ventricular muscle.

coronary and non-coronary cusps (fig. 4.29). Parts of the non-coronary and left coronary cusps are usually in fibrous continuity with the mitral valve, the precise areas of each cusp varying as indicated above. The non-coronary cusp is in fibrous continuity with the central fibrous body and the membranous septum in its posterior part (fig. 4.12). The anterior part of this cusp, together with the right coronary cusp and part of the left coronary cusp, take origin from the muscular aortic outlet but are additionally supported by an annulus derived from the fibrous skeleton of the heart (fig. 4.12; see Chapter 5). The area of the aorta containing the semilunar cusps is the aortic root. It is arranged in clover leaf fashion at the site of the cusps to produce the aortic sinuses. The valve leaflets are apposed to the sinus wall when the valve is open (fig. 4.30).

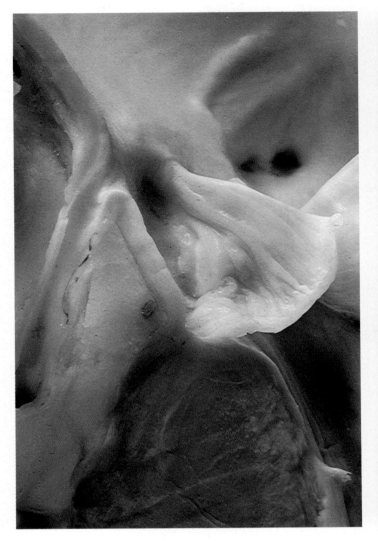

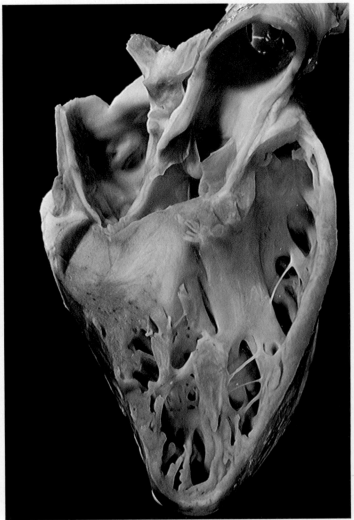

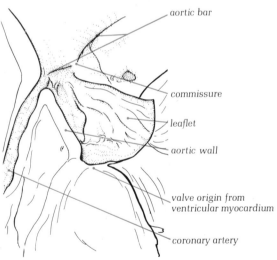

aortic bar

commissure

leaflet

aortic wall

valve origin from
ventricular myocardium

coronary artery

Fig. 4.31   Bisection of the aorta through the
origin of a coronary artery. Note that the
valve leaflet closes against the aortic bar and
that the coronary artery ostium is beneath the
bar.

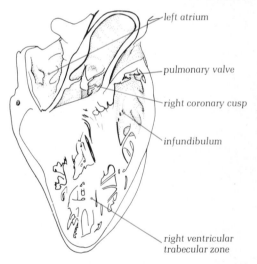

left atrium

pulmonary valve

right coronary cusp

infundibulum

right ventricular
trabecular zone

Fig. 4.32   Section through the aortic outflow
tract from the right side showing how the
right coronary cusp is related to the
infundibulum of the right ventricle.

The proximal boundary of the
sinus is therefore the transition of
aortic wall with the left ventricular
outlet portion. Its distal boundary
is the rim against which the valve
leaflet opens, sometimes called the
aortic bar (fig. 4.31). Above the
aortic sinuses is the ascending aorta.

By virtue of its central position, the
aortic valve is related to all other
cardiac chambers. The right coronary
cusp is overlaid by the infundibulum
of the right ventricle (fig. 4.32). Its more
posterior part is related to the anterior
wall of the right atrium at its junction
with the atrial appendage (fig. 4.33).

The non-coronary cusp is wedged in
the interatrial fold and has a variable
relationship to both atrial
chambers. Via the membranous
septum, it has a direct relationship
to the right ventricle and an intimate
relationship with the right atrium
(fig. 4.34). The atrioventricular

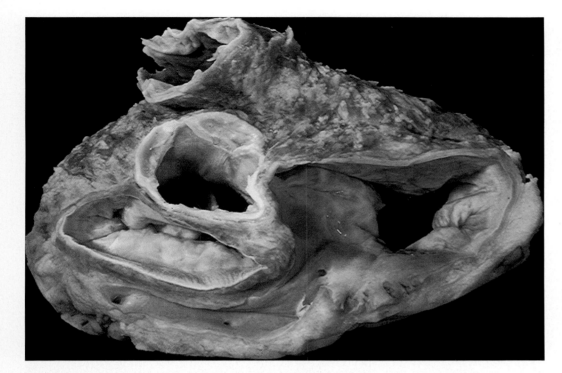

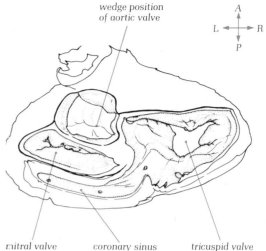

Fig. 4.33   A dissected atrioventricular junction viewed from above showing how the aortic valve wedges itself between the mitral and tricuspid valves.

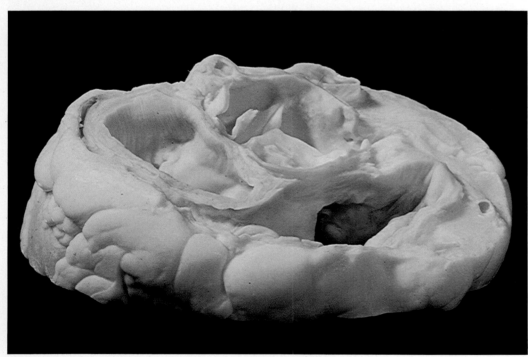

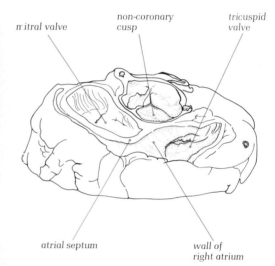

Fig. 4.34   Section through the atrioventricular junction viewed from above and behind showing the relationship of the non-coronary cusp to the right atrium.

bundle penetrates the central fibrous body beneath the non-coronary cusp. The left coronary cusp has a relation to the left atrial cavity and also to the transverse sinus, a good portion of this cusp forming part of the intervalvar fibrosa with the mitral valve (fig. 4.12).

Like the pulmonary valve, the cusps of the aortic valve show variations in their dimensions within the same person (fig. 4.30) and it is rare to find valves with cusps of the same size (Vollebergh & Becker, 1977).

Differentiation of Morphologically Right and Left Ventricles

As with the atria, it is vital for the paediatric cardiologist to distinguish the two ventricles one from the other. Such distinction is considerably easier than with the atrial chambers (see Chapter 2). The morphologically right ventricle has a characteristically coarse trabecular zone and has the trabecula septomarginalis on its septal surface. Its inlet and outlet

portions are separated by the crista supraventricularis, and its atrioventricular valve, the tricuspid valve, has chordal attachments to the inlet septum. The shape of its cavity is triangular. In contrast, the morphologically left ventricle has fine trabeculations with a smooth septal surface; its inlet and outlet portions are in fibrous continuity and its atrioventricular valve, the mitral valve, does not have direct chordal attachments to the inlet septum. Its cavity shape is conical.

The Interventricular Septum

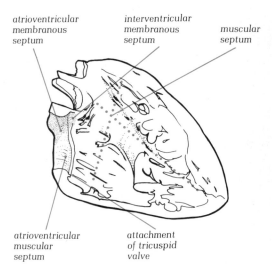

atrioventricular membranous septum

interventricular membranous septum

muscular septum

atrioventricular muscular septum

attachment of tricuspid valve

Fig. 4.35   The ventricular septum viewed from its right aspect after removal of the atria and the parietal wall of the right ventricle and transillumination of the fibrous part of the ventricular septum.

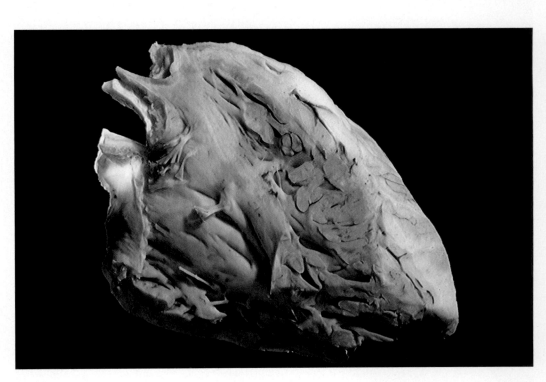

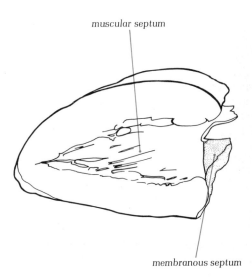

muscular septum

membranous septum

Fig. 4.36   The isolated ventricular septum viewed from its left aspect after removal of the atrial septum and transillumination of the membranous part.

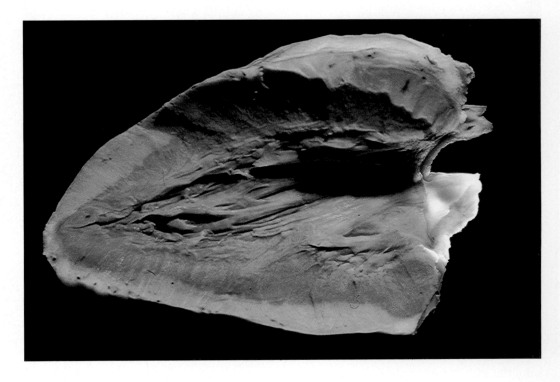

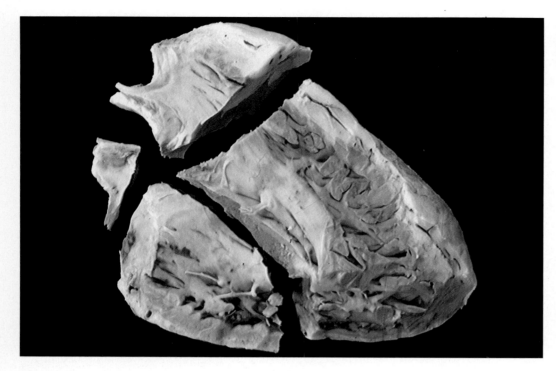

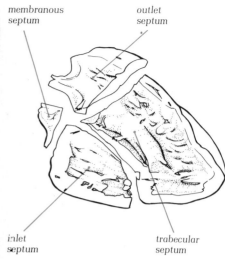

Fig. 4.37 The same septum as in figs. 4.35 & 4.36 following separation into its constituent parts. These are the membranous septum and the inlet, trabecular and outlet components of the muscular septum.

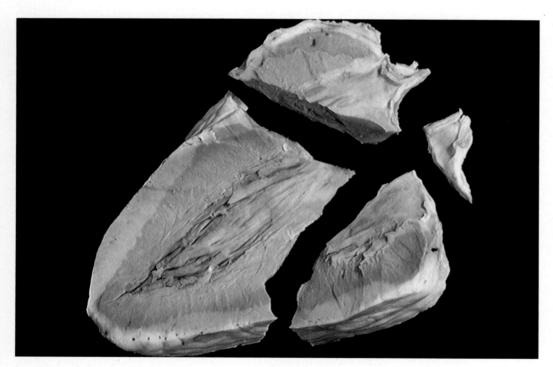

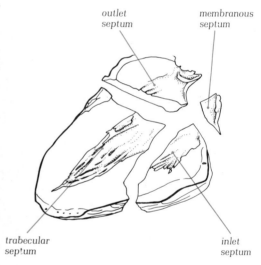

Fig. 4.38 The septum viewed from the left after division into its constituent parts.

The interventricular septum is comprised for its most part of muscle, but is completed by a small fibrous portion, the membranous septum (figs. 4.35 & 4.36). The muscular septum itself is divisible into inlet, trabecular and outlet portions (figs. 4.37 & 4.38).

The inlet part of the muscular septum separates the ventricular inlet portions and extends to the crux cordis. It is orientated more or less in the sagittal plane at an angle of 45° to the vertical plane. Because the leaflets of the tricuspid valve are attached to the septum more apically than those of the mitral valve, part of this septum interposes between the left ventricle and the right atrium (fig. 4.39). This is the atrioventricular muscular septum, not to be confused with the atrioventricular component of the membranous septum (figs. 4.40 & 4.41). On its right ventricular aspect, the inlet septum is limited by the attachments of the chordae of the tricuspid valve septal leaflet.

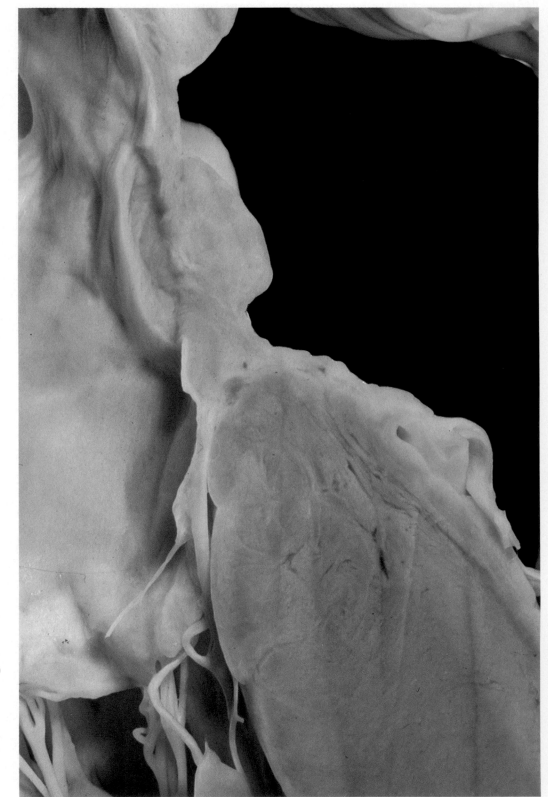

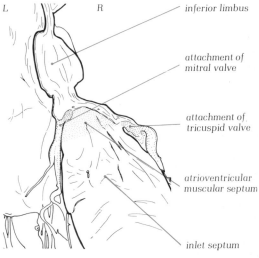

L   R

inferior limbus

attachment of
mitral valve

attachment of
tricuspid valve

atrioventricular
muscular septum

inlet septum

Fig. 4.39   Section through the atrial and
ventricular septum viewed from behind
showing the atrioventricular muscular
septum.

On the left ventricular side, this line
corresponds with the posterior extent
of the smooth septum (figs. 4.42 & 4.43;
compare with figs. 4.37 & 4.38).
The inlet septum merges beyond these
points with the trabecular septum,
which extends from the membranous
septum to the apex running at an
angle of about 45° (fig. 4.42). It widens
considerably when viewed en face
as it passes apically (figs. 4.37 & 4.38).
Its basal portion is smooth in the left
ventricular aspect (fig. 4.44) with the
left bundle branch fibres on its
surface, and is overlaid on its right

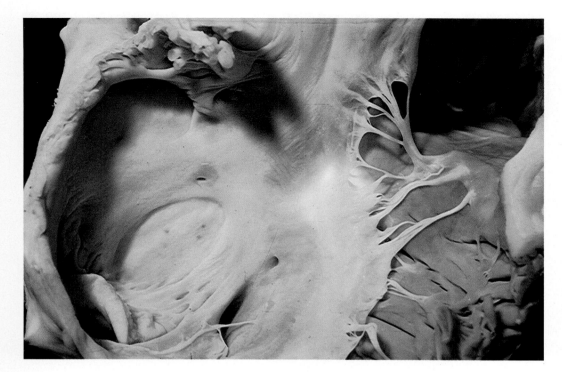

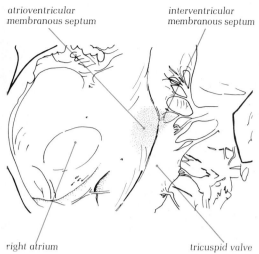

Fig. 4.40 The right side of the heart transilluminated from the left ventricle, showing the membranous septum. The attachment of the tricuspid valve separates this into atrioventricular and interventricular portions.

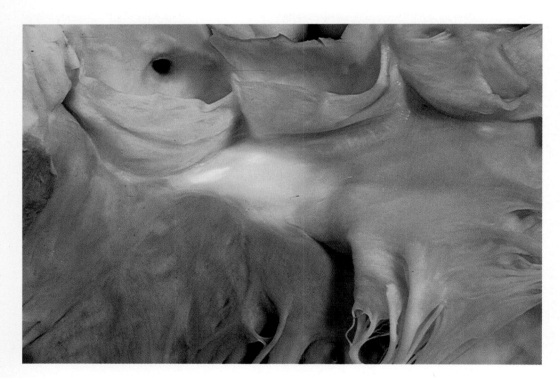

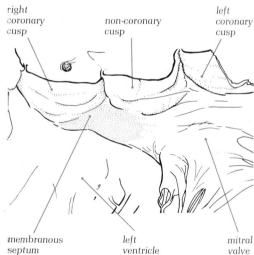

Fig. 4.41 The left ventricular aspect of the heart shown in fig. 4.40 showing the extent of the membranous septum.

ventricular side by the trabecula septomarginalis (*fig. 4.45*). The posterior part of the trabecular septum is in line with the inlet septum (see *fig. 4.46*). As it passes towards the apex its plane changes significantly, and it becomes orientated in a more horizontal plane with a curvature into the frontal plane (*fig. 4.47*). The apical parts of the trabecular septum have fine trabeculations on their left ventricular aspect and coarse trabeculations on their right aspect (*figs. 4.37 & 4.38*). The outlet part of

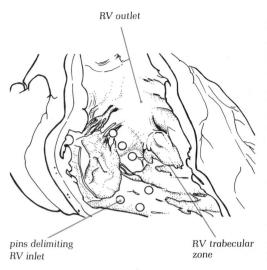

RV outlet

pins delimiting
RV inlet

RV trabecular
zone

Fig. 4.42   Pins introduced into the right
ventricular aspect of the muscular septum
to show the extent of its inlet portion. The
left ventricular aspect is shown in fig. 4.43.

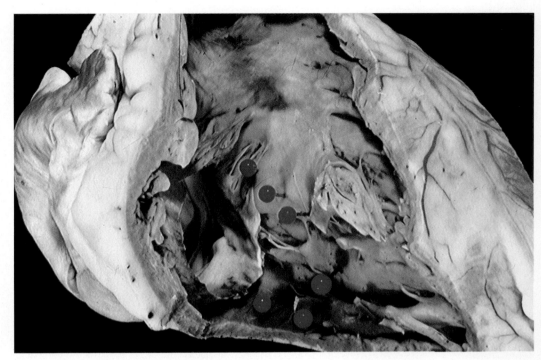

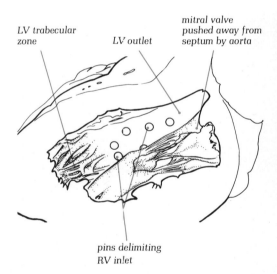

LV trabecular
zone

LV outlet

mitral valve
pushed away from
septum by aorta

pins delimiting
RV inlet

Fig. 4.43   The position of the pins introduced
into the septum shown in fig. 4.42 viewed from
the left ventricular aspect.

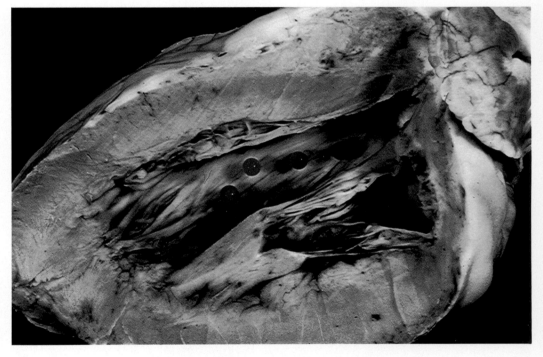

the septum is small, merging
imperceptibly with the upper frontally-
orientated part of the trabecular
septum (figs. 4.37 & 4.38). As indicated
before, the posterior wall of the
infundibulum immediately beneath
the facing cusps of the pulmonary
valve is not a septal structure,
separating the infundibulum instead
from the outside of the heart. The
outlet septum is below the distal part
of the infundibulum and separates
the ventricular outlets. It follows
from this description that the
muscular ventricular septum is a

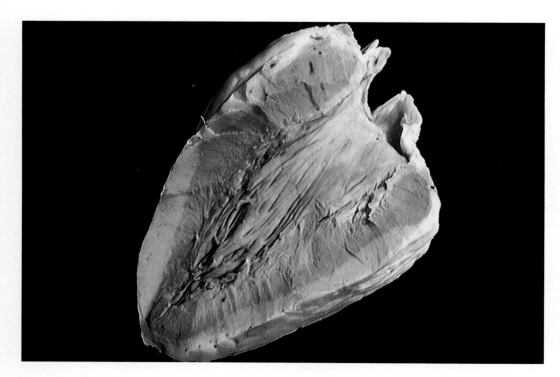

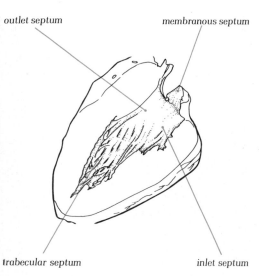

Fig. 4.44   The right side of the septum shown in figs. 4.35 – 4.38 without transillumination.

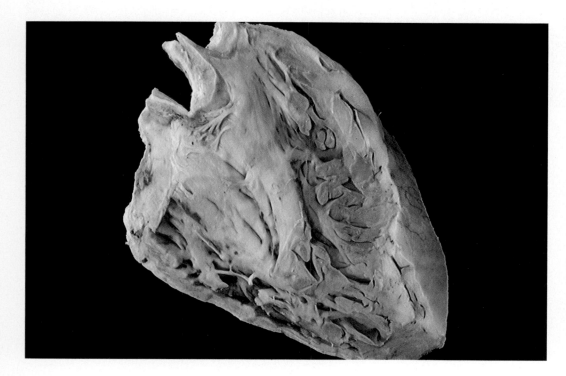

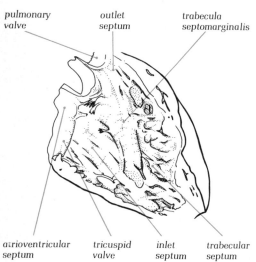

Fig. 4.45   The left side of the septum shown in figs. 4.35 – 4.38 without transillumination.

complex structure, its components subtending considerable angles one to the other. At the level of the fibrous skeleton the inlet and outlet portions are at nearly a right angle (fig. 4.48). Additionally, the trabecular septum itself extends from a near-vertical and near-sagittal position posteriorly to a near-horizontal and near-frontal position anteriorly and superiorly (fig. 4.47). This configuration is due to the 'twisting' interrelationship of the ventricular chambers.

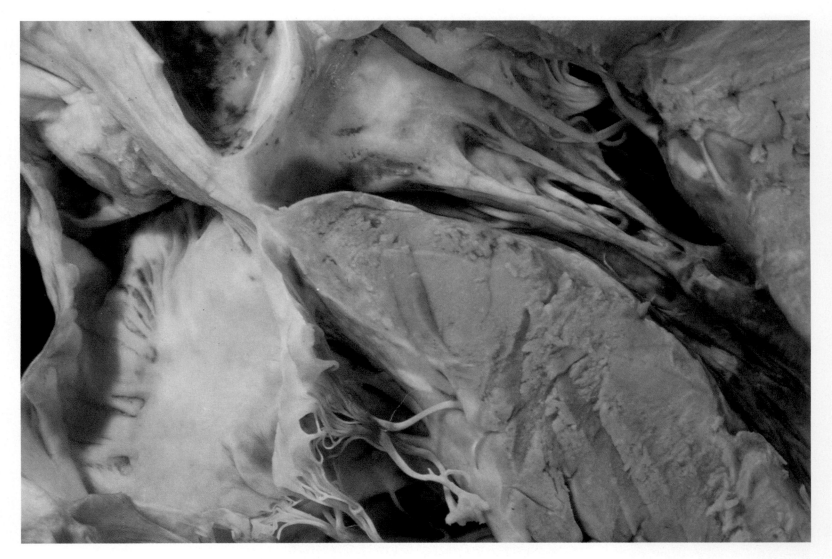

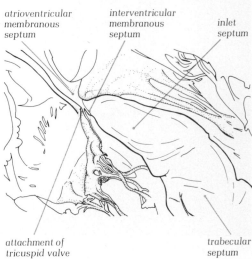

atrioventricular *interventricular* *inlet*
membranous *membranous* *septum*
septum *septum*

attachment of *trabecular*
tricuspid valve *septum*

Fig. 4.46 *A frontal section through the posterior inlet part of the ventricles showing the membranous septum separated by the tricuspid valve attachment into atrioventricular and interventricular portions.*

The membranous septum is a very small structure located at the junction of the inlet, trabecular and outlet components of the muscular septum (*figs. 4.35 & 4.36*). In reality, the membranous septum is part of the cardiac fibrous skeleton (see *Chapter 5*). Because the septal tricuspid attachment is more apical than that of the mitral valve, it crosses the area of the membranous septum dividing it into atrioventricular and interventricular components (*fig. 4.40*). The area of membranous septum which is

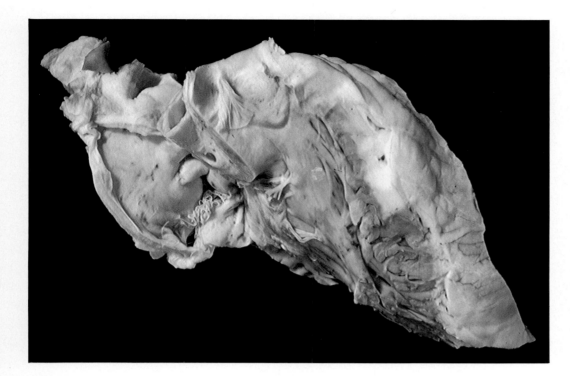

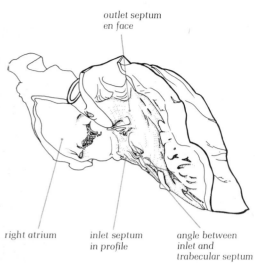

Fig. 4.47   The septum shown in figs. 4.35 – 4.38 orientated in its in situ position prior to removal of the atria.

outlet septum en face

right atrium   inlet septum in profile   angle between inlet and trabecular septum

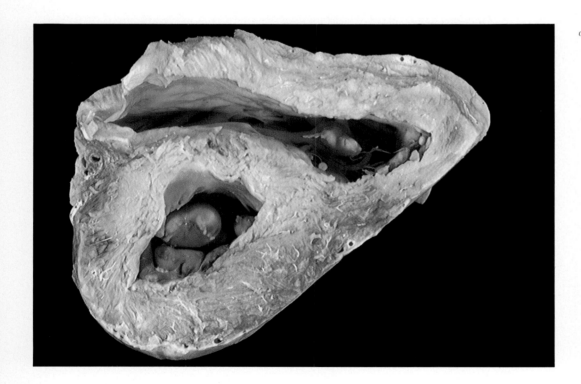

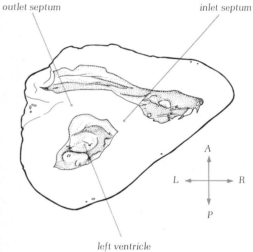

outlet septum   inlet septum

A
L ← → R
P

left ventricle

Fig. 4.48   The base of the heart seen from its atrial aspect following removal of the atria and fibrous skeleton showing the difference in orientation of the inlet and outlet parts of the septum.

atrioventricular or interventricular depends upon the precise attachment of the tricuspid septal leaflet. In infants this is usually towards the ventricle, placing most if not all of the membranous septum in atrioventricular position (*Allwork* *& Anderson, 1979*). With increasing age and the development of a more sigmoid septum, the area of the membranous septum increases, the increase being seen as production of a large interventricular component (fig. 4.40).

5 The Cardiac Skeleton and Musculature

The Fibrous Skeleton of the Heart

The Orientation of Fibres within the Ventricular Mass

The Fibrous Skeleton of the Heart

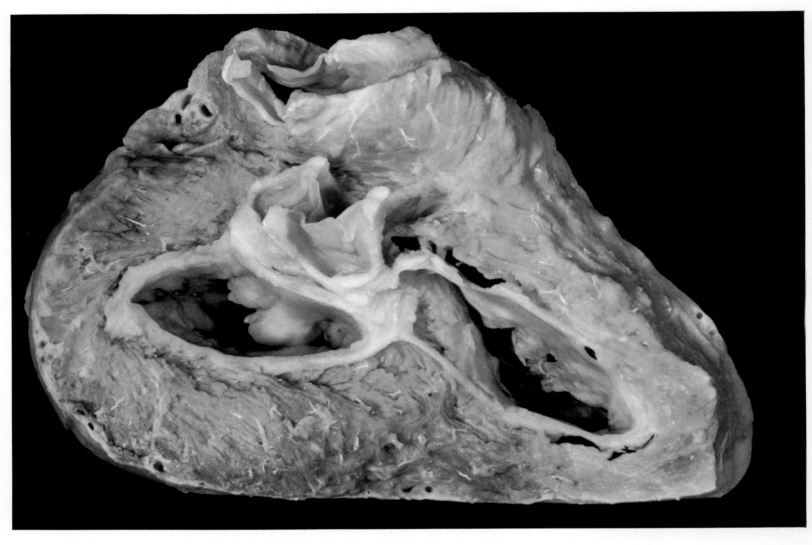

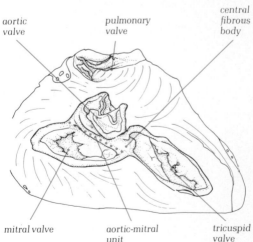

aortic valve

pulmonary valve

central fibrous body

mitral valve

aortic-mitral unit

tricuspid valve

Fig. 5.1   The atrioventricular junction viewed from above and behind following removal of the atria and the great arteries. Note the firm aortic-mitral unit which constitutes the greater part of the fibrous skeleton.

Many accounts are given which ascribe to the cardiac skeleton the function of separating the atrial and ventricular musculatures (*Verduyn Lunel, 1972*) and of acting as a skeleton for insertion and origin of the ventricular myocardial fibres (*MacCallum, 1900; Mall, 1911*). However, when observing the bulk of myocardium present at the

atrioventricular junction, it is evident that all this musculature cannot be attached to the fibrous skeleton. Moreover, the skeleton itself is more pronounced in some parts of the atrioventricular junctions than in others, and is not always positioned between atrial and ventricular musculatures, although these musculatures are separated by either

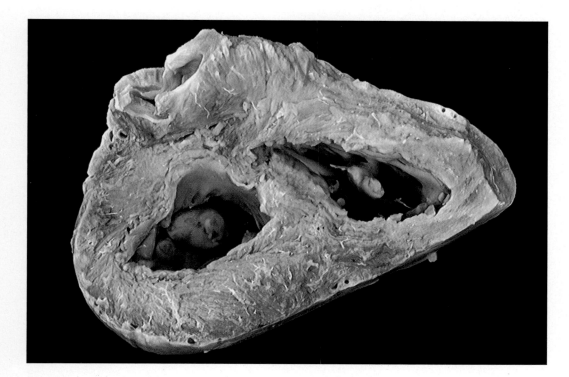

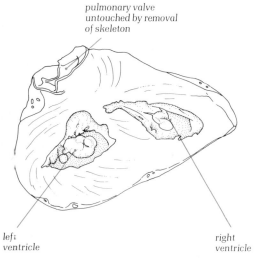

Fig. 5.2 The same heart following removal of the fibrous skeleton.

pulmonary valve untouched by removal of skeleton

left ventricle

right ventricle

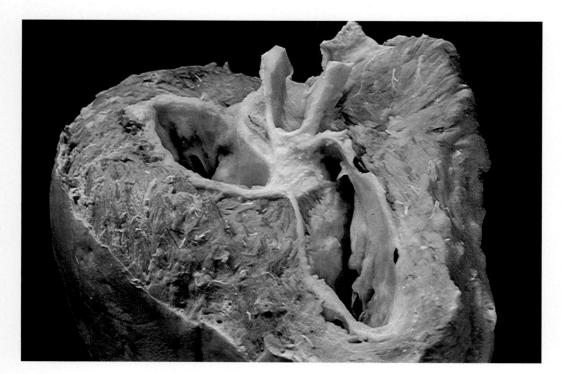

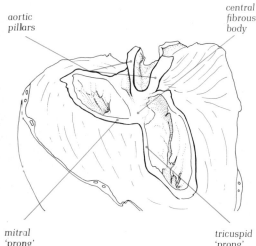

aortic pillars

central fibrous body

mitral 'prong'

tricuspid 'prong'

Fig. 5.3 The same heart viewed from above and the right showing the two posterior prongs from the central fibrous body and the pillars of the aortic valve.

fibrous or adipose tissue planes. By observing the morphology and attachments of the fibrous skeleton, it seems to us that its major function is to support the atrioventricular valves and to anchor them to the ventricular mass. The skeleton includes the aortic valve in its structure (fig. 5.1) but has no direct attachment to the pulmonary valve orifice (fig. 5.2). Indeed, the pulmonary valve does not have an annulus comparable to those of the other valves. Its leaflets are supported by the muscular infundibulum of the right ventricle and are separated by the posterior wall of the infundibulum from the aortic annulus (fig. 5.2). A tendon has been reported to extend from the skeleton into this area (MacCallum, 1900), but we have been unable to locate this structure, observing only a fibrous raphe. The mitral, tricuspid and aortic valves are set together within the fibrous skeleton, but the skeleton is by no means of uniform dimensions around all three valves (fig. 5.3). The strongest parts of the

5.3

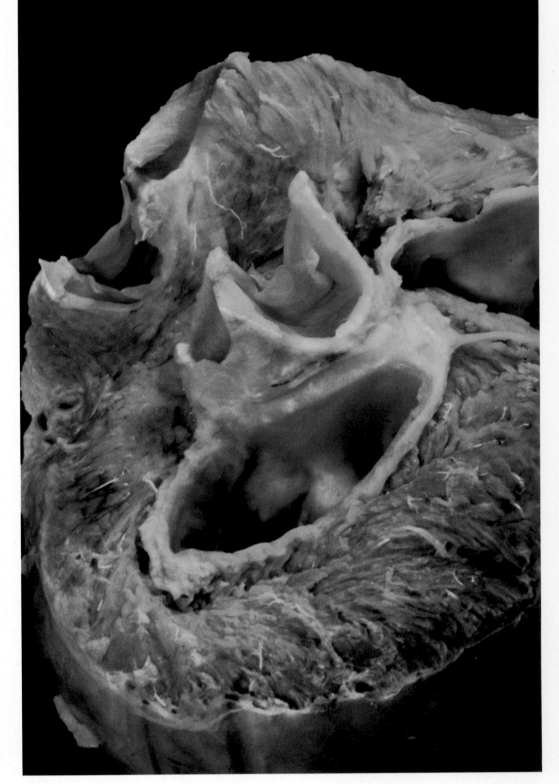

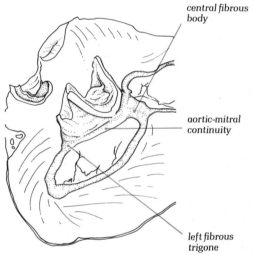

central fibrous
body

aortic-mitral
continuity

left fibrous
trigone

Fig. 5.4   *The same heart viewed from above and the left showing the area of fibrous continuity between the left fibrous trigone and the central fibrous body.*

skeleton are the annuli supporting the mitral and aortic valves, both continuous rings of collagenous tissue *(figs. 5.4 & 5.5)*. These two annuli are continuous in the area of aortic-mitral fibrous continuity *(fig. 5.6)*. They are additionally thickened at the margins of this junction to form the left and right fibrous trigones *(fig. 5.7)*. Since

the aortic valve is an arterial valve, its cusps are attached to the fibrous skeleton in semilunar fashion. Thus, three struts arise from the fibrous skeleton, being part of the skeleton, to support the commissures of the aortic valve *(figs. 5.3 & 5.4)*. The anterior strut faces the posterior

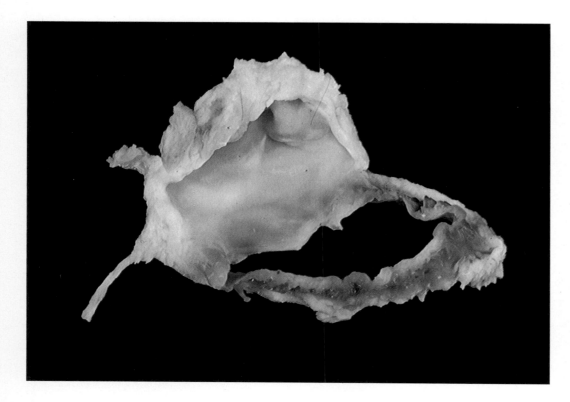

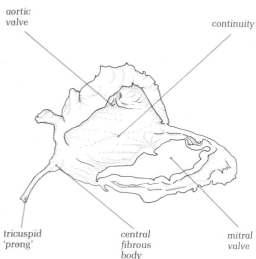

aortic valve

continuity

tricuspid 'prong'

central fibrous body

mitral valve

Fig. 5.5 *Fibrous skeleton removed from the heart shown in figs. 5.1–5.4 and viewed from beneath. It shows only the strong mitral unit with the area of aortic-mitral fibrous continuity.*

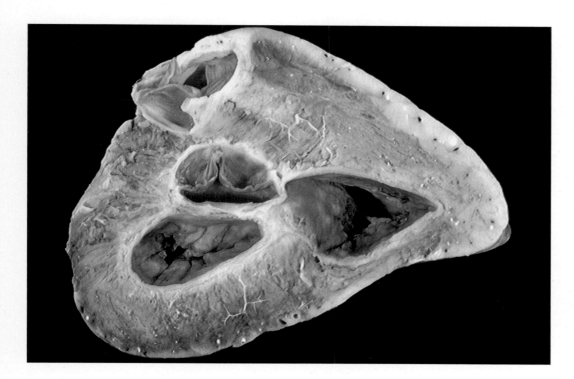

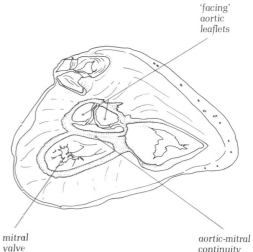

'facing' aortic leaflets

mitral valve

aortic-mitral continuity

Fig. 5.6 *A separate heart dissected to show the aortic-mitral fibrous unit following removal of the aortic leaflets.*

commissure of the pulmonary valve; the right strut is just anterior to the junction of mitral and tricuspid annuli *(vide infra)* and the left strut is along the area of aortic-mitral continuity, its precise position depending upon the interrelationships of the aortic and mitral valves. The area from the mitral annulus, therefore, tents up to the strut of the commissure of the left coronary and non-coronary cusps, placing part of the left ventricular outflow tract as part of the intervalvar fibrous area *(fig. 5.4)*, and thus as part of the fibrous skeleton. In the 'septal' area of

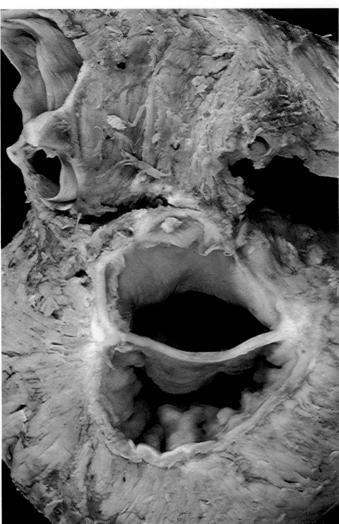

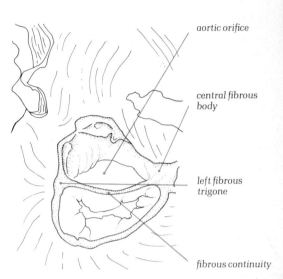

aortic orifice

central fibrous body

left fibrous trigone

fibrous continuity

Fig. 5.7　Detail of the heart shown in fig. 5.6 showing the aortic-mitral fibrous continuity stretching between the left fibrous trigone and the central fibrous body.

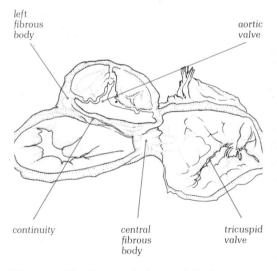

left fibrous body

aortic valve

continuity

central fibrous body

tricuspid valve

Fig. 5.8　The fibrous skeleton of the heart together with the valve leaflets removed from the same heart as in figs. 5.1–5.4 and shown in its entirety.

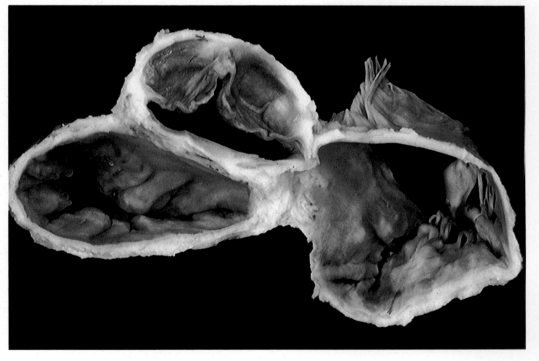

the atrioventricular junction, the aortic-mitral unit of the fibrous skeleton is also continuous with the annulus of the tricuspid valve (fig. 5.8). This area of the fibrous skeleton is the central fibrous body (figs. 5.3 & 5.6). It includes the right fibrous trigone and the membranous septum. The attachment of the tricuspid annulus to the right side of the central

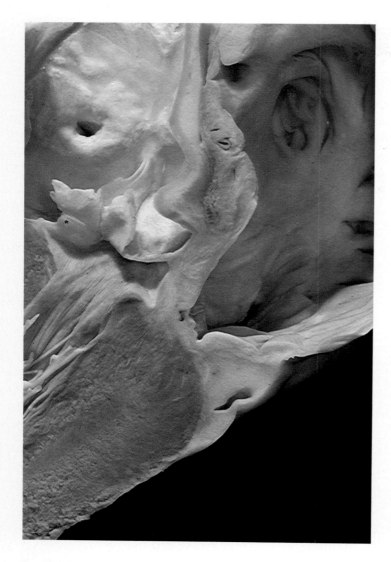

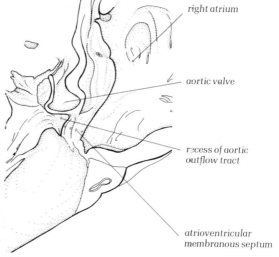

right atrium

aortic valve

recess of aortic outflow tract

atrioventricular membranous septum

Fig. 5.9   Section through the aortic outflow tract showing how the membranous septum separates the posterior recess of the aortic outflow tract from the right atrium.

fibrous body swings upwards from a more apical posterior attachment (apical in comparison to the attachment of the mitral valve) to a more basal anterior attachment in relation to the aortic annulus (fig. 5.3). This places part of the membranous septum beneath the tricuspid annulus (the interventricular component, fig. 5.5); and part above the tricuspid annulus (the atrioventricular component, fig. 5.4). The annuli of the tricuspid and mitral valves diverge from the posterior margin of the central fibrous body, the tricuspid annulus rapidly veering away towards the ventricular apex (fig. 5.3). In this area, therefore, part of the inlet ventricular septum is overlaid by

fibres of the atrial wall and interposes between the left ventricle and the right atrium. This is the muscular atrioventricular septum (see fig. 2.28). It is difficult on purely morphological grounds to distinguish precisely the muscular part of the atrioventricular septum from its membranous component. A section through the area shows that all this part of the fibrous skeleton is interposed between the left ventricle and the right atrium (fig. 5.9). In contrast, not all of the area transilluminates (see fig. 4.40), and not all forms a thin fibrous partition without overlying atrial musculature on its superior aspect. It is the latter partition which is usually described as the

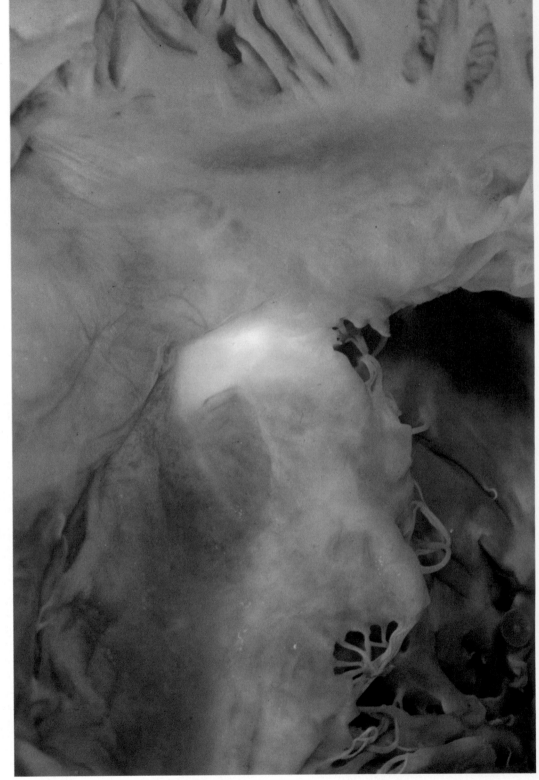

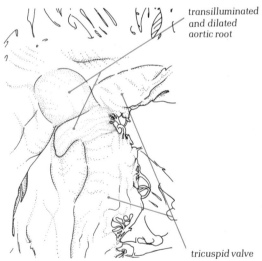

transilluminated
and dilated
aortic root

tricuspid valve

Fig. 5.10   Transilluminated heart which has dilatation of the aortic root showing the large area of aorta related to the right atrium.

atrioventricular membranous septum, and in hearts in which ageing has produced dilatation of the aortic root the area can become huge *(fig. 5.10)*. Nonetheless, from the standpoint of morphology, the entire central fibrous body is an atrioventricular structure. The central fibrous body is firmly adherent on its ventricular aspect to the ventricular fibres, inserting and taking origin from the fibrous tissue.

Similarly, the annular parts supporting the aortic and mitral valves have ventricular muscle fibres attached to their ventricular surfaces.

The tricuspid annulus, as indicated, diverges away from the central fibrous body and encircles and supports the tricuspid leaflets. It is far less well formed than the mitral annulus and is composed mostly of

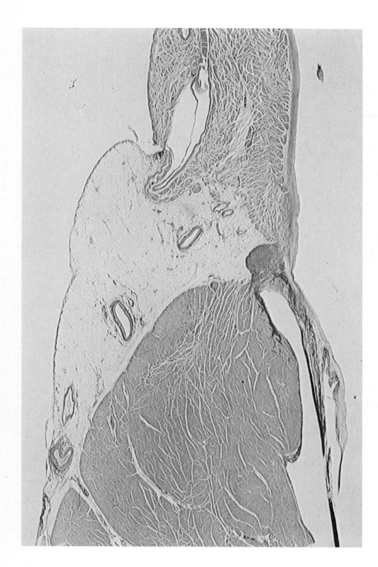

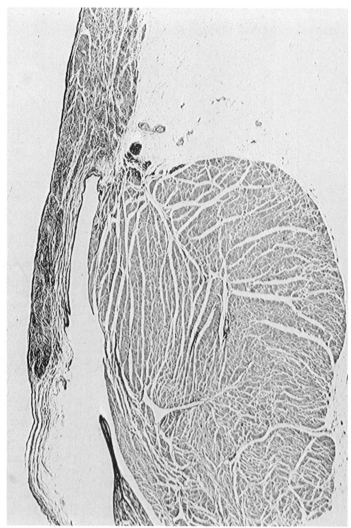

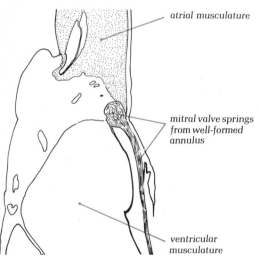

atrial musculature

mitral valve springs
from well-formed
annulus

ventricular
musculature

Fig. 5.11   Histological section showing the
firm and strong mitral annulus.

atrial musculature

fibrous tissue

ventricular
musculature

tricuspid valve

Fig. 5.12   Histological section of the
tricuspid annulus which is much less well
formed than the mitral annulus (fig. 5.11).

the conjoined valve leaflets, without a
complete thickened collagenous ring
such as is seen in the mitral annulus
(figs. 5.11 & 5.12). In places,
collagenous segments can be found
reinforcing the ring composed of the
conjoined leaflets, but it is rarely, if
ever, a complete collagenous annulus.
The tricuspid leaflet apparatus can be
removed as one unit along with the

mitral and aortic valves (fig. 5.8), and
the annulus is attached to the base of
the right ventricle, albeit less firmly
than is the mitral annulus attached to
the left ventricle. The atrial and
ventricular musculature have
important relationships to the
fibrous skeleton. In the left atrium, the
atrial fibres attach to the annulus
posteriorly and laterally (fig. 5.6). In

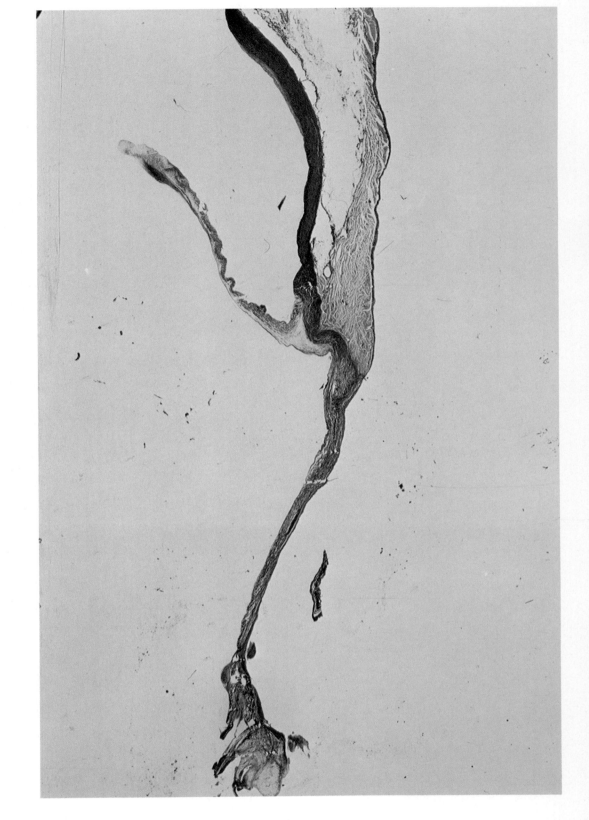

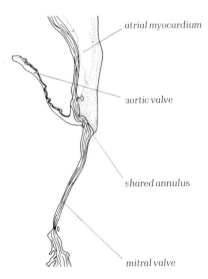

atrial myocardium

aortic valve

shared annulus

mitral valve

Fig. 5.13   Section through the area of
aortic-mitral fibrous continuity showing how
the two valves share the same annular
structure.

the area of aortic-mitral continuity,
the atrial fibres are attached to the
intervalvar fibrous area (fig. 5.13). In
the septal area, the atrial fibres insert
into the atrial aspect of the central
fibrous body, particularly in the area

of the atrioventricular node.
Nonetheless, the central fibrous body
does not occupy the entire area of the
apparent atrial septum. As has been
indicated, the floor of the coronary
sinus does not constitute part of the
septum (fig. 5.14). In this area, a tissue

plane extends forwards to the
atrioventricular node carrying the
nodal artery (fig. 5.15). This plane,
containing adipose tissue, is the only
structure to separate the atrial and
ventricular musculatures between the
diverging posterior groups of the

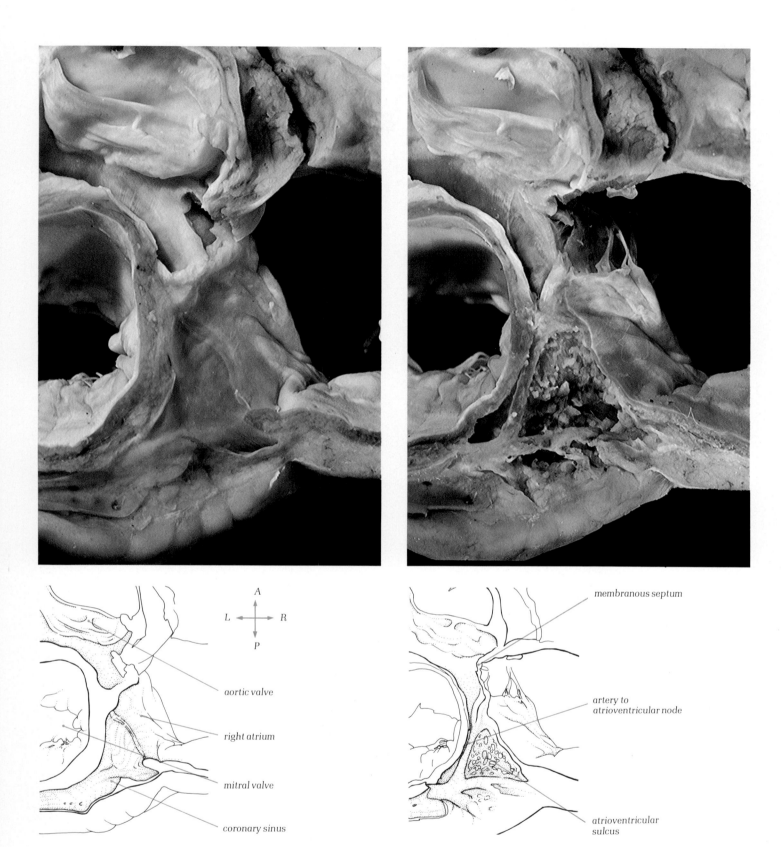

Fig. 5.14 Cross-section through the atrioventricular junction showing the floor of the coronary sinus and its relation to the aortic outflow tract.

Fig. 5.15 Further dissection of the heart shown in fig. 5.14 demonstrating how the floor lies above the posterior atrioventricular sulcus.

atrioventricular annuli (fig. 5.16). The atrioventricular bundle is the continuation into the ventricles of the axis of the atrioventricular node, and this structure passes through the central fibrous body to reach the ventricular conduction tissues (see Chapter 6). In the right atrioventricular annulus, the atrial fibres continue further down into the atrialis of the tricuspid valve than do the left atrial fibres in the mitral valve, particularly in the septal leaflet of the tricuspid valve. Here the basal aspect of the valve leaflets, themselves continuous with the atrioventricular sulcus, forms the plane of separation of atrial and ventricular musculatures, reinforced by the collagenous annulus where present (fig. 5.11).

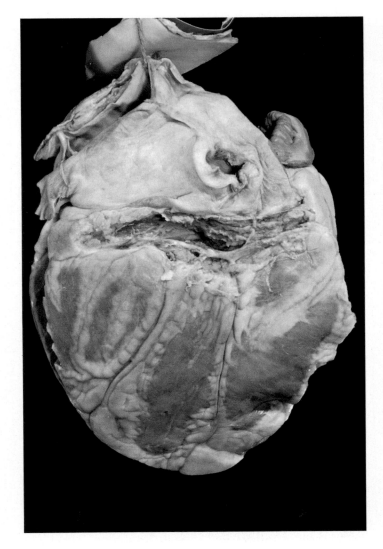

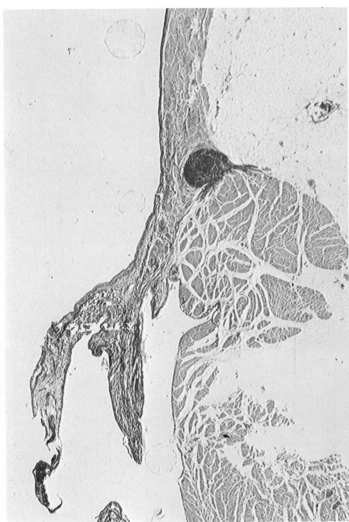

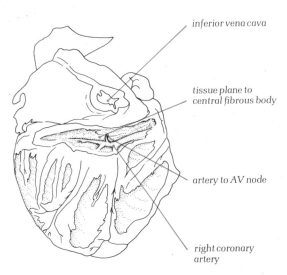

inferior vena cava

tissue plane to central fibrous body

artery to AV node

right coronary artery

Fig. 5.16   Dissection of the tissue plane shown in fig. 5.15 opened from behind showing the plane which passes forwards towards the central fibrous body and through which runs the artery to the atrioventricular node.

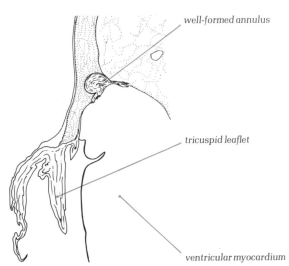

well-formed annulus

tricuspid leaflet

ventricular myocardium

Fig. 5.17   Section through the tricuspid valve annulus showing that, in some places around the ring, this is a better-formed structure.

On the ventricular side, the muscular fibres of the left ventricle are firmly attached to the underside of the collagenous fibrous skeleton, albeit that, by necessity, this applies only to the small part of the ventricular basal surface adjacent to the annulus. In this area, the mitral annulus truly interposes between atrial and ventricular musculatures (fig. 5.11). In contrast, on the right side, the ventricular fibres in some places have no apparent attachment to the valve leaflets (fig. 5.12) while in other places in the same heart, segments of collagenous annulus may support the leaflet and be attached to the ventricular myocardium (fig. 5.17). Nonetheless, even in these areas, the atrial muscle inserts further into the valve than on the mitral side and the

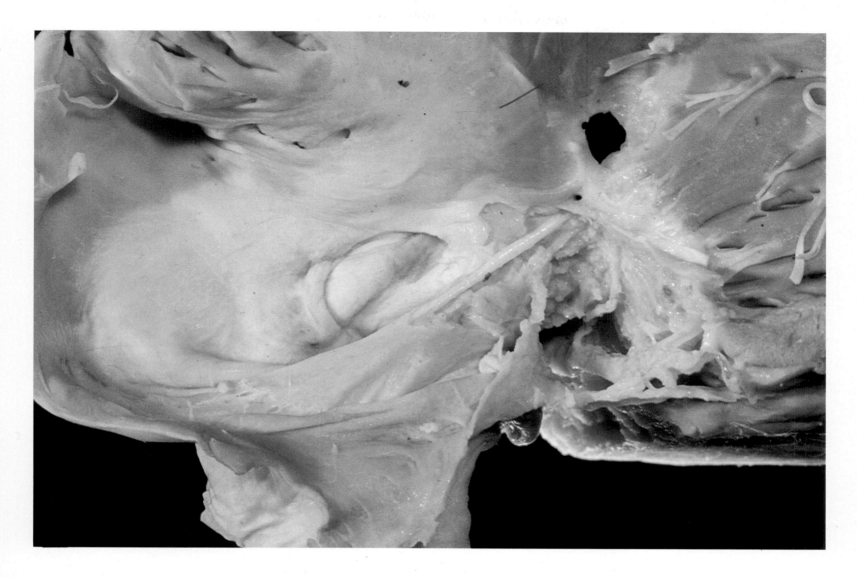

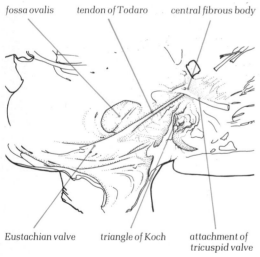

fossa ovalis   tendon of Todaro   central fibrous body

Eustachian valve   triangle of Koch   attachment of
tricuspid valve

Fig. 5.18   Dissection of the triangle of Koch
showing the tendon of Todaro (continuation
of the valve) inserting into the central fibrous
body.

separation of atrial and ventricular
musculatures is accomplished mostly
by the plane of the atrioventricular
sulcus, continuous with the fibrosa of
the tricuspid valve leaflets.

An important extension from the
fibrous skeleton, as far as the
conduction system is concerned (see
Chapter 6), is the tendon of Todaro.
This structure is the fibrous
continuation of the commissure of the
valves of the inferior vena cava and
coronary sinus. It passes
intramyocardially through the sinus
septum and inserts into the central
fibrous body (fig. 5.18). It is the
superior landmark to the triangle of
Koch, which marks the site of the
atrioventricular conduction tissue.

The Orientation of Fibres within the Ventricular Mass

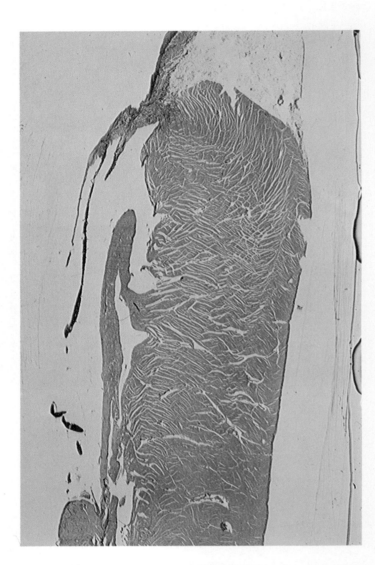

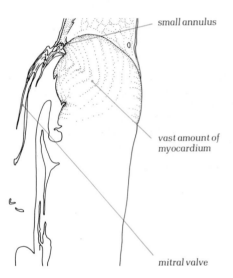

small annulus

vast amount of
myocardium

mitral valve

Fig. 5.19   Histological section through the
left atrioventricular junction illustrating how
few of the myocardial fibres insert into the
annulus.

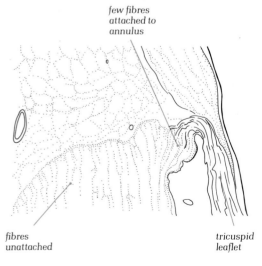

few fibres
attached to
annulus

fibres
unattached

tricuspid
leaflet

Fig. 5.20   Similar section through the right
atrioventricular junction illustrating similar
findings.

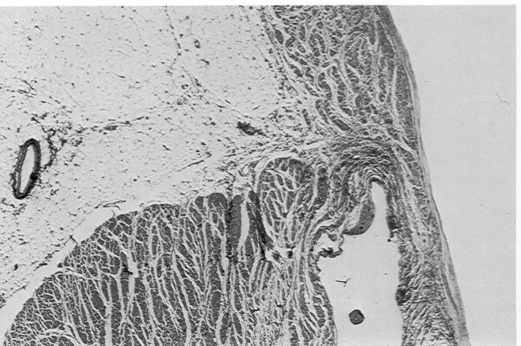

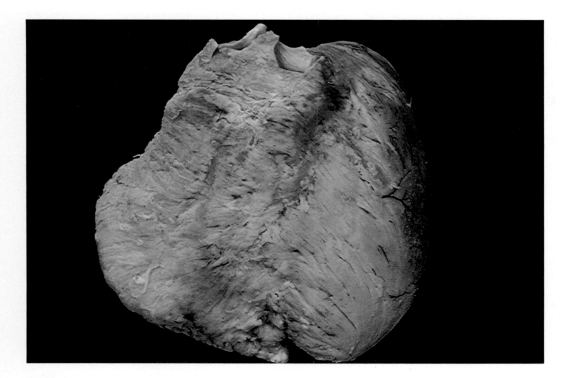

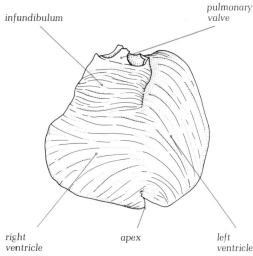

Fig. 5.21 *Anterior view of the dissected heart (see text) following removal of the atria and pericardium.*

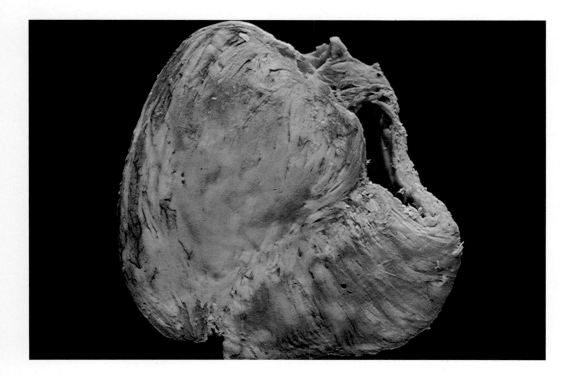

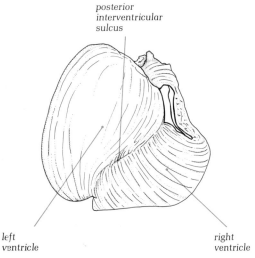

Fig. 5.22 *Posterior view of dissected heart after removal of the atria and pericardium.*

The generally accepted view of the fibres of the ventricular muscle mass is that they take origin from and insert into the fibrous skeleton or chordae tendineae of the valves, much as voluntary muscles have their own origins and insertions. It is also widely quoted that the superficial fibres of one ventricle, taking origin from the fibrous annulus of the atrioventricular valve, spiral round the ventricles and penetrate at the apex of the opposite ventricle to insert into the papillary muscles of that ventricle. These concepts are based primarily on the original works of MacCallum and Mall, themselves extensions of the work of German investigators in the previous century (*Ludwig, 1849; Krehl, 1891*). However, all the illustrations of MacCallum, which are widely reproduced, represent dissections of the hearts of embryo pigs. MacCallum did not state precisely how many human hearts he studied, merely indicating that the results in 'several' were comparable. We have some degree of difficulty in conceptualizing the fibre orientation as described by MacCallum and confirmed by others (*Robb & Robb, 1942*). Although it is stated that all ventricular fibres

5.15

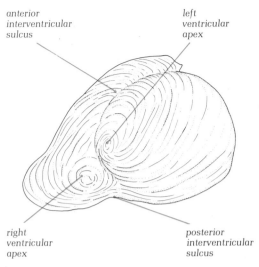

anterior interventricular sulcus

left ventricular apex

right ventricular apex

posterior interventricular sulcus

Fig. 5.23 *Apical view of the ventricular mass shown in figs. 5.21 and 5.22.*

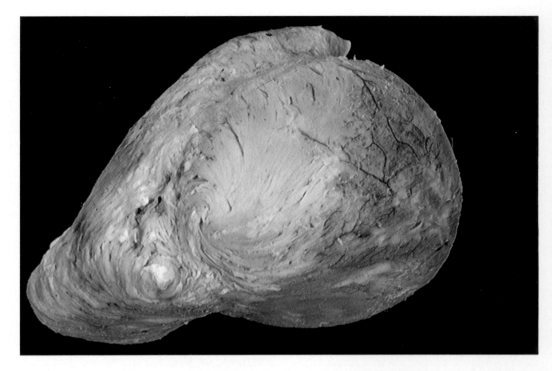

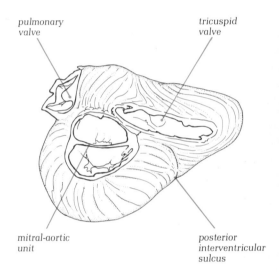

pulmonary valve

tricuspid valve

mitral-aortic unit

posterior interventricular sulcus

Fig. 5.24 *The same ventricular mass viewed from the aspect of the atrioventricular junction.*

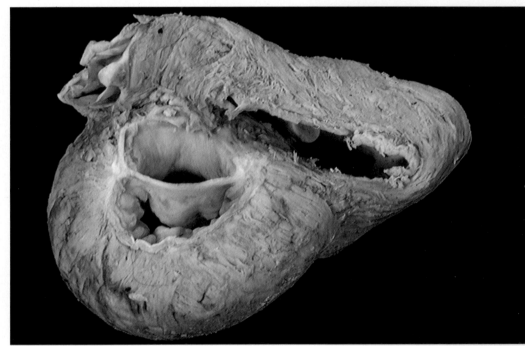

originate from or insert into the fibrous skeleton, this structure seems to be grossly inadequate in terms of size to cope with such a task. Furthermore, study of histological sections *(figs. 5.19 & 5.20)* reveals that very little of the ventricular musculature obtains a direct attachment to the atrioventricular fibrous rings, particularly on the

tricuspid side. We have therefore attempted to evaluate the disposition of muscle fibres in the ventricular mass of a three-year-old child, the heart having been preserved in formalin. Clearly, this work requires further substantiation; but the findings in this single heart are of considerable interest and possible functional significance.

When the epicardium is removed, the orientation of the superficial fibres is easily apparent. Both anterior and posterior interventricular sulci are well seen with minimal cross-over of fibres anteriorly *(fig. 5.21)*, but more extensive cross-over posteriorly *(fig. 5.22)*. The anterior sulcus, with fibres being predominantly confined to their own ventricle, is shown in the

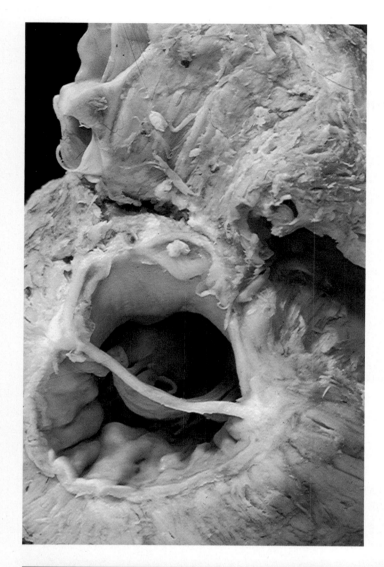

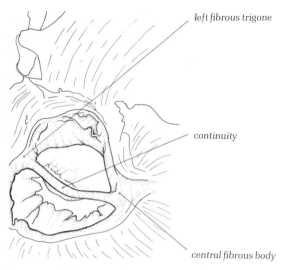

Fig. 5.25   Detail of fig. 5.24 showing the area
of aortic-mitral fibrous continuity, the left
fibrous trigone and the central fibrous body.

left fibrous trigone

continuity

central fibrous body

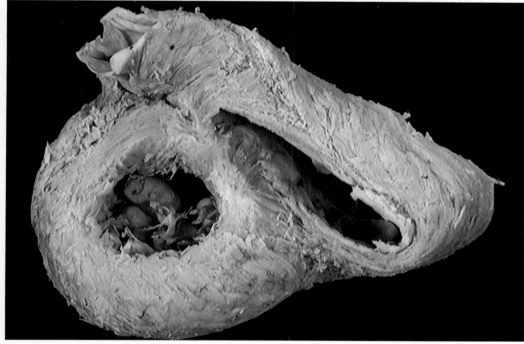

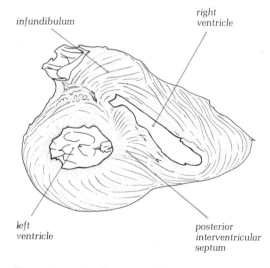

infundibulum

*right
ventricle*

*left
ventricle*

*posterior
interventricular
septum*

Fig. 5.26   Atrial aspect of the ventricular
mass shown in fig. 5.24 following removal of
the fibrous skeleton.

apical view, which also demonstrates
that each ventricle has its own apex
with a vortex effect constructed by
the fibres running from superficial to
deep layers at this point. However, it
can be seen that the posterior fibres
extend from left ventricle to right
(*fig. 5.23*). The basal view of the

ventricular mass illustrates that the
superficial left ventricular fibres
radiate from the mitral annulus. The
basal fibres of the right ventricle
originate mostly from the central
fibrous body and swing
circumferentially round the tricuspid
orifice, which itself gives rise to few

fibres (*figs. 5.20 & 5.24*).
    Anteriorly, these circumferential
right ventricular fibres decussate
with fibres from the infundibulum
before turning down the anterior
surface to curl into the anterior sulcus
and the apex (*fig. 5.24*). Further
dissection in the area of the central

5.17

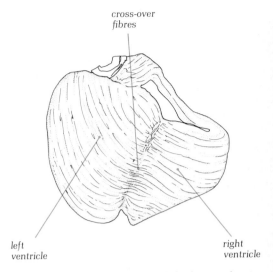

cross-over
fibres

left
ventricle

right
ventricle

Fig. 5.27 *Posterior aspect of the heart after minimal dissection showing cross-over fibres in the posterior interventricular sulcus.*

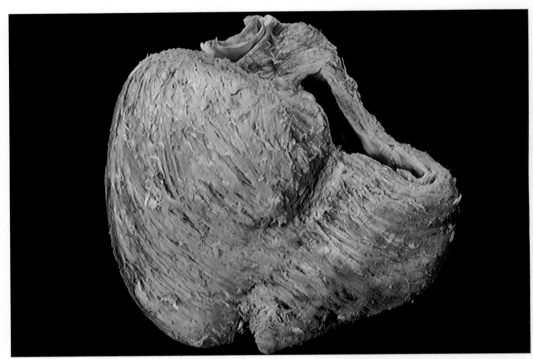

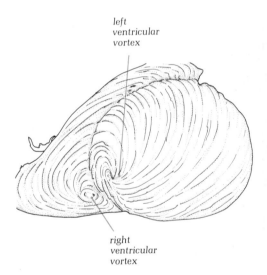

left
ventricular
vortex

right
ventricular
vortex

Fig. 5.28 *The apical view of the same heart showing separate vortices for the right and left ventricles.*

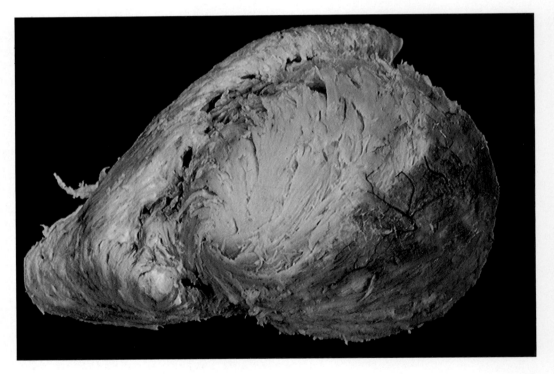

fibrous body *(fig. 5.25)* shows that the septal fibres run downwards, completing the circle of radial fibres of the left ventricle from the aortic-mitral unit. The infundibular fibres pass rightwards and leftwards from a raphe between the posterior pulmonary commissure and the anterior margin of the tricuspid valve.

This raphe is representative of the 'conus tendon' *(MacCallum, 1900)*. With continuing superficial dissection at the base, it is easy to remove the aortic-mitral fibrous skeleton *(fig. 5.26)*. This manoeuvre illustrates how little the skeleton contributes to muscle attachments, since the appearance of the muscle mass is altered little by its removal (compare

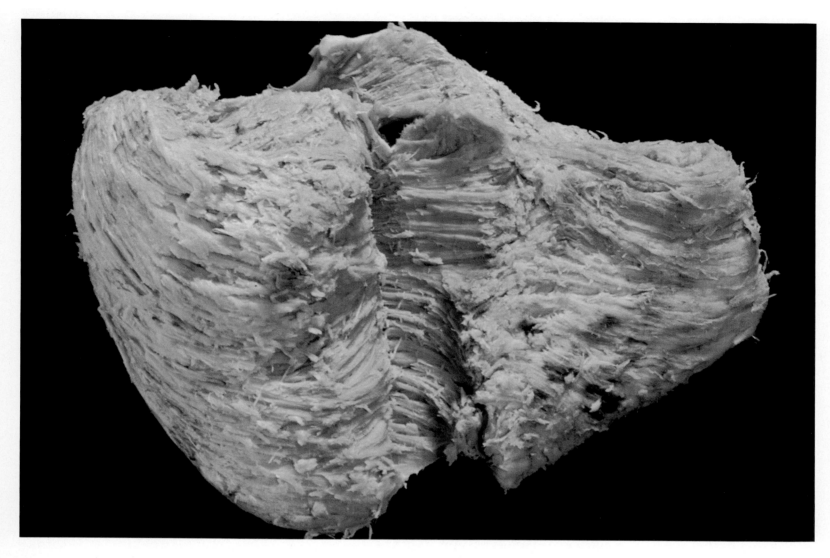

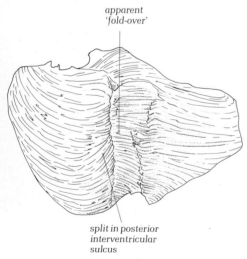

apparent
'fold-over'

split in posterior
interventricular
sulcus

Fig. 5.29   The ventricular mass after being
split along the posterior interventricular
sulcus. There is an apparent 'fold-over' of
fibres from right to left.

figs. 5.24 & 5.26). What is evident is
that the anterior fibres of the left
ventricle which are immediately
beneath the superficial layer run a
circular course round the ventricular
lumen.

Continuing dissection of the
superficial layer of the posterior
surface shows that the cross-over

fibres between the ventricles are
themselves superficial and limited in
number (figs. 5.27 & 5.28). Dissection
into the posterior groove then permits
the ventricles to be 'peeled open',
giving the impression of a discrete
cleavage between the ventricles from
behind (fig. 5.29). Careful attention
shows this to be spurious, the peeled
fibres belonging to the left ventricle.

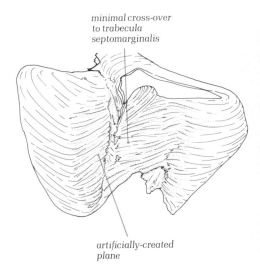

minimal cross-over
to trabecula
septomarginalis

artificially-created
plane

Fig. 5.30   Further dissection from the stage
shown in fig. 5.29 shows this to be spurious
as the 'fold-over' fibres belong to the left
ventricle. Only minimal fibres cross from
right to left and these pass down the trabecula
septomarginalis.

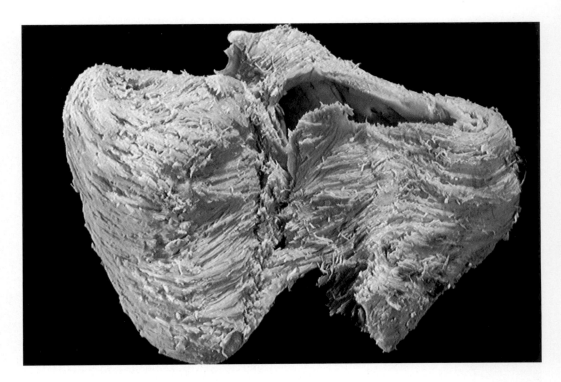

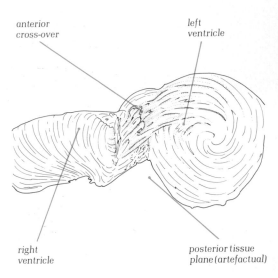

anterior
cross-over

left
ventricle

right
ventricle

posterior tissue
plane (artefactual)

Fig. 5.31   Further dissection showing the
fibres which pass anteriorly from the right
ventricle into the left ventricle near the
trabecula septomarginalis.

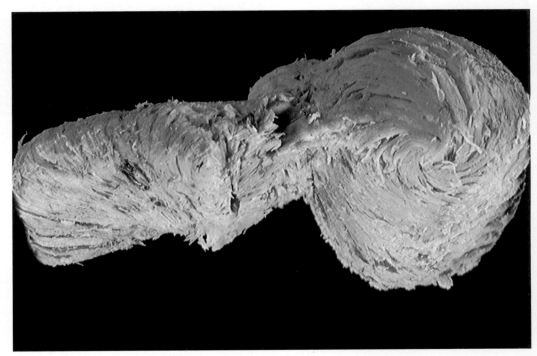

Removal of these fibres (fig. 5.30)
demonstrates that the right
ventricular fibres originate from the
left ventricle, swinging posteriorly
and round the back of the right
ventricular cavity. This is well
demonstrated by the apical view
(fig. 5.31). Further removal of fibres in
this decussatory area then shows
that the left ventricular fibres cross
into the papillary muscle and
trabecula septomarginalis of the right
ventricle. There is a double cross-over
since the superior fibres pass down
from the central fibrous body into the
trabecula septomarginalis and the
inferior fibres swing up from the left

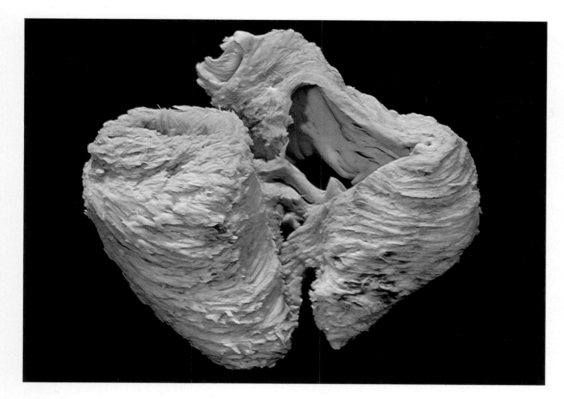

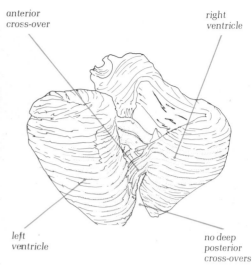

Fig. 5.32 Further dissection reveals that the posterior cross-over fibres were superficial structures.

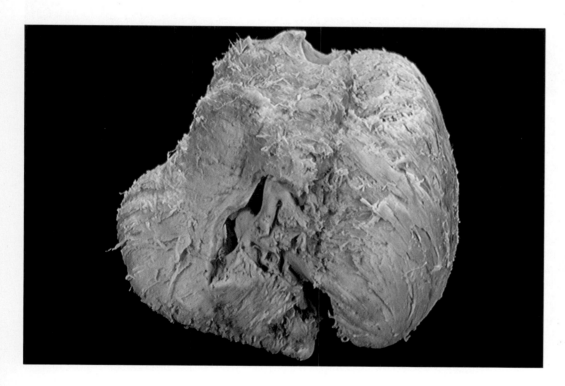

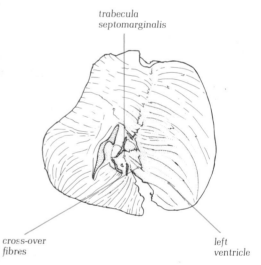

Fig. 5.33 Anterior view of cross-over fibres.

ventricular apex into the anterior papillary muscle. These are reinforced by apical right ventricular fibres which swing into the muscle grouping from the right (figs. 5.32 & 5.33). This dissection shows that the septum belongs very much to the left ventricle and the fibre orientation is such that the septal trabeculations and papillary muscles of the right ventricle are bound into the left ventricular structure. Further dissection of the right ventricle reveals that the muscles are orientated mostly in the same direction throughout the thickness of the walls.

5.21

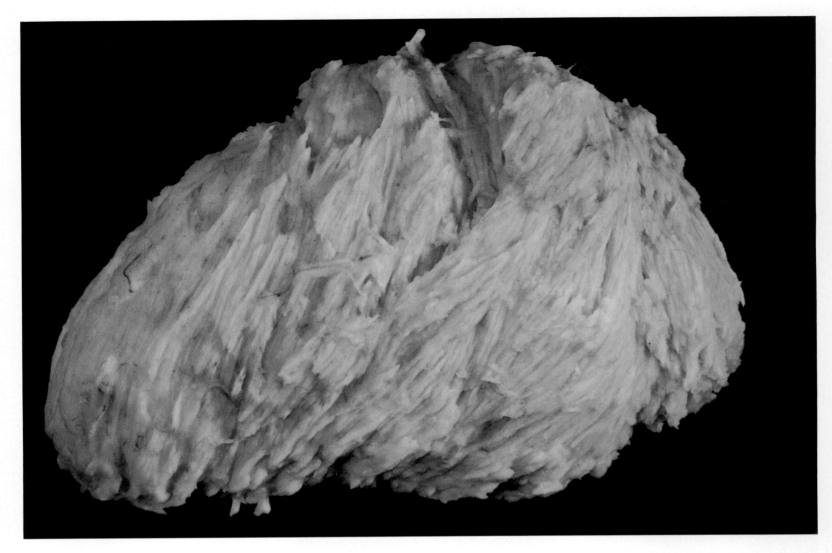

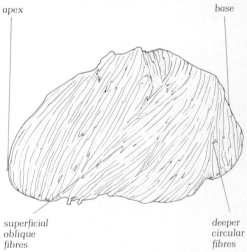

apex   base

superficial   deeper
oblique   circular
fibres   fibres

Fig. 5.34   The isolated left ventricle showing
the superficial oblique fibres.

This is far from the case in the left
ventricle. Here, removal of the
superficial fibres shows a large
circumferential mass of fibres at the
base enclosing the aortic-mitral unit
(fig. 5.34). This 'bulbo-spiral' muscle

has been well documented (Mall,
1911). The fibres on the surface spiral
down from the base and turn in at the
apical vortex; but just below these
fibres there is a more general circular

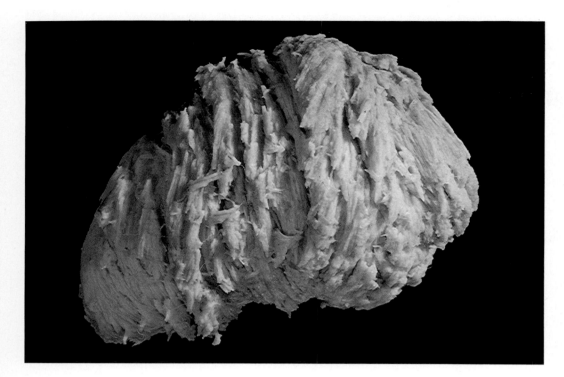

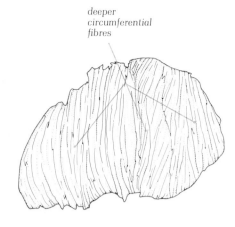

Fig. 5.35 Deeper dissection of the left ventricle shows how the fibres become circumferential.

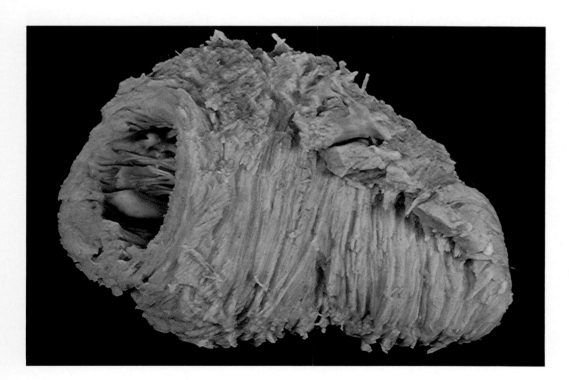

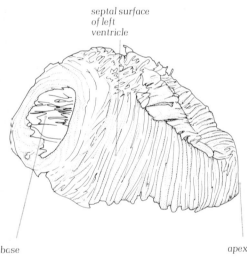

Fig. 5.36 Dissection of the septal surface of the left ventricle.

arrangement. This is illustrated by further dissection which shows loss of spiralling and conversion to a general circular arrangement (fig. 5.35).

On the septal surface a rather different arrangement is seen. The fibres to the right side are circular, with the anterior fibres swinging over and backwards into the right ventricular trabeculae (fig. 5.36).

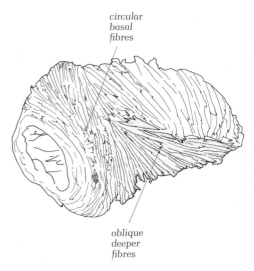

circular
basal
fibres

oblique
deeper
fibres

Fig. 5.37   Deep dissection of the left ventricle
shows how the fibres run obliquely from
apex towards the base.

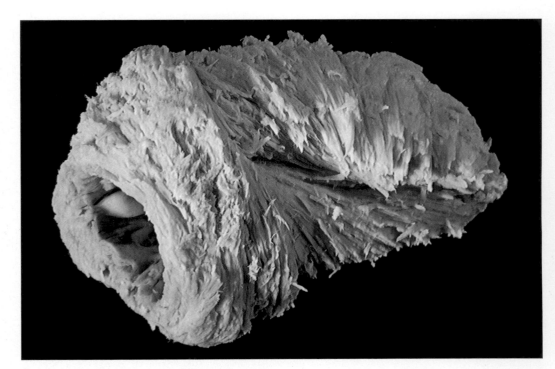

cavity of
left ventricle

'bulbo-spiral'
muscle

Fig. 5.38   This dissection shows the
circumferential fibres around the mitral
annulus (the bulbo-spiral muscle).

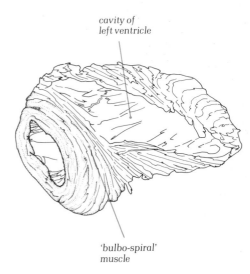

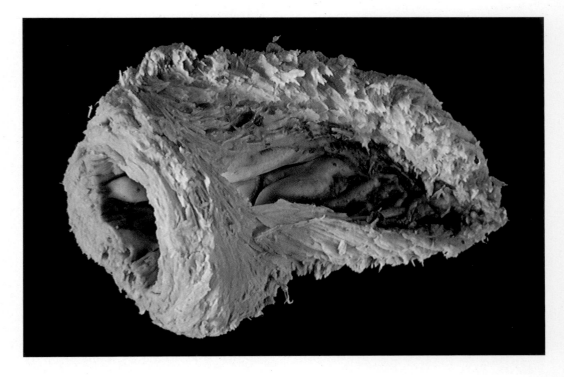

Deeper dissection shows that the
fibres from the apex turn in and are
orientated in an apex-base direction
(fig. 5.37), swinging round to join the
basal circular fibres. These fibres are
subendocardial, since further

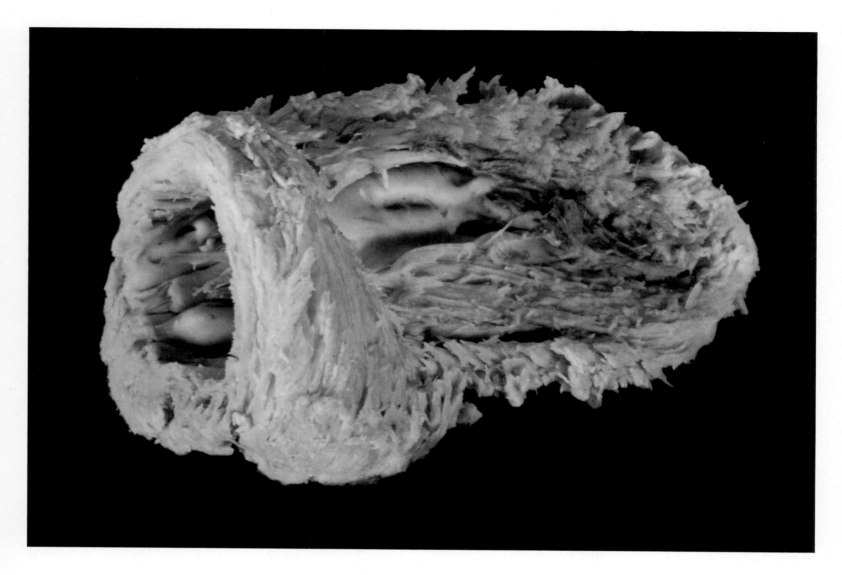

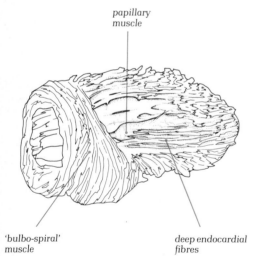

papillary
muscle

'bulbo-spiral'
muscle

deep endocardial
fibres

Fig. 5.39   The deep fibres of the left ventricle
pass into the papillary muscles from the
endocardial surface.

dissection swiftly reveals the cavity of
the ventricle (fig. 5.38). The papillary
muscles are mounted on the lateral
wall of the ventricular mass and
apical fibres turn upwards to form the
posteromedial group (fig. 5.39). The

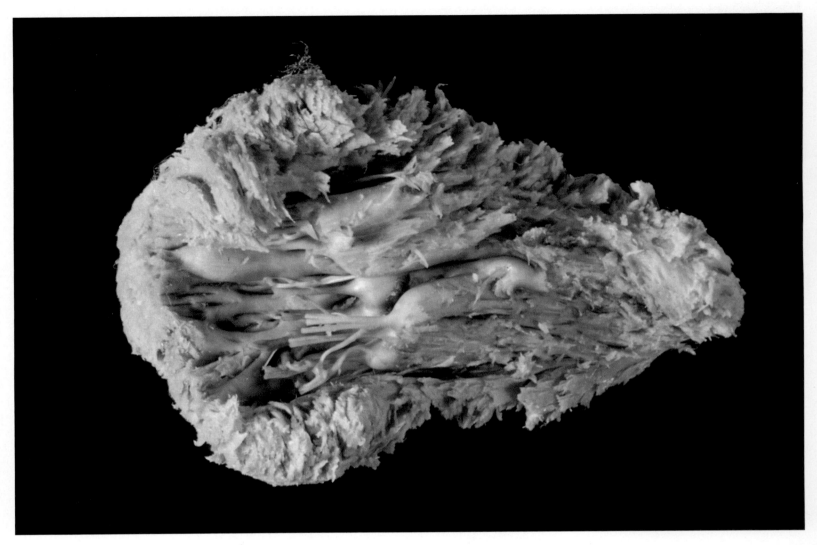

anterolateral group is formed by an intermixing of the circumferential fibres, which then reorientate themselves in apex-base fashion (fig. 5.40).

Thus, our findings by gradual dissection of a single heart show many features in common with the 'classical' view but other features which are incongruent. There is a general orientation into superficial, middle and deep layers; but the zones are in no way clear cut. Through all layers, fibres seem to belong mostly to their own ventricle, superficial cross-overs being primarily limited in this heart to the posterior surface and also far less than generally described. As with Lev and Simkins (1956), we were unable to distinguish the complicated pathways described whereby muscles start in the annuli and end in papillary muscles. Indeed, our overall impression is that the fibrous skeleton has been grossly overemphasized as having a skeletal role. The heart is not comparable to a skeletal muscle; rather, it is a modified blood vessel.

As such, should we expect muscles to have origins and insertions? As we have indicated above, it seems to us that the major purpose of the cardiac fibrous skeleton is to support the atrioventricular valves. The muscle fibres seem to attach to the fibres next to them, using the term 'fibre' in a gross rather than a microscopic respect. The muscular architecture in the single heart studied demonstrated a primary role for the left ventricle, the septum belonging to the left ventricle and the right ventricular papillary muscles being integrated into the left ventricular fibre system. The left ventricular fibres themselves were spiral superficially with a vertical apex but circular in the main mass of muscle with a tendency for fibres to run in the ventricular long axis in the deep layers, particularly in the papillary muscles. This account is an endorsement of that of Thane (1894), taking cognizance of a decreased role for the fibrous skeleton. More work is needed on this topic but one thing is certain; much information can be obtained

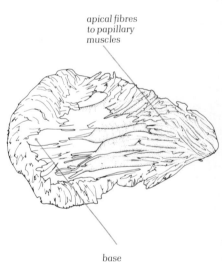

apical fibres
to papillary
muscles

base

Fig. 5.40 Final dissection of the endocardial surface shows the apical fibres passing up into the papillary muscles.

merely by careful dissection of formalin-fixed material, and preliminary findings in our laboratory confirm this initial experience Indeed, in our hands, attempts to use macerating fluids (that suggested by MacCallum sounded frighteningly explosive!) hindered, rather than helped, our efforts.

6 Cardiac Sub-systems

The Coronary Circulation
The Conduction System
The Nervous System

The Coronary Circulation

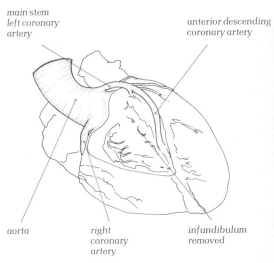

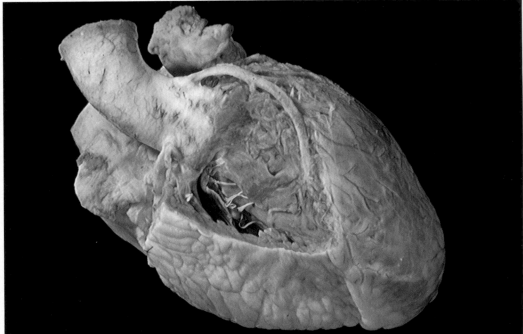

Fig. 6.1   A heart dissected from the front by removal of the infundibulum of the right ventricle showing the origin of the coronary arteries from the root of the aorta.

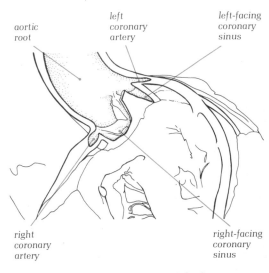

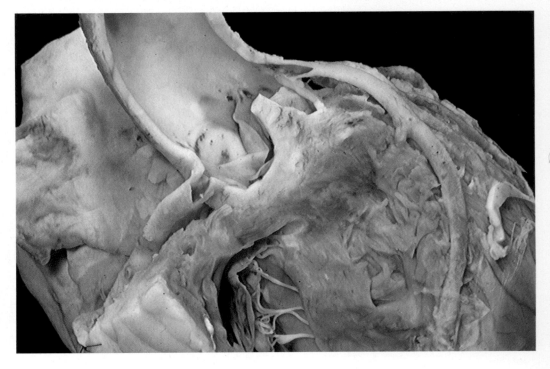

Fig. 6.2   Further dissection of the heart shown in fig. 6.1 showing that the coronary arteries take origin above the facing leaflets of the aortic valve.

The coronary circulation consists of the coronary arteries (the first branches of the aorta) which run into the myocardium. The circulation continues through a capillary network to the coronary veins which drain for their most part into the coronary sinus of the right atrium.

The Coronary Arteries

There are two main coronary arteries, right and left, which have each classically been considered to be end arteries. That is to say that the tributaries of the right coronary artery do not anastomose with those of the left coronary artery. This

concept has now been disproven and it has been shown that collateral pathways may exist from birth onwards which are not necessarily an expression of a pathological condition.

The coronary arteries originate from the aortic sinuses which face the pulmonary valve, the so-called right

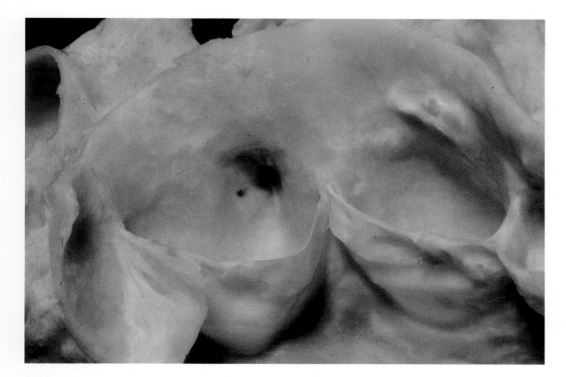

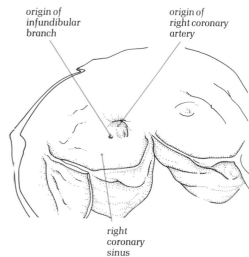

Fig. 6.3   View of the origin of the right coronary artery. In this heart, there is a separate orifice for the infundibular branch.

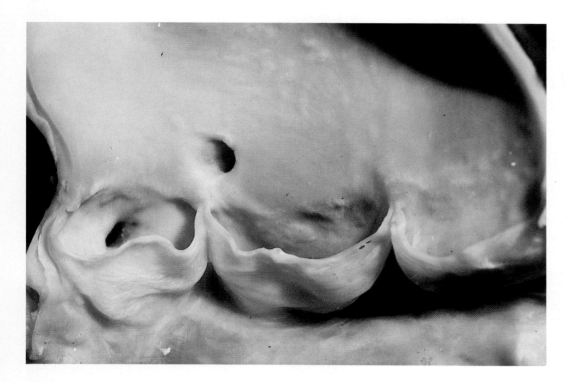

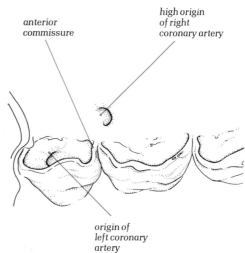

Fig. 6.4   A heart showing a high origin of the right coronary artery above the anterior commissure. The left coronary artery originates in a more usual position.

and left coronary sinuses (fig. 6.1). Usually, the coronary arteries arise from within the sinus below the aortic bar (fig. 6.2) and from between two commissures (fig. 6.3). In the left coronary sinus, there is usually one ostium only; in contrast, it is usual to find multiple ostia in the right coronary sinus (fig. 6.3). The major ostium supplies the main right coronary artery. Minor ostia when present supply the early tributaries which in the presence of a single ostium take origin from the main artery. The most frequent additional ostium is to be found anterior to the main ostium giving rise to the infundibular or conal branch.

Although usually the coronary ostia arise from within the aortic sinuses, they may arise from above the level of the aortic bar (fig. 6.4) and the ostium may be located close to an aortic commissure (fig. 6.4). In the latter situation, the coronary artery will usually have an oblique course through the aortic wall.

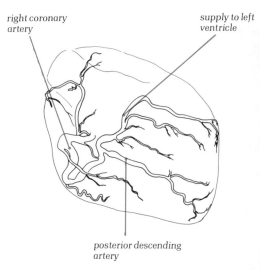

right coronary artery ——— ——— supply to left ventricle

posterior descending artery

Fig. 6.5   A post mortem coronary arteriogram showing injection of the right coronary artery. The artery supplies the posterior descending artery and also most of the posterior surface of the left ventricle.

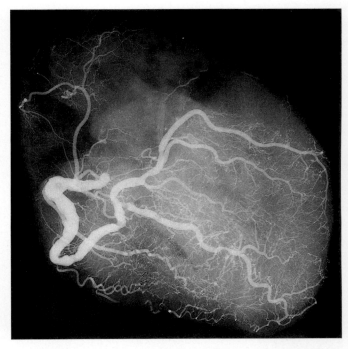

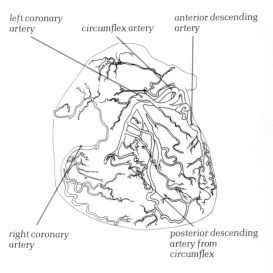

left coronary artery   circumflex artery   anterior descending artery

right coronary artery   posterior descending artery from circumflex

Fig. 6.6   A post mortem coronary arteriogram in a heart with left dominance. The injection into the left coronary artery shows that it supplies the posterior descending coronary artery.

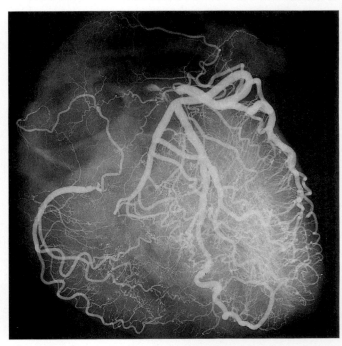

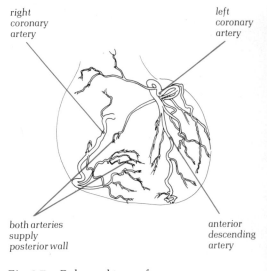

right coronary artery   left coronary artery

both arteries supply posterior wall   anterior descending artery

Fig. 6.7   Balanced type of coronary circulation showing how right and left coronary arteries supply the posterior aspects of the heart.

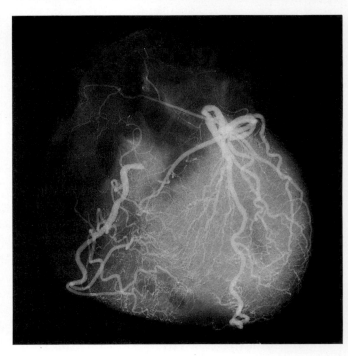

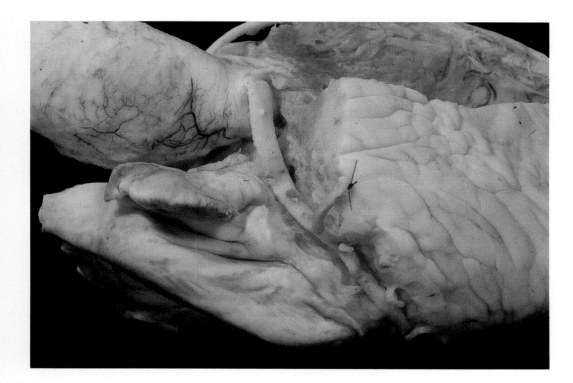

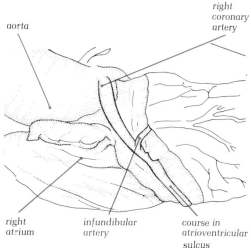

aorta

right coronary artery

right atrium

infundibular artery

course in atrioventricular sulcus

Fig. 6.8 Dissection of the right coronary artery showing how it passes immediately into the atrioventricular sulcus.

The major coronary arteries all occupy a subepicardial position, being found in the atrioventricular sulcus and in the interventricular sulcus. Minor branches from the subepicardial arteries in the atrioventricular sulcus ascend into the atria or descend into the ventricles round the circumference of the sulcus. The branches of the major arteries in the interventricular sulcus penetrate to supply the ventricular septum. The extent of the myocardium supplied by the right and left arteries varies from heart to heart. The most frequent pattern is for the right coronary artery to encircle the tricuspid orifice and supply the posterior descending coronary artery. This arrangement, termed right dominance, is found in approximately 90% of hearts (fig. 6.5). In approximately 10% of hearts, the circumflex branch of the left coronary artery supplies the posterior descending artery, a left dominant pattern (fig. 6.6). In a few remaining hearts, branches of both the right coronary and the left circumflex artery give off parallel descending branches close to the interventricular groove, a so-called balanced pattern of coronary supply (fig. 6.7). This arrangement is significant because the dominant coronary artery usually supplies the artery to the atrioventricular node. In a balanced pattern, this artery most frequently arises from the right coronary artery.

The right coronary artery emerges from the right coronary sinus directly into the atrioventricular sulcus (fig. 6.8). It immediately gives off the infundibular artery (conal branch) if this artery does not have a separate ostium from the sinus (fig. 6.3). The infundibular artery ramifies over the right ventricular outflow tract and usually has a small branch which encircles the pulmonary valve orifice to join with a branch from the left coronary artery.

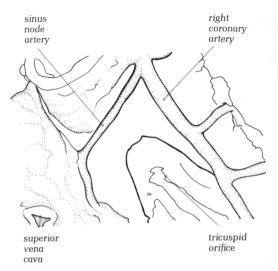

sinus node artery

right coronary artery

superior vena cava

tricuspid orifice

Fig. 6.9   Dissection of the artery to the sinus node which in this heart originates immediately from the right coronary artery.

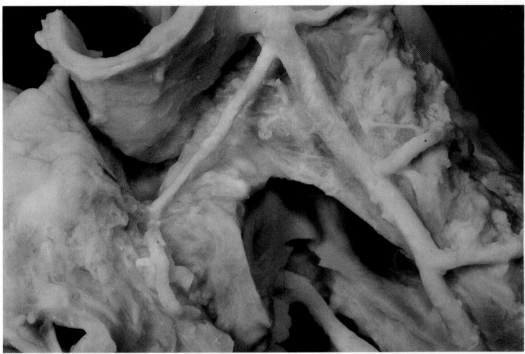

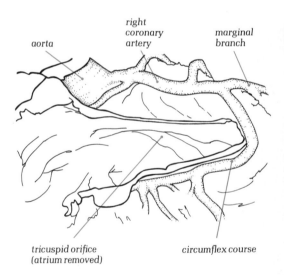

aorta

right coronary artery

marginal branch

tricuspid orifice (atrium removed)

circumflex course

Fig. 6.10   Dissection showing the circumflex course of the right coronary artery as illustrated by removal of the right atrium.

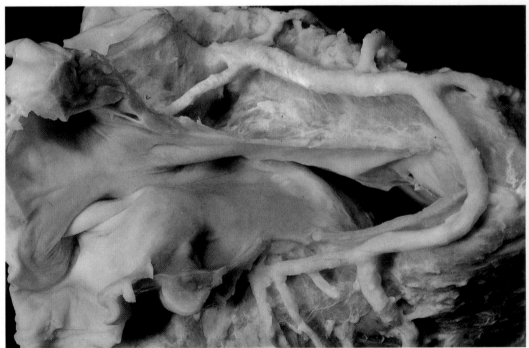

In much the same area, the sinus node artery arises from the right coronary artery in about 55% of individuals (fig. 6.9). This artery ascends through the interatrial groove along the anteromedial wall of the right atrium and passes either in front of, or behind, or branches and passes both in front of and behind to form a circle around the orifice of the superior vena cava to supply the sinus node lying in the sulcus terminalis (Anderson et al., 1979). The right coronary artery continues in the anterior atrioventricular sulcus and its next major tributary is the marginal branch which runs along the acute margin of the heart towards the apex (fig. 6.10). The right coronary then turns down the posterior atrioventricular sulcus and extends to the crux cordis. In cases of right dominance, the posterior descending coronary artery is given off at the crux (fig. 6.11). The continuation of the right coronary artery then forms a U-loop along the inlet septum which

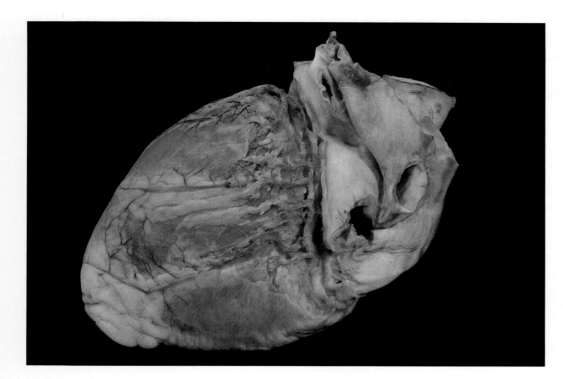

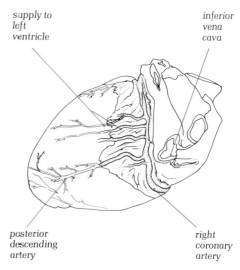

Fig. 6.11 Posterior view of a heart which has a dominant right coronary circulation.

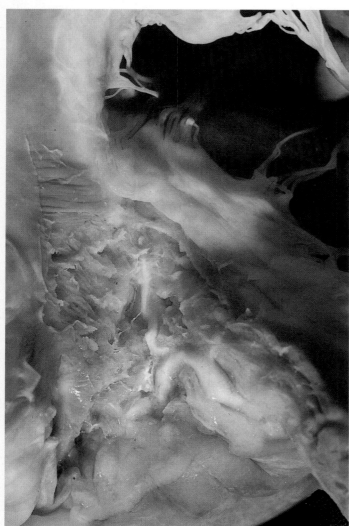

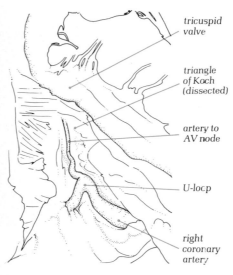

tricuspid
valve

triangle
of Koch
(dissected)

artery to
AV node

U-loop

right
coronary
artery

Fig. 6.12 Dissection showing the origin of the artery to the atrioventricular node from a U-loop on the right coronary artery.

gives rise to the atrioventricular nodal artery at its apex (fig. 6.12). This passes forwards into the fibrous and adipose tissue plane beneath the coronary sinus to reach the nodal area (fig. 2.31). The termination of the right coronary artery beyond the loop usually supplies the inferior wall of the left ventricle and part of the posteromedial papillary muscle group of the mitral valve. The extent of supply of the left ventricular wall by such a dominant right coronary artery varies considerably in different individuals. Throughout its circumflex course, the right coronary artery gives additional branches to both the right atrial and right ventricular walls which do not have specific names (fig. 6.10). A dominant right coronary artery may also terminate in a branch which extends onto the posterior surface of the left atrium.

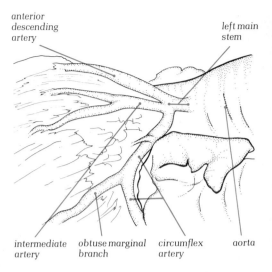

anterior descending artery

left main stem

intermediate artery

obtuse marginal branch

circumflex artery

aorta

Fig. 6.13 Dissection showing the short main branch of the left coronary artery which divides into the anterior descending and circumflex branches.

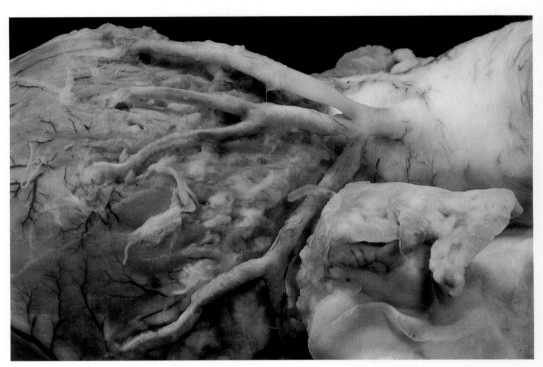

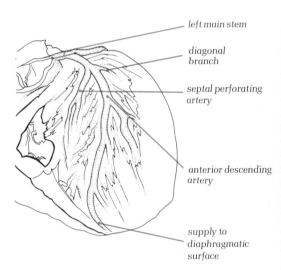

left main stem

diagonal branch

septal perforating artery

anterior descending artery

supply to diaphragmatic surface

Fig. 6.14 Dissection illustrating the course of the anterior descending coronary artery and its septal perforating branches. The coronary angiogram is of the same heart.

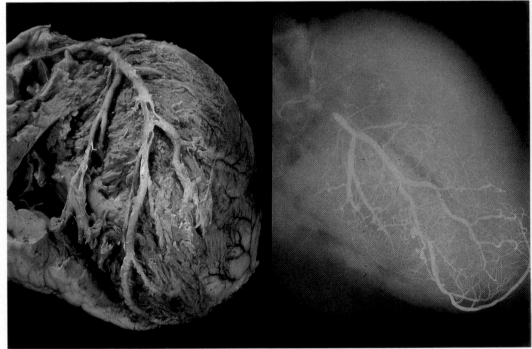

The left coronary artery emerges from the left aortic sinus into the left side of the atrioventricular sulcus (fig. 6.13). The main stem of the left coronary artery is of variable length but is usually short, rarely exceeding 1cm in length before branching into anterior descending and circumflex coronary arteries. In approximately 30% of cases, there is a third branch originating at the site of division of the right main stem. This branch, termed the intermediate artery, crosses obliquely over the parietal ventricular wall. The anterior descending coronary artery turns downwards towards the apex in the anterior interventricular groove. Its

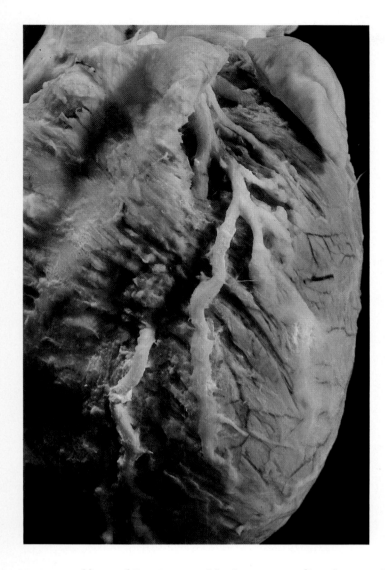

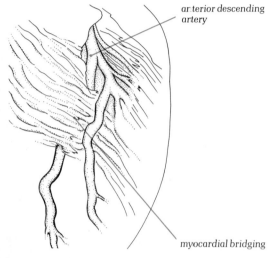

Fig. 6.15   A heart in which the anterior descending coronary artery is bridged by myocardial tissue.

pattern of branching is variable, but frequently, a diagonal branch arises close to its origin from the left main stem *(fig. 6.13)*. This diagonal artery, however, or additional diagonal arteries, may originate more distally from the anterior descending artery, passing backwards to supply the obtuse margin of the heart. As the anterior descending artery passes towards the apex, it gives off a series of branches which pass perpendicularly into the anterior interventricular septum *(fig. 6.14)*. The first perforating branch usually originates within 1cm of the origin of the anterior descending artery and is the largest artery *(fig. 6.14)*. It gives important tributaries to the ventricular conduction system. These perforating branches are intramyocardial, rather than epicardial, branches. However, the anterior descending artery itself, although usually an epicardial structure, can pass intramyocardially for some distance before returning to its epicardial position. This is called myocardial bridging *(fig. 6.15)*. The

distal part of the anterior descending artery usually dips round the ventricular apex and continues in the posterior interventricular groove *(fig. 6.14)*. The extent of the posterior supply depends upon the size of the posterior descending artery and varies considerably.

The circumflex branch of the left coronary artery is the other branch of the left main arterial stem *(fig. 6.13)*. In approximately 45% of cases, it immediately gives rise to the sinus node artery which runs along the anterior interatrial furrow and then takes a similar course to the sinus node when it arises from the right coronary artery. The circumflex artery continues its course in the left atrioventricular sulcus, its extent depending upon whether the artery will become the dominant artery. When the left coronary artery is not dominant, its area of supply depends upon the extent of the right coronary artery *(compare figs. 6.5 & 6.6)*. A marginal branch usually originates from the proximal segment of the left circumflex coronary artery. This

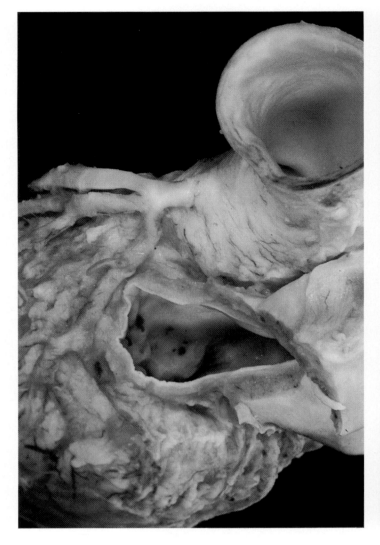

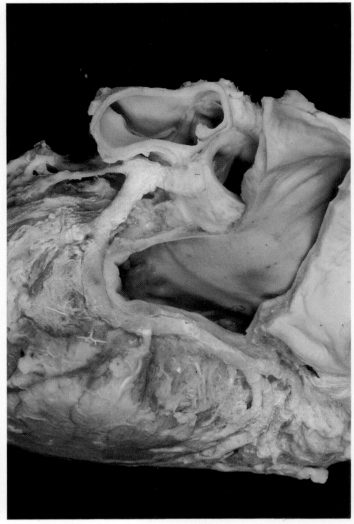

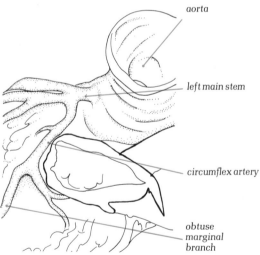

aorta

left main stem

circumflex artery

obtuse
marginal
branch

Fig. 6.16   Dissection showing the course of
the left circumflex coronary artery in a heart
with right dominance.

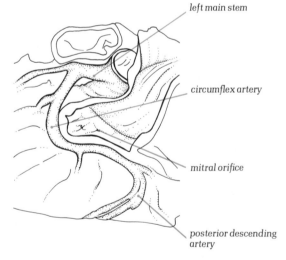

left main stem

circumflex artery

mitral orifice

posterior descending
artery

Fig. 6.17   The course of the left coronary
artery in another heart with left dominance.
The circumflex artery is much more closely
related to the mitral annulus.

marginal branch may take a more
peripheral course along the obtuse
margin of the heart. In cases of
extreme right dominance, this branch
may be the termination of the left
circumflex artery. The proximity of
the circumflex artery to the mitral
annulus varies considerably. It is

much closer to the annulus,
particularly the intervalvar fibrous
area, when the main stem is short;
and it follows the annulus for a
greater distance when the left
coronary artery is dominant (compare
figs. 6.16 & 6.17). When the left
circumflex supplies most or all of the
diaphragmatic surface, it gives

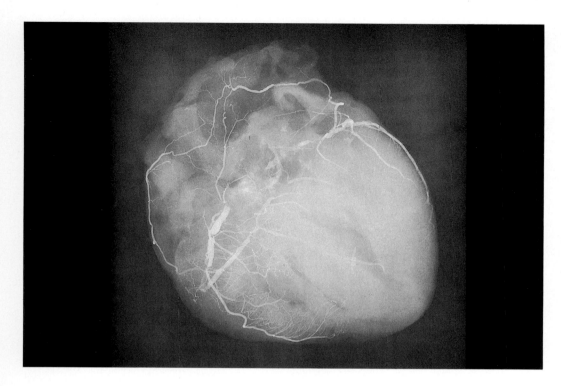

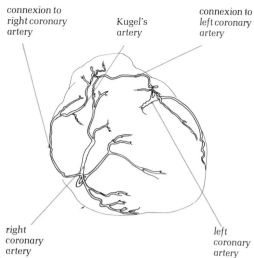

connexion to
right coronary
artery

Kugel's
artery

connexion to
left coronary
artery

right
coronary
artery

left
coronary
artery

Fig. 6.18   A post mortem angiogram
illustrating the course of Kugel's artery.

additional branches to the atrial and
ventricular musculature, including
the supply to the posteromedial
papillary muscle group.

The myocardial supply from the
epicardial coronary arteries is usually
derived from perpendicular branches
which then penetrate the myocardium
and course towards the endocardium.
During their course, these arteries
ramify again perpendicularly, these
branches themselves ramifying
amongst the myocardial fibre bundles.
In the subendocardial layer, an
extensive network of
intercommunicating branches is
present, running parallel to the
endocardial surface. The mitral
papillary muscles are vascularized by
arteries which take a separate course
and do not contribute to the
remainder of the left ventricular
myocardium. The number of arteries
depends upon the architecture of the
papillary muscle: a pillar muscle has
a single artery; finger-like groups
have multiple arteries. The arteries
penetrate the myocardial wall
perpendicularly from the epicardium
to the base of the papillary muscle
and then ascend through its
substance in corkscrew fashion,
giving off branches to supply the
muscle. They are unusually thick-
walled and have extensive
longitudinally-arranged medial
muscle fibres.

As stated previously, collateral
networks exist between the right and
left coronary artery networks. Some
of these are present at precapillary
level, while other pathways may
utilize larger calibre vessels. Among
the latter category, two major
pathways are recognized. The first is
the communication between septal
perforating branches of the anterior
and posterior descending arteries.
A second important route exists
through atrial branches. When
present, this circuit most frequently
comprises a large artery, originating
from the right coronary artery, which
communicates with an additional
large branch from the left circumflex
artery. This communicating artery
runs along the anterior atrial wall and
is termed the arteria auricularis
magna (Kugel's artery, fig. 6.18).

The Coronary Veins

The coronary arterial blood, having
passed through the capillary network,
is collected by venules which drain to
the cardiac veins. Two major groups
of veins exist: those draining to the
coronary sinus, and those draining
directly to the cardiac chambers, the
venae cordae minimis. A further
group of larger veins runs over the
anterior aspect of the heart, cross
superficially over the right coronary
artery, and drain blood directly to the
right atrium. These veins are the
anterior cardiac veins.

The veins which drain to the
coronary sinus run together with the

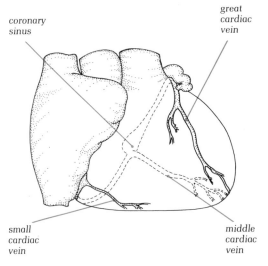

coronary sinus

great cardiac vein

small cardiac vein

middle cardiac vein

Fig. 6.19   Diagram of the anterior surface of the heart showing the position of the cardiac veins.

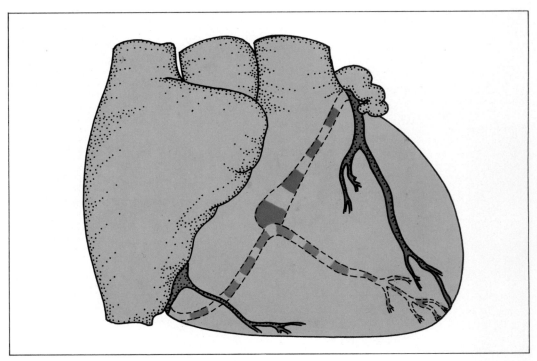

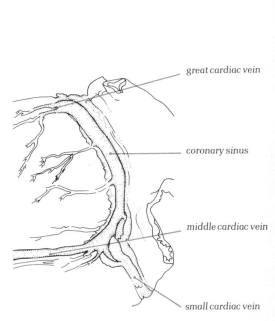

great cardiac vein

coronary sinus

middle cardiac vein

small cardiac vein

Fig. 6.20   Posterior view of the heart in its in situ position showing how the coronary sinus collects the venous tributaries before draining into the right atrium.

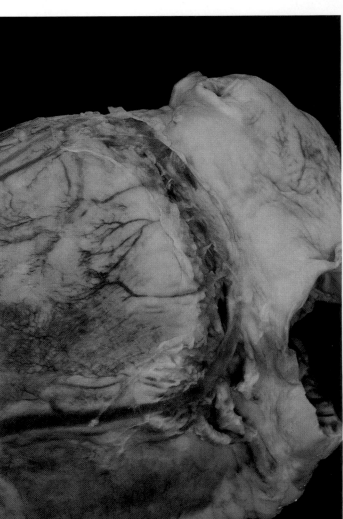

coronary arteries. The great cardiac vein ascends along the anterior descending artery and runs along the left atrioventricular sulcus, where it receives venous channels from the obtuse margin (fig. 6.19). In the posterior atrioventricular sulcus, it becomes the coronary sinus which runs along the wall of the left atrium to drain into the right atrium (fig. 6.20). Near its entrance to the right atrium (fig. 6.21), the coronary sinus receives the venous blood draining through the middle cardiac vein which ascends in the posterior interventricular groove, and the small cardiac vein which ascends alongside the marginal coronary artery and turns into the posterior atrioventricular sulcus with the right coronary artery (fig. 6.22). Veins from the atria also drain down into the coronary sinus. The oblique vein of the left atrium is the vestige of the left

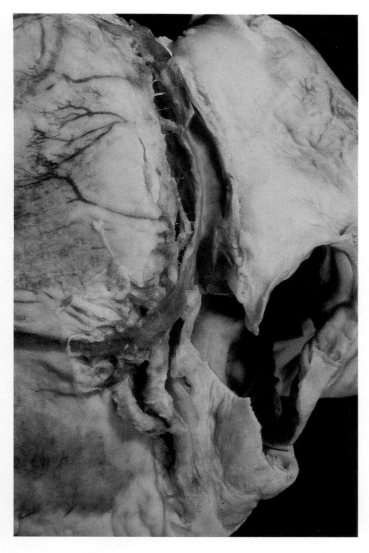

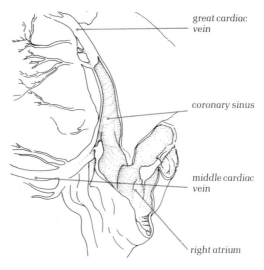

Fig. 6.21 Dissection of the coronary sinus showing the way it receives the cardiac veins and drains to the right atrium.

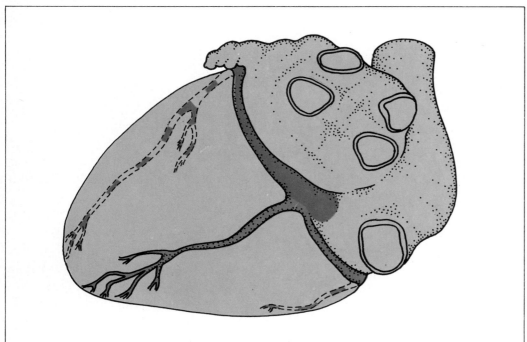

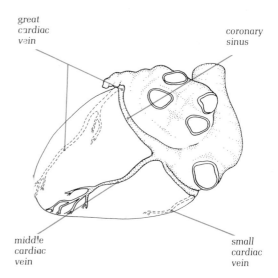

Fig. 6.22 Diagram of the posterior surface of the heart showing the position of the cardiac veins draining to the coronary sinus.

sinus horn. It is a large channel in the presence of a left superior vena cava, draining the left superior cava to the coronary sinus (fig. 2.21).

Apart from these major channels, there are smaller outlets which drain through the Thebesian foraminae directly into the cardiac chambers, particularly the right atrium and ventricle. It is possible that these are sinusoids, rather than true venous channels.

In addition to the arteries and veins, there is an extensive lymphatic network in the heart. This network is divided into a deep endocardial, a middle and a superficial epicardial network. These channels all drain eventually into collecting channels which follow an epicardial course, accompanying the major arterial stems. The primary lymph nodes draining the heart are found in the anterior mediastinum.

6.13

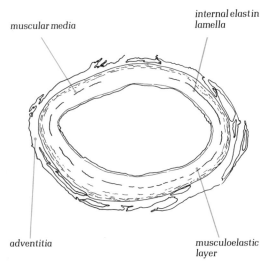

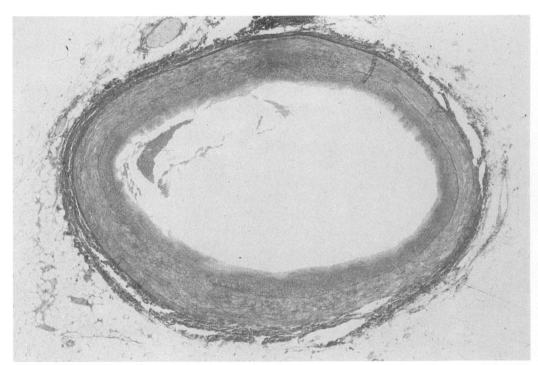

Fig. 6.23   Cross-section of a coronary artery showing the medial layer composed mostly of circular muscular tissue.

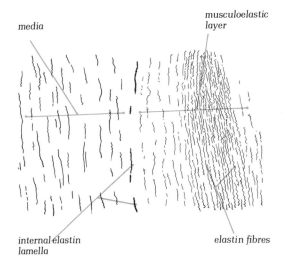

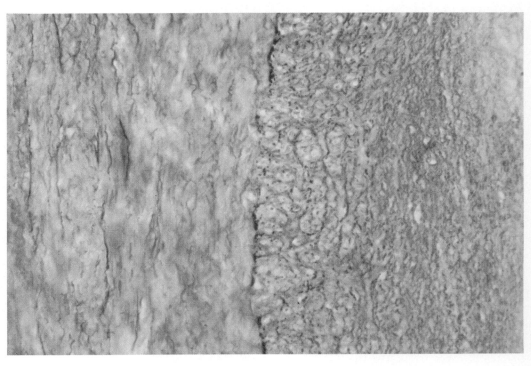

Fig. 6.24   Detail of the junction between the media and musculoelastic layer. The latter is composed of longitudinal muscle cells with intervening elastin fibres.

Histology of Coronary Arteries

At their origin from the ascending aorta, the coronary arteries are elastic arteries. However, they change immediately into muscular arteries, characterized by a media which, for its major part, is composed of smooth muscle cells arranged in a more or less circular fashion (fig. 6.23). Elastin and collagen fibres are present, but these do not dominate the histological picture as they do in the aorta.

At the junction of the media with the adventitia, a condensation of elastin fibres occurs which intermingles with the collagen fibres that form the major constituent of the adventitia. A distinctive outer elastin lamella is not present, although superficial examination at low magnification may give this impression.

Towards the intima, the media is delineated by a distinct membrane, the so-called internal elastin lamella (fig. 6.24). In neonates and infants, this membrane may already exhibit local fenestrations and reduplications of elastin fibres. In such areas, smooth muscle cells are present, most likely derived from proliferating medial smooth muscle cells. With increasing age, this phenomenon may intensify and ultimately produce a distinctive intimal layer composed of smooth muscle cells with intervening collagen and elastin fibres (fig. 6.24). This newly-created intimal layer is called the musculoelastic layer (Neufeld, 1974). By the end of the first year of life, this layer can almost always be identified, although its extent may vary considerably. It may present as discrete localized intimal cushions; or, in other instances, it may present as a fully circumferential layer. Neither its precise mode of origin nor its potential significance is, at present, fully understood.

The Conduction System

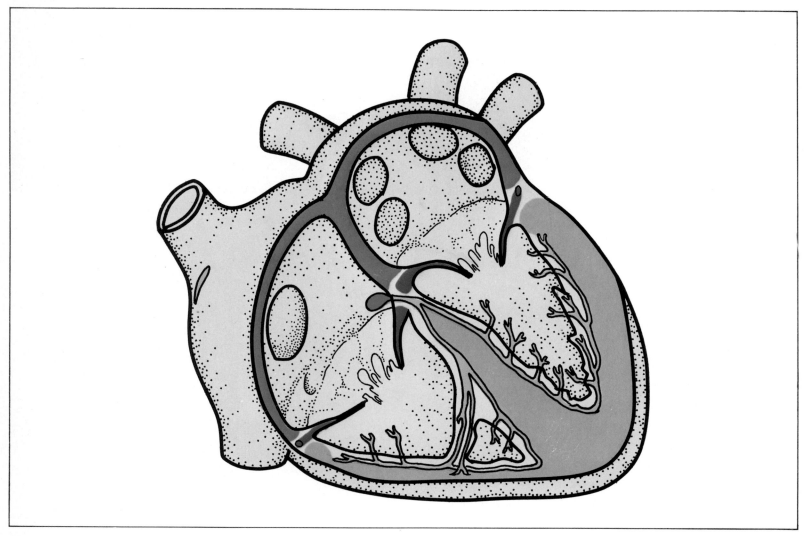

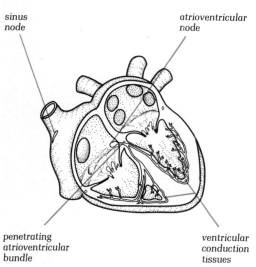

sinus node

atrioventricular node

penetrating atrioventricular bundle

ventricular conduction tissues

Fig. 6.25   A stylized diagram of the components of the conduction system.

The conduction tissues are responsible for the initiation and conduction of the heartbeat. They are composed of myocardial tissues, but myocardial tissues which can be distinguished histologically from the 'working' atrial and ventricular myocardium. For this reason, they are frequently referred to as the 'specialized tissues' of the heart. The structures made of conduction tissue are the sinus node, the atrioventricular node, the atrioventricular bundle and the ventricular conduction tissues (Anderson & Becker, 1978; fig. 6.25). That part of the conduction system which carries the impulse through the fibrous skeleton is also called the atrioventricular specialized junctional area.

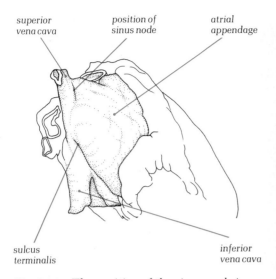

superior
vena cava · position of
sinus node · atrial
appendage

sulcus
terminalis · inferior
vena cava

Fig. 6.26   The position of the sinus node in
the normal heart.

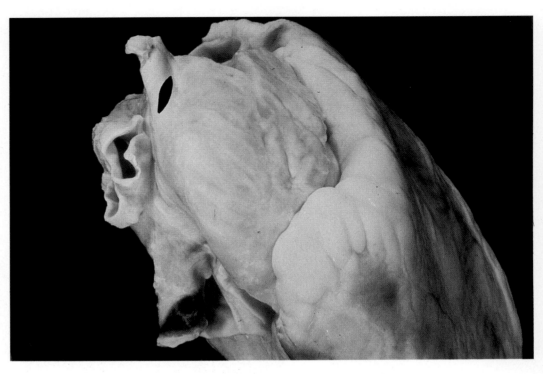

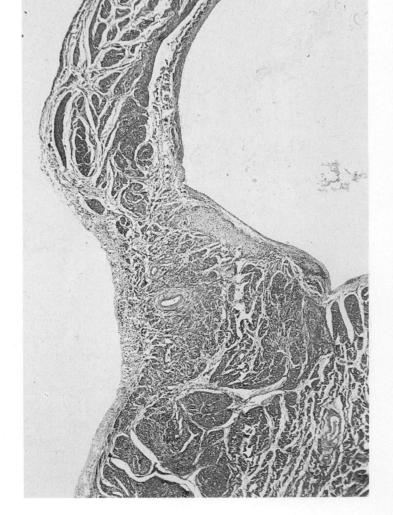

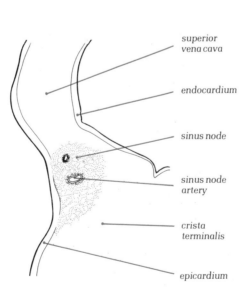

superior
vena cava

endocardium

sinus node

sinus node
artery

crista
terminalis

epicardium

Fig. 6.27   Histological section of an infant
sinus node. Trichrome stain.

The sinus node, or pacemaker, is situated in the sulcus terminalis at the lateral junction of the superior vena cava with the right atrium (fig. 6.26). It is a spindle-shaped structure with an extensive tail, the cauda, which runs down the sulcus terminalis towards the orifice of the inferior vena cava. It is rare to find a node which extends medially to the superior caval orifice in horseshoe fashion (Hudson, 1967). The node is usually arranged around a prominent artery which is a branch of the right coronary artery in 55% of persons, and the left circumflex artery in the remainder. Whatever its origin, the artery to the node may run into the nodal tissue in front of the superior vena cava, behind it, or as an arterial circle enclosing the caval orifice

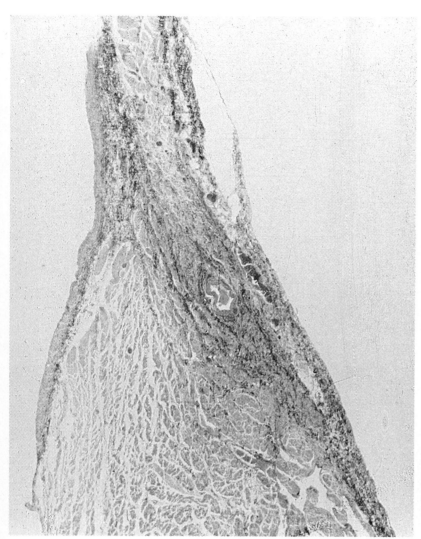
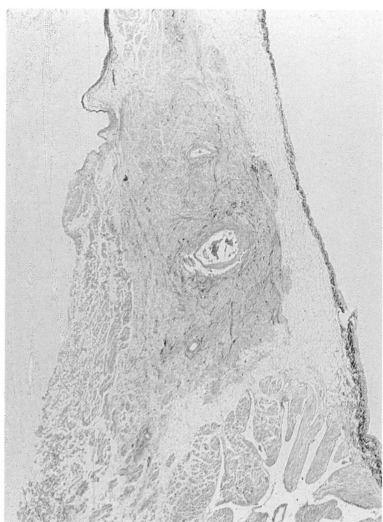

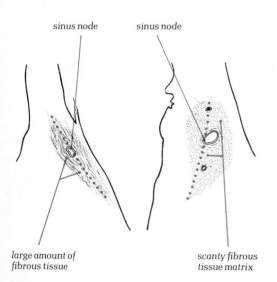

sinus node   sinus node

large amount of   scanty fibrous
fibrous tissue   tissue matrix

Fig. 6.28   Histological section of adult sinus node (left). Note the increase in connective tissue (stained purple) in comparison to the infant node (right). Fibrous tissue stain.

(*Anderson et al., 1979*). Although usually a single large artery passes through the node, multiple small arteries may be observed. The node is made up of densely-packed small nodal cells arranged in interweaving fasciculi, all of it set in a dense fibrous tissue matrix (*fig. 6.27*). With increasing age, the amount of fibrous tissue increases relative to the area occupied by nodal cells, a phenomenon which does not indicate nodal pathology *per se* (*fig. 6.28*). At the nodal margins, there is a fairly sharp distinction between nodal cells and working myocardial cells with only a very minimal transitional zone, that zone being most marked on the crista terminalis. When the topography of the node is studied, its transitional junctions with the surrounding myocardium are limited.

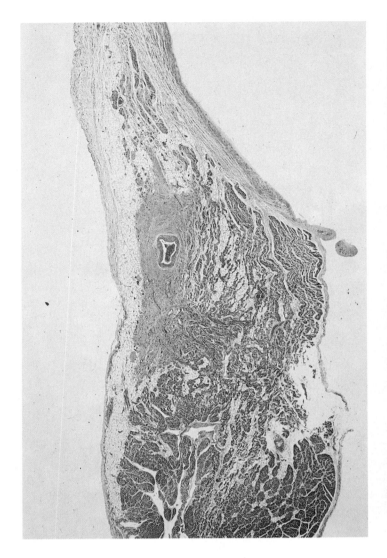

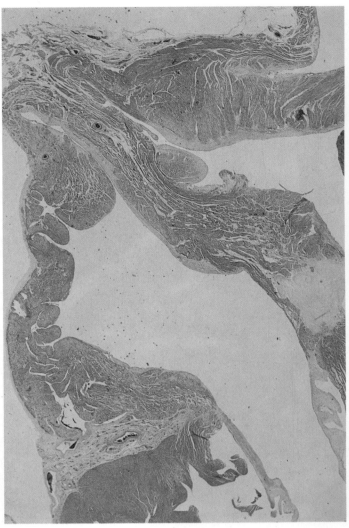

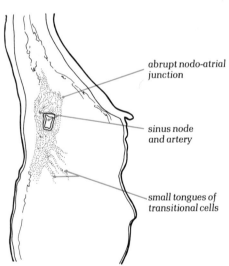

abrupt nodo-atrial
junction

sinus node
and artery

small tongues of
transitional cells

sinus node

'working' atrial
myocardium

right atrium

atrioventricular
node

atrioventricular
ring tissue

tricuspid valve

Fig. 6.29   Section through the sinus node
showing the tongues of nodal tissue
extending into the crista terminalis.
Trichrome stain.

Fig. 6.30   Section through the entire right
atrial tissues showing how the internodal
myocardium lacks any insulated tracts.
Trichrome stain.

Although continuous with the crista
terminalis over a broad front, there
are relatively few areas where
'streaming' of fibres from node to
atrial myocardium can be identified
(fig. 6.29). There are numerous
autonomic ganglia and nerves
adjacent to the sinus node; and
presumably, these give a rich plexus

to the nodal cells. Such rich plexuses
are the rule in animal species but have
not as yet been unequivocally
demonstrated in the human node.

The question of how the sinus
impulse reaches the atrioventricular
node is at the present time
controversial. Some authorities have
suggested that 'specialized tracts' run

between the nodes (James, 1963). Our
own studies have not substantiated
this claim (Janse & Anderson, 1974;
Becker & Anderson, 1976). We find the
muscle bands and bundles of the right
atrium and the interatrial septum to
be composed of working myocardium,
and we are unable to identify any
'tracts' isolated within the muscular

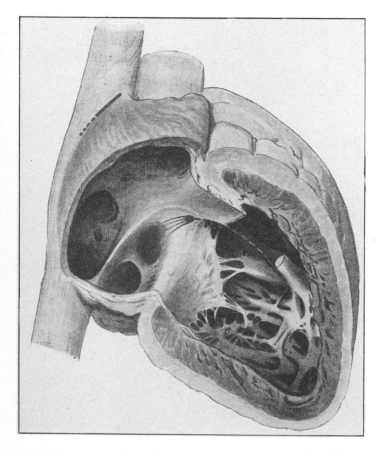

Fig. 6.31   Reproduction of the diagram from the publication of Koch (1909) illustrating the triangle which now bears his name.

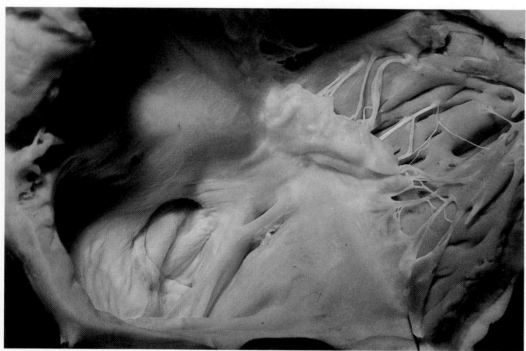

right atrium

attachment of tricuspid valve

site of tendon of Todaro

commissure of venous valve

triangle of Koch

Fig. 6.32   The septal surface of the right atrium showing the landmarks of the triangle of Koch.

bands delimited by the orifices of the right atrium together with the fossa ovalis. We have found parallel and closely-packed bundles of working myocardium in the crista terminalis and the limbus of the fossa, an observation which could well be the morphological counterpart of the preferential pathways demonstrated unequivocally by electrophysiologists (*Spach et al., 1969*). However, these areas are histologically 'unspecialized' (*fig. 6.30*).

The atrioventricular node is found in the base of the atrial septum at the apex of the triangle of Koch (*1909*) (*fig. 6.31*). This triangle is delimited by the tendon of Todaro (the continuation of the Eustachian valve), and the annulus of the tricuspid valve, the two meeting at the central fibrous body to produce the apex of the triangle (*fig. 6.32*). The node is made

6.19

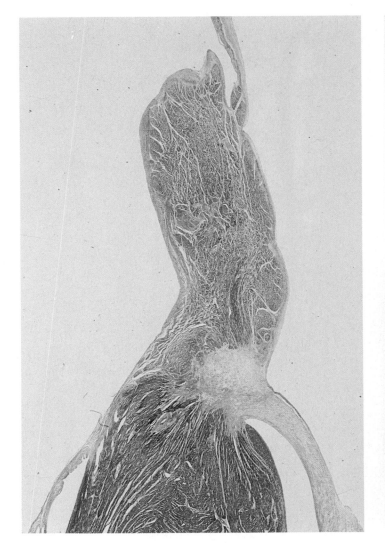

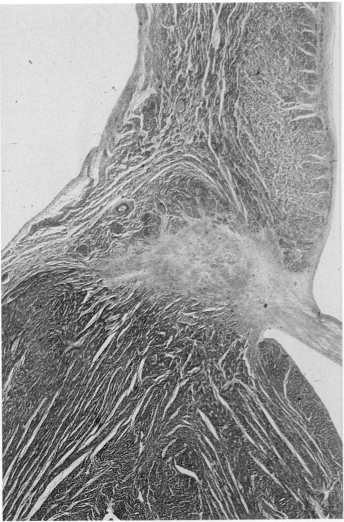

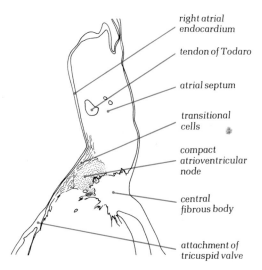

right atrial
endocardium

tendon of Todaro

atrial septum

transitional
cells

compact
atrioventricular
node

central
fibrous body

attachment of
tricuspid valve

Fig. 6.33   Section through the atrial septum
showing the position of the compact
atrioventricular node. Trichrome stain.

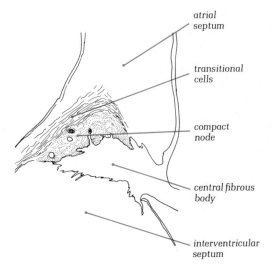

atrial
septum

transitional
cells

compact
node

central fibrous
body

interventricular
septum

Fig. 6.34   Detail of the posterior extent of the
compact atrioventricular node showing how
it is a half oval of cells closely applied to the
fibrous body (green stain) with transitional
cells streaming over its surface. Trichrome
stain.

up of a half oval of small densely-
packed nodal cells set with its flat
surface against the central fibrous
body (fig. 6.33). Extensions fan out
posteriorly from the compact node
hugging the mitral and tricuspid
annuli (fig. 6.34). Transitional atrial

fibres run into the node between these
extensions and also form a
circumferential layer around the
compact node (fig. 6.34). The
superficial atrial cells stream over the
nodal axis to enter the base of the
septal leaflet of the tricuspid valve

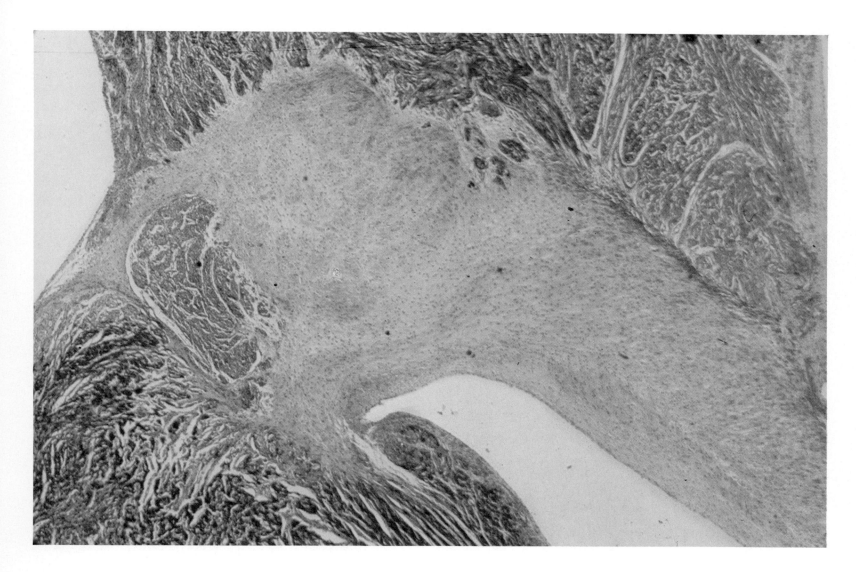

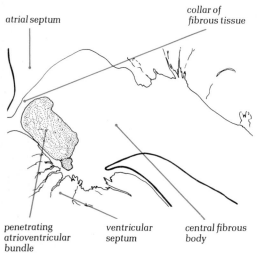

atrial septum

collar of
fibrous tissue

penetrating
atrioventricular
bundle

ventricular
septum

central fibrous
body

*Fig. 6.35   Section through the penetrating
atrioventricular bundle. Trichrome stain.*

(overlay fibres, fig. 6.33). The left
surface of the compact node is
separated from the left atrial side of
the septum by transitional fibres so
that the node is an interatrial, rather
than a right atrial, structure (fig. 6.34).
At the apex of the triangle of Koch, the
axis of the compact node gathers

itself together and runs into the
central fibrous body, becoming the
penetrating atrioventricular bundle
(fig. 6.35). Histologically, the bundle
is composed of similar cells to the
node, the junction of the two being the
point where the axis enters the central
fibrous body and becomes sealed off

from atrial input fibres. Having
entered the central fibrous body, the
interweaving pattern of the node
gradually disappears, the fibres
becoming realigned in parallel fashion.
Having penetrated the annulus, the
conduction tissue axis reaches the
crest of the trabecular septum
beneath the membranous septum
where it commences to branch. This

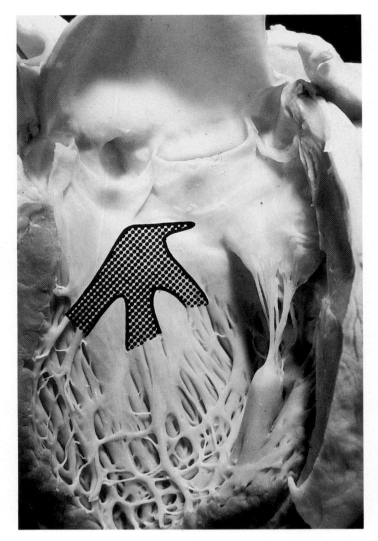

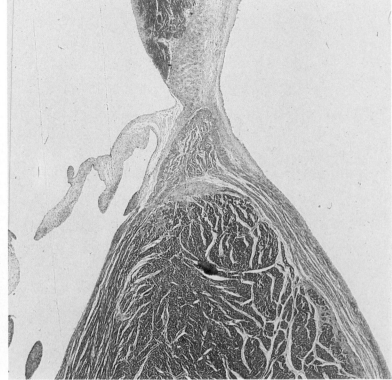

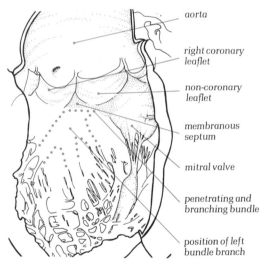

aorta

right coronary
leaflet

non-coronary
leaflet

membranous
septum

mitral valve

penetrating and
branching bundle

position of left
bundle branch

Fig. 6.36   The left ventricular outflow tract
showing the position of the left bundle branch
in relation to the membranous septum.

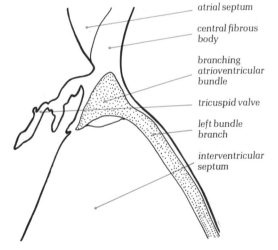

atrial septum

central fibrous
body

branching
atrioventricular
bundle

tricuspid valve

left bundle
branch

interventricular
septum

Fig. 6.37   Cross-section of the branching
atrioventricular bundle showing the sheet-
like left bundle branch cascading down the
left septal surface. Trichrome stain.

point, when viewed from the aortic
outflow tract, is beneath the
commissure between the right and
non-coronary cusps of the aortic
valve (fig. 6.36). The branching bundle
is placed on the crest of the septum

and the left bundle branch fibres
cascade as a continuous fan from the
branching bundle, forming an
interweaving subendocardial sheet
(fig. 6.37). The right bundle branch
continues anteriorly beyond the end

of the branching portion (fig. 6.38),
usually dipping downwards to pass
as a thin cord which then enters the
substance of the trabecula
septomarginalis, and tending to run

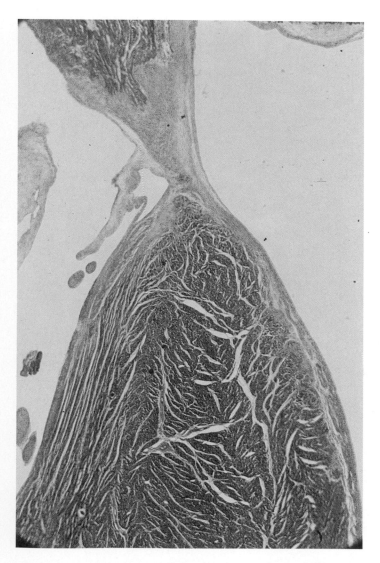

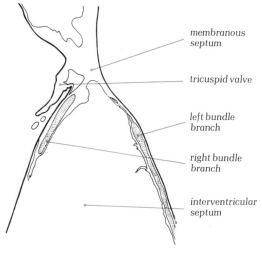

Fig. 6.38 Cross-section through the septum showing the descending right bundle branch and left bundle branches.

membranous septum

tricuspid valve

left bundle branch

right bundle branch

interventricular septum

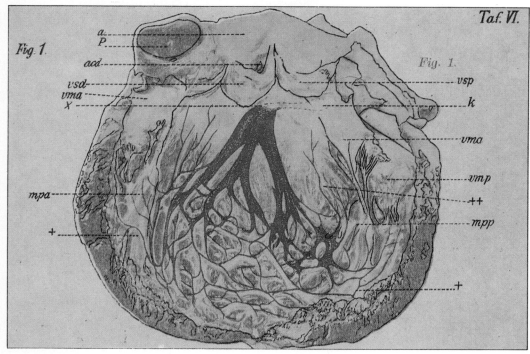

Fig. 6.39 Reproduction of illustration from Tawara's original publication (1906) showing the tripartite division of the left bundle branch.

beneath the medial papillary muscle complex.

The pattern of branching of the left bundle within the left ventricle has been controversial of late (Rosenbaum et al., 1970). Our own findings endorse the original study of Tawara (1906) which demonstrated a fan-like bundle branch with three major radiations: anterior, middle and posterior (fig. 6.39). The right bundle branch passes down within the substance of the trabecula septomarginalis as a narrow cord, part of which crosses the cavity of the right ventricle within the moderator band. Both right and left bundle

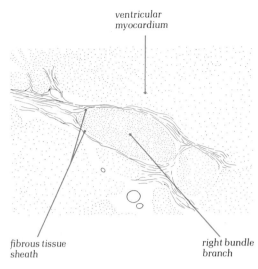

ventricular
myocardium

fibrous tissue
sheath

right bundle
branch

Fig. 6.40   Histological section of the right
bundle branch showing how the cells are only
minimally differentiated from the
surrounding myocardial tissue but are
isolated from these tissues by connective
tissue sheaths. Haematoxylin and eosin stain.

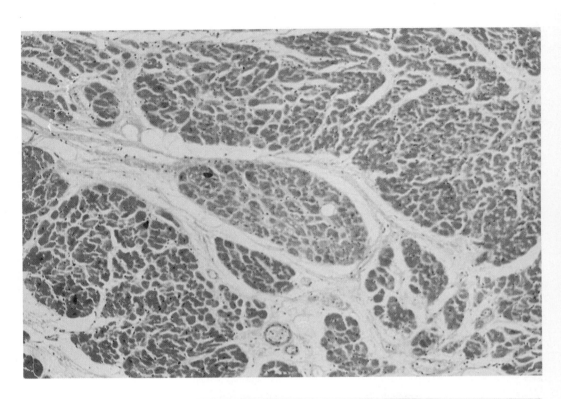

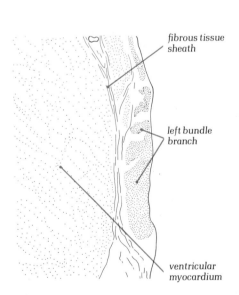

fibrous tissue
sheath

left bundle
branch

ventricular
myocardium

Fig. 6.41   Histological section of the left
bundle branch. Compare with fig. 6.40.
Haematoxylin and eosin stain.

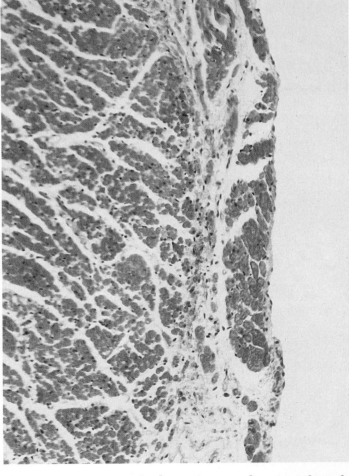

branches are isolated from the septal
surface as they descend by fibrous
tissue sheaths. They are composed of
cells minimally differentiated from the
ventricular myocardium in terms of
either size or staining affinity (figs.
6.40 & 6.41). Consequently, when they
lose their insulating sheath at the
ventricular apices, we have not found
it possible to trace the transitions
which presumably occur between the
conduction tissues and the working
myocardium.

As the atrioventricular conduction
axis descends through the annulus
fibrosus, multiple extensions of

7 Clinical Cardiac Anatomy I

Angiographic Anatomy

by Sally P. Allwork

Angiographic Anatomy

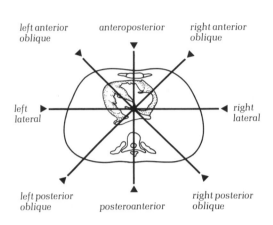

left anterior oblique   anteroposterior   right anterior oblique

left lateral   right lateral

left posterior oblique   posteroanterior   right posterior oblique

Fig. 7.1 Transverse section of thorax from above showing radiological projections. Arrows indicate direction of X-ray beam.

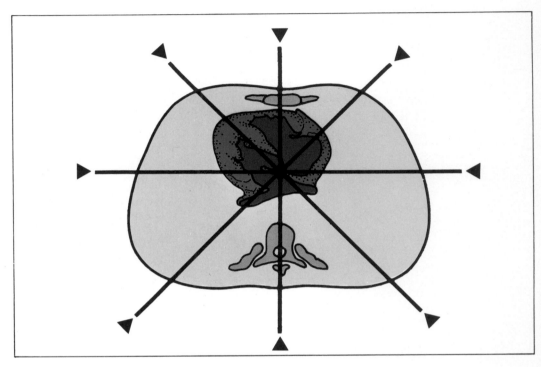

The importance of understanding cardiac morphology is well-exemplified by angiocardiograms and coronary arteriograms. The morphologist examines the walls of the chambers and the superficial disposition of the arteries while the radiologist looks at the spatial morphology of the chambers and arteries themselves. Corrosion casts of the chambers and the vasculature represent the solids of the radiographic shadows and demonstrate how these shadows are cast *(Raphael & Allwork, 1974, 1976; Raphael, Hawtin & Allwork, 1979).*

The projections most commonly used for coronary arteriography are right anterior oblique, left anterior oblique and left lateral *(fig. 7.1).* The anteroposterior view preferred at

post mortem arteriography is seldom helpful because of the opacity of the sternum and vertebrae. It is necessary to examine the anatomy in more than one projection: firstly, because of the complexity of the three-dimensional network; and secondly, because in disease, some branches enlarge greatly and may be difficult to identify in one view alone.

When the chambers are opacified, the preferred views are anteroposterior, left lateral, left anterior oblique and right anterior oblique. When cases of congenital cardiac malformations are studied, craniocaudal tilt (of either the X-ray tube or the patient) may be helpful. The projections thus produced are called 4-chamber or long-axis views *(Bargeron et al., 1977).* A tilted view is

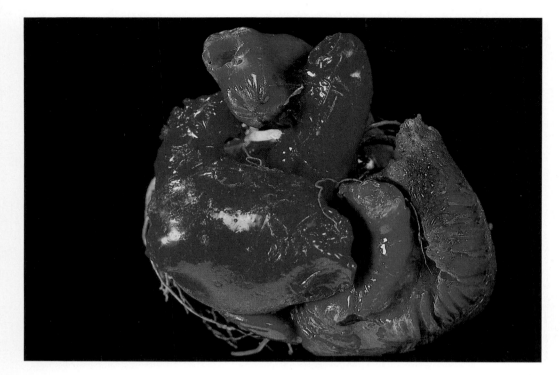

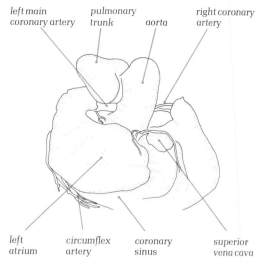

left main   *pulmonary*   *right coronary*
coronary artery   *trunk*   *aorta*   *artery*

left   *circumflex*   *coronary*   *superior*
atrium   *artery*   *sinus*   *vena cava*

Fig. 7.2   *Heart cast from above, angled approximately 10° posterior to the vertical. The right heart is blue, the left red; the left main coronary artery, the anterior descending branch and its ramifications are white; the circumflex artery and its branches yellow; the right coronary artery and its branches green.*

sometimes helpful also in elucidating the origin of the circumflex coronary artery and its branches. Because the radiographic anatomy of the heart is usually described spatially, slightly different names may be applied to familiar structures.

If a cast of the heart is studied from above, the four chambers and the arteries are clearly seen (fig. 7.2). The right ventricle is anterior and extends to the left. The right atrium is on the right and forms the anterolateral border. The left atrium is posteroinferior to it. The left ventricle forms the inferolateral border of the cast. Part of it is hidden by the sigmoid curve of the right ventricle. When the cast is viewed in such a way that the sigmoid curve of the right ventricle is avoided, it can be seen that two major planes exist within the heart itself, both obliquely orientated, which intersect. The plane of the atrioventricular valves, or short-axis plane, is more or less vertical. The plane of the septa, in contrast, is at right angles to the short axis. The septal plane occupies

different positions when viewed from the back as opposed to the front. When seen from the back (fig. 7.3), the septal plane crosses the valvar plane between the atrioventricular valves; this site is the crux or cross of the heart. In contrast, when seen from the front, the septal plane crosses the valvar plane between the arterial valves, this being eccentrically-positioned towards the left edge of the cardiac silhouette (fig. 7.4). These planes are the atrioventricular and interventricular sulci respectively. They are important because they are occupied by the major branches of the coronary arteries (figs. 7.2-7.4).

Thus, branches of the two coronary arteries occupy all four sulci. The right coronary artery, originating in the anteromedial (right-facing) aortic sinus, traverses the right atrioventricular sulcus until it reaches the crux, when it usually gives the posterior descending branch. This occupies the posterior interventricular sulcus, vascularizing the posterior part of the ventricular septum.

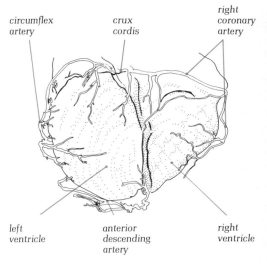

circumflex artery   crux cordis   right coronary artery

left ventricle   anterior descending artery   right ventricle

Fig. 7.3   The same cast as in fig. 7.2 from the back to show the crux of the heart.

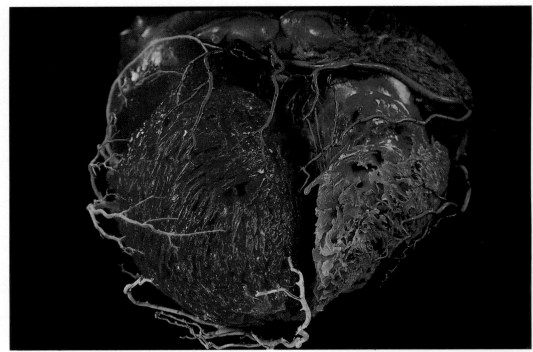

The left coronary artery arises from the anterolateral (left-facing) aortic sinus and passes in the fat between the pulmonary artery and left atrial appendage to divide into two branches. The anterior descending branch traverses the anterior interventricular sulcus and gives branches to the anterior ventricular septum. Identification of this artery automatically identifies the plane of the anterior ventricular septum. The circumflex branch encircles the left atrioventricular sulcus and may terminate either as a muscular artery on the obtuse (posterolateral) margin or as a posterior descending artery in the posterior interventricular sulcus.

The obtuse marginal branch or branches and posterolateral continuations of the right coronary artery vascularize the papillary muscles of the mitral valve as well as left ventricular muscle. This is of major importance, since disease proximal to these branches can lead to ischaemia and mitral valve dysfunction.

The Angiographic Anatomy of the Coronary Arteries

The precise origin of the coronary arteries from their respective aortic sinuses varies considerably among individuals, as does the degree of rotation of the heart within the thorax; so identical projections do not give identical images.

The main coronary arteries are subepicardial, as described in Chapter 6. However, they can vary very considerably in depth, relative to the epicardial fat. As age advances, the fat layer increases in thickness; this accretion is aggravated by ischaemic disease. When the coronary arteries are deeply embedded in the fat, they may be very difficult to find at surgical operation. The coronary arteriogram may be a guide to location because tortuous arteries are always superficial and do not penetrate the muscle. The converse, however, is not always true! Straight arteries may be superficial or deep. When they originate from the epicardial surface of the main artery, they usually do penetrate the muscle.

General Morphology

If a cast of the arteries is viewed in the anteroposterior projection, the arteries overlap and obscure one another (fig. 7.4). Nevertheless, some important features are evident. Although there are only two coronary arteries originating from the aorta, three major arterial branches are generally considered, namely, the right coronary artery together with

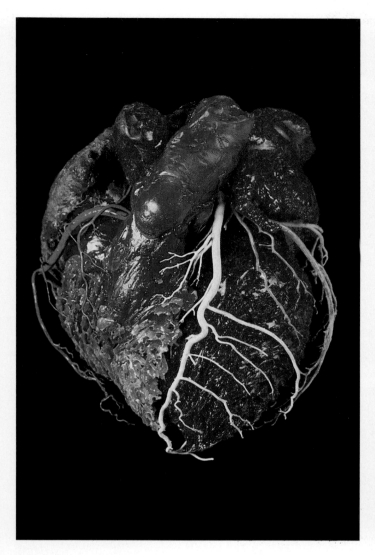

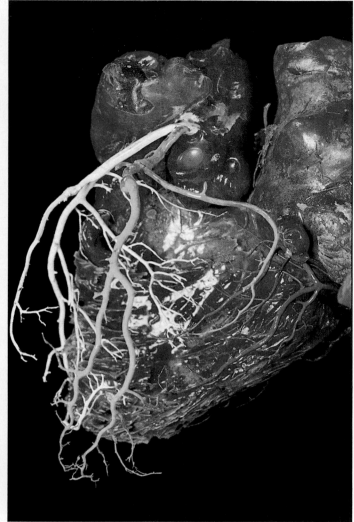

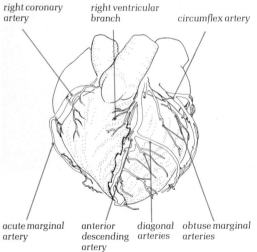

Fig. 7.4   The same cast viewed from the front with slight angulation. The coronary arteries traverse both atrioventricular and interventricular sulci.

right coronary artery

right ventricular branch

circumflex artery

acute marginal artery

anterior descending artery

diagonal arteries

obtuse marginal arteries

Fig. 7.5   Right heart cast, lateral view, showing a dominant right circulation. Note the characteristically straight septal branches of the anterior descending artery which supply the anterior septum.

anterior descending artery

septal arteries

circumflex artery

diagonal artery

obtuse marginal arteries

the anterior descending and circumflex branches of the left coronary artery. These are the arteries discussed in 'three-vessel disease'. When considering disease processes, a fourth artery* is also named. This is the proximal undivided portion of the left coronary artery and is called the left main coronary artery. It varies in length from about 6-26mm in adults and is present in most individuals (fig. 7.2). Separate origins of the anterior descending and circumflex coronary arteries is an uncommon type of normal anatomy (see Chapter 6).

* It should be clearly recognized, however, that there are two coronary arteries, left and right. The left separates into two, sometimes three, branches. Single coronary artery is rare in otherwise congenitally normal hearts (Allwork, 1979).

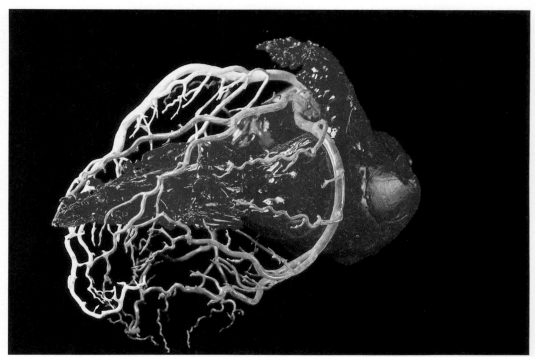

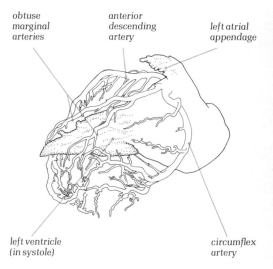

obtuse
marginal
arteries

anterior
descending
artery

left atrial
appendage

left ventricle
(in systole)

circumflex
artery

Fig. 7.6   Left heart cast, lateral projection,
showing a dominant left circulation.

right
coronary
artery

arterial
branch to
sinus node

anterior
descending
artery

posterior
descending
arteries

first
septal
artery

Fig. 7.7   Left heart cast, right anterior
oblique projection, showing balanced
circulation. Both right and left coronary
arteries supply the posterior septum.
N.B. It is very rare for a septal artery to
continue as a posterior descending artery.

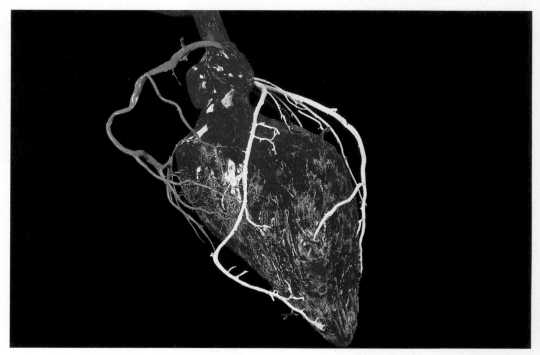

Dominance

The artery giving the posterior descending coronary artery is said to be the dominant, or preponderant, coronary artery. In the majority of people, this artery is the continuation of the right coronary artery (fig. 7.5) so that 'right dominance' is present. In about 10% of people, 'left dominance' exists, as the posterior descending artery is the continuation of the circumflex artery (fig. 7.6); while the circulation is said to be 'balanced' in a small percentage of people in whom both left and right arteries contribute (fig. 7.7). The respective branches which supply the sinus and atrioventricular nodes generally arise from the 'dominant' artery. However, in about 40% of 'dominantly right' individuals, the sinus node artery takes origin from the circumflex branch of the left coronary. The atrioventricular branch is usually from the right in 'balanced circulation' subjects. These anatomical facts are of importance in the interpretation of arrhythmias associated with myocardial infarction.

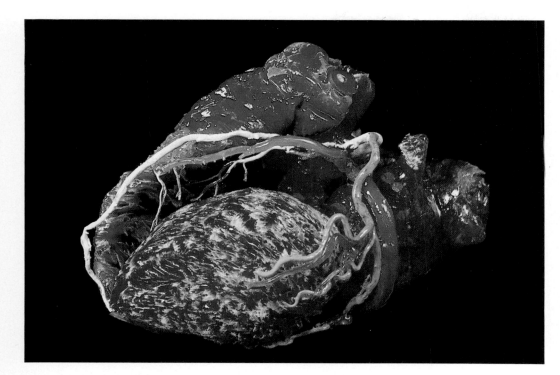

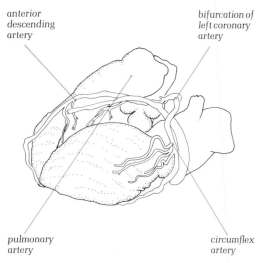

anterior descending artery

bifurcation of left coronary artery

pulmonary artery

circumflex artery

Fig. 7.8 Cast of the whole heart, lateral projection. The veins have also been cast and overlap the proximal part of the anterior descending artery.

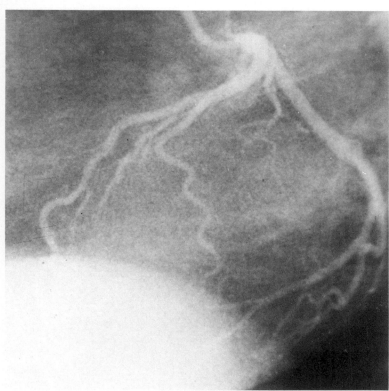

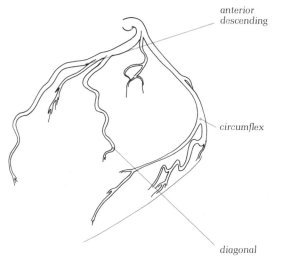

anterior descending

circumflex

diagonal

Fig. 7.9 Left coronary arteriogram, left lateral projection. The apical part of the anterior descending artery is not well seen in this individual.

Coronary Anatomy in Radiological Projections

Lateral Projection – The Left Coronary Artery

The left main stem is seen 'end-on' so no conclusions about its origin or length may be drawn, due to foreshortening (figs. 7.8 & 7.9). In contrast, the bifurcation into anterior descending and circumflex branches is optimally shown. The long course of the anterior descending artery is well seen and is always recognizable as the most anterior artery in this projection. Depending on the depth of inspiration achieved by the patient, its ascension within the inferior interventricular sulcus may be visible (compare figs. 7.6 & 7.9). On the debit side, the proximal part of the artery is overlapped by its first diagonal branch. The circumflex artery is well profiled as it passes inferoposteriorly in the left atrioventricular sulcus. It, too, is overlapped by its obtuse marginal branch, but the 'true'* circumflex may be identified by its tighter curve as it passes inferiorly in its sulcus.

*When surgical treatment is discussed, the usual site of a 'circumflex' bypass graft is the obtuse marginal artery. This artery is often incorrectly referred to as the circumflex. The 'true' circumflex artery is surgically inaccessible in the left atrioventricular sulcus.

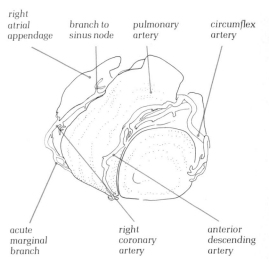

right atrial appendage

branch to sinus node

pulmonary artery

circumflex artery

acute marginal branch

right coronary artery

anterior descending artery

Fig. 7.10 The same heart as in fig. 7.8 in steep left anterior oblique projection. The ostium is obscured by the pulmonary outflow tract but the branch to the sinus node is visible.

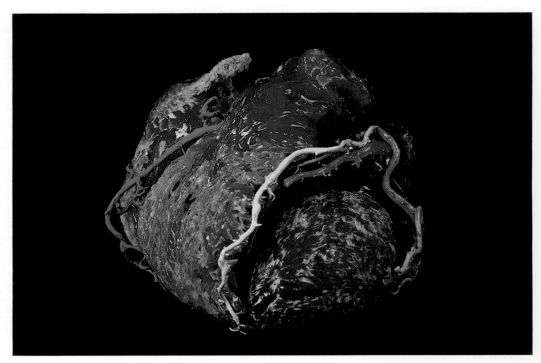

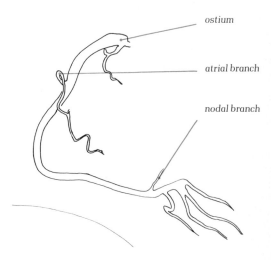

ostium

atrial branch

nodal branch

Fig. 7.11 Right coronary arteriogram in steep left anterior oblique projection which corresponds to the lateral projection for this artery.

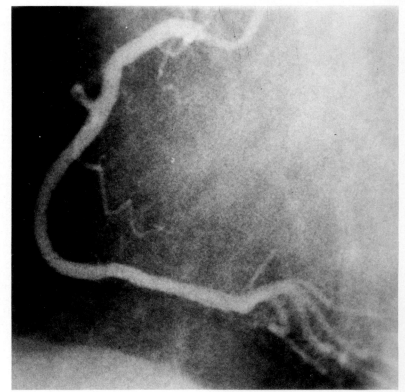

Lateral Projection – The Right Coronary Artery

The right coronary artery is more usually examined (for logistic reasons) from a steep left anterior oblique view which corresponds to lateral for this vessel. The ostium is in good profile and the wide curve of the artery as it traverses the right atrioventricular sulcus is well seen (figs. 7.10 & 7.11). Right ventricular branches pass to the right and atrial branches to the left. The branch to the

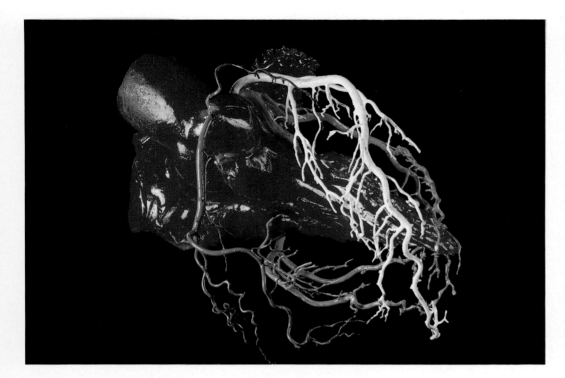

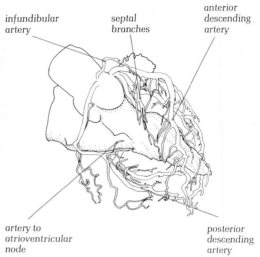

infundibular artery   septal branches   anterior descending artery

artery to atrioventricular node

posterior descending artery

Fig. 7.12   The same cast as in fig. 7.6, right anterior oblique projection to illustrate the termination of the right coronary artery in a dominant left circulation.

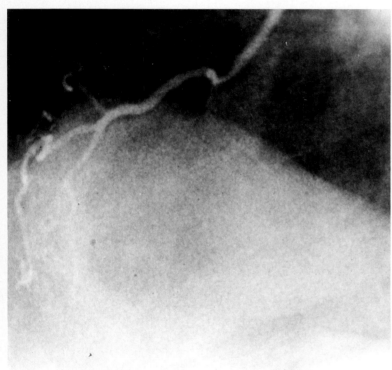

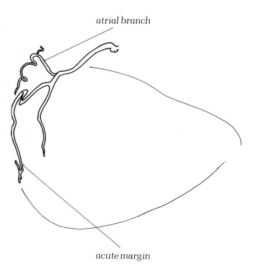

atrial branch

acute margin

Fig. 7.13   Right coronary arteriogram, right anterior oblique projection. The right coronary artery in this individual does not reach the crux cordis.

atrioventricular node passes vertically upwards from the crux (fig. 7.11) but the posterior descending and posterolateral branches are too foreshortened for much information to be derived from them.

If the left coronary artery is dominant, the right is a small artery which does not usually reach the crux of the heart. It gives a few muscular branches to the right ventricle before terminating at or near the acute margin (figs. 7.12 & 7.13).

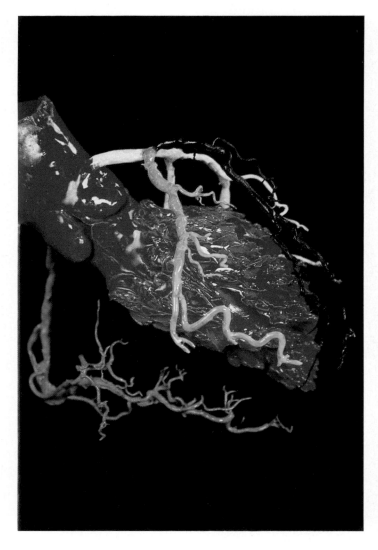

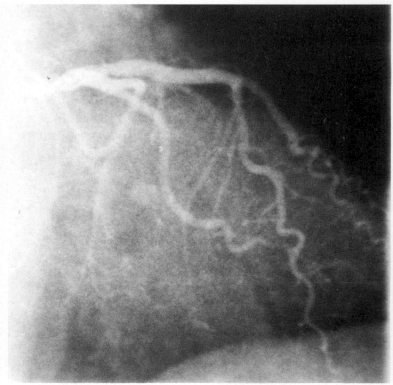

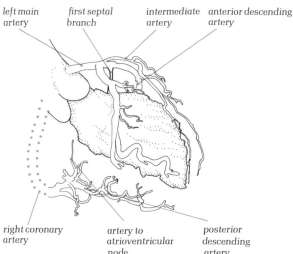

left main artery | first septal branch | intermediate artery | anterior descending artery

right coronary artery | artery to atrioventricular node | posterior descending artery

Fig. 7.14   Cast of the left coronary artery in right anterior oblique projection. The picture is printed in reverse so that the position of the circumflex artery corresponds to the arteriogram.

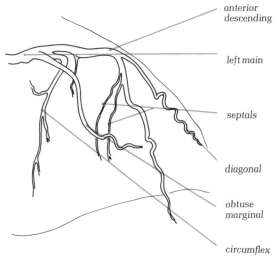

anterior descending

left main

septals

diagonal

obtuse marginal

circumflex

Fig. 7.15   Left coronary arteriogram in right anterior oblique projection.

Right Anterior Oblique Projection – The Left Coronary Artery

The left main coronary artery (figs. 7.14 & 7.15) may either have optimal profile or be rather indistinct in this view, according to the individual (figs. 7.16 & 7.17). The anterior descending artery is well seen without foreshortening as it passes in the anterior interventricular sulcus. The origin of the diagonal branch or branches may overlap and so be obscured. Septal branches are recognized as they descend vertically into the muscle in their characteristically straight fashion. The position of the first branch is relatively constant, but the number varies among individuals. As in the lateral view, the anterior descending artery is recognized throughout its length by its length (it may be seen to

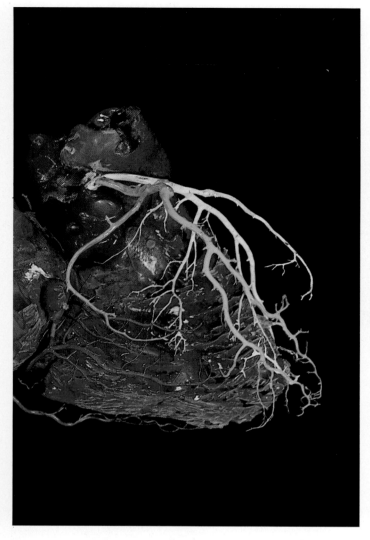

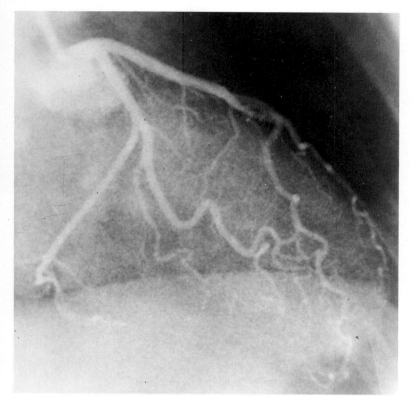

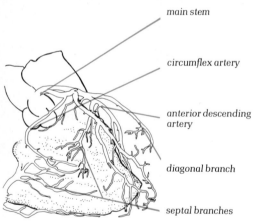

main stem

circumflex artery

anterior descending
artery

diagonal branch

septal branches

Fig. 7.16   Same cast as fig. 7.5 photographed
in right anterior oblique projection. In this
cast, the main stem is not well seen.

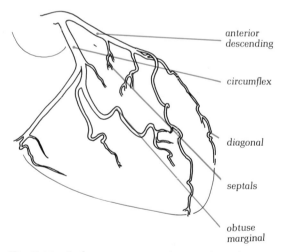

anterior
descending

circumflex

diagonal

septals

obtuse
marginal

Fig. 7.17   Left coronary arteriogram in right
anterior oblique projection in which the main
stem is indistinct.

ascend for a variable distance), its
angled curve and its septal branches.

The origin of the circumflex artery
is usually excellently seen in this
view (figs. 7.14 & 7.15), but, like the
anterior descending branch, not
always. It originates at an angle of

about 40° and passes forwards and
downwards in the atrioventricular
sulcus giving its big branch, often
multiple, to the obtuse margin (the
free wall of the left ventricle, fig. 7.9).
These arteries are often tortuous,
indicating that they are superficial;

but equally often they are straight and
buried in muscle. The 'true' (in the
atrioventricular sulcus) circumflex
artery angles gently backwards to
terminate either in the inferior
interventricular sulcus (fig. 7.15) or as
a little posterolateral branch (fig. 7.17).   7.11

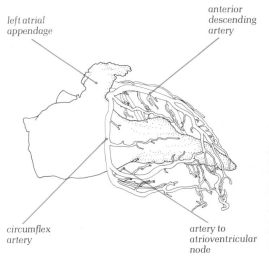

left atrial appendage

anterior descending artery

circumflex artery

artery to atrioventricular node

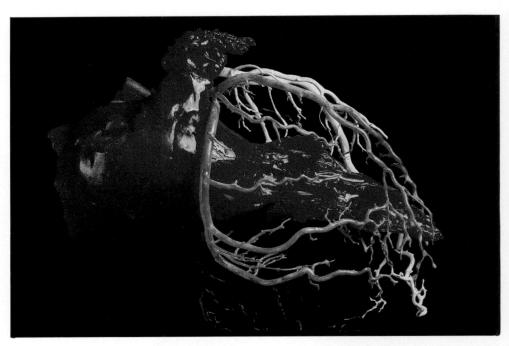

Fig. 7.18   The same cast as in figs. 7.6 & 7.12 reversed photographically to reproduce right anterior oblique projection of the left coronary artery.

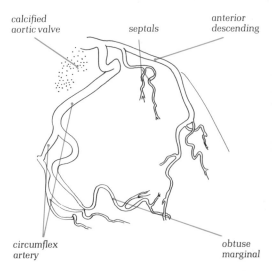

calcified aortic valve

septals

anterior descending

circumflex artery

obtuse marginal

Fig. 7.19   Left coronary arteriogram in right anterior oblique projection showing dominant left circulation.

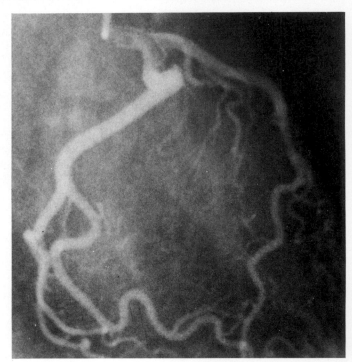

When the left coronary artery is dominant (*figs. 7.18 & 7.19*), the circumflex is usually the bigger artery and supplies the posterior descending coronary artery (recognized by septal arteries arising upwards from its upper surface) and often a right posterolateral branch (*fig. 7.18*). This is foreshortened as it 'approaches' the camera.

Right Anterior Oblique Projection – The Right Coronary Artery

The ostium and proximal parts 'face' the camera and are not, therefore, profiled (*figs. 7.20 & 7.21*). Ventricular branches passing forwards are readily distinguished from atrial branches passing backwards. The artery passes, still in the atrioventricular sulcus, around the acute margin of the heart, where there is usually an acute marginal artery, and loops into the atrioventricular septal junction (the crux cordis) like an inverted letter 'U'. The 'U' is foreshortened but recognizable, as is the artery to the atrioventricular node which arises from the summit of the 'U'. The posterior descending artery is optimally profiled but is overlapped by posterolateral branches. In subjects with marked right dominance, the artery passes over the crux cordis to occupy the left atrioventricular sulcus (*fig. 7.22*).

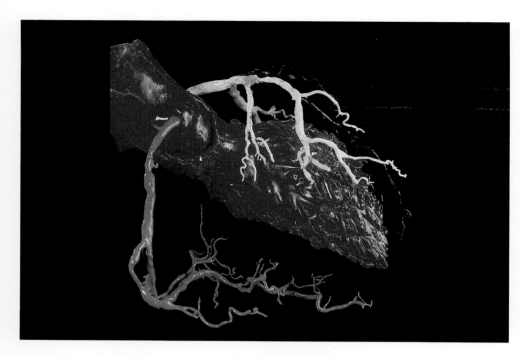

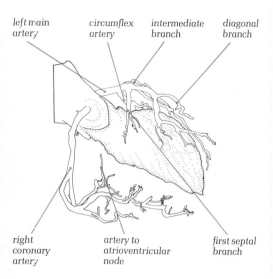

Fig. 7.20   The same left heart cast as in fig. 7.14 photographed in right anterior oblique projection.

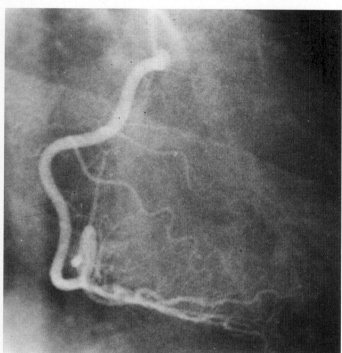

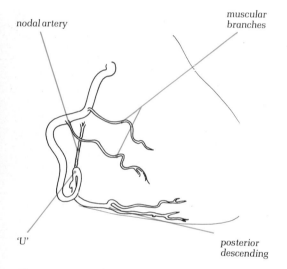

Fig. 7.21   A right coronary arteriogram in right anterior oblique projection.

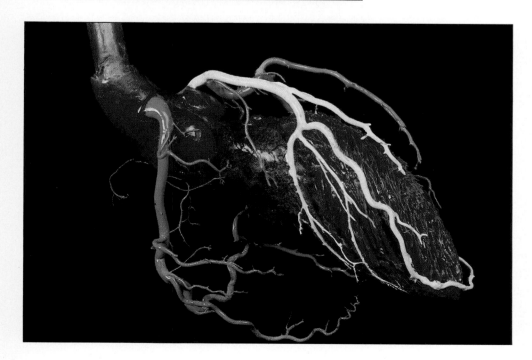

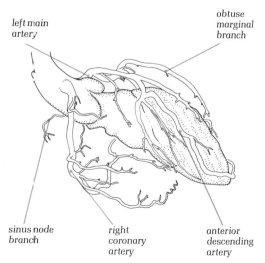

Fig. 7.22   Left heart cast with high take-off and markedly dominant right coronary artery photographed in right anterior oblique projection.

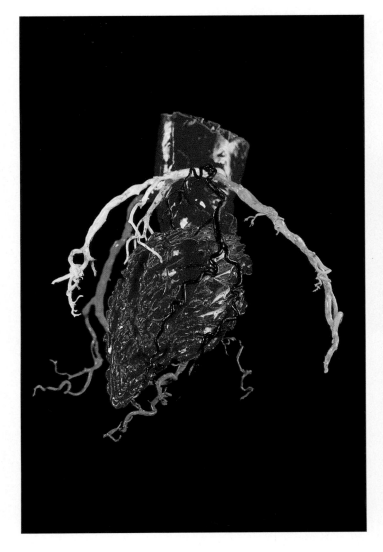

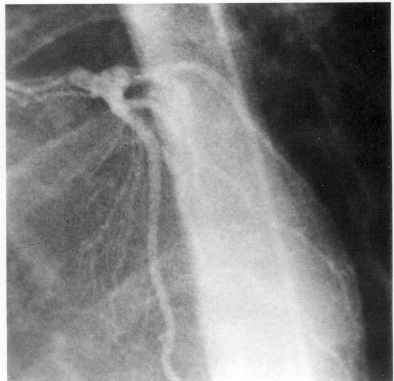

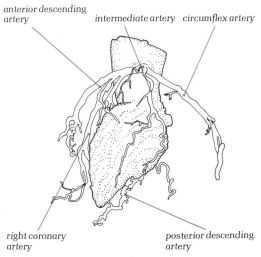

anterior descending
artery   intermediate artery   circumflex artery

right coronary
artery   posterior descending
                         artery

Fig. 7.23   The same left heart cast as in
figs. 7.14 & 7.20 photographed in left anterior
oblique projection. The left main stem is not
well seen in this view.

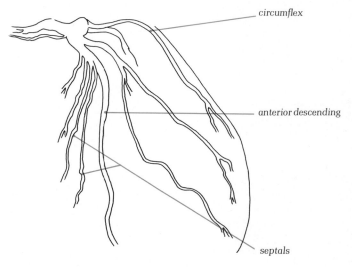

circumflex

anterior descending

septals

Fig. 7.24   Left coronary arteriogram in left
anterior oblique projection. The left main
stem is well seen.

Left Anterior Oblique Projection –
The Left Coronary Artery

In most people, a moderate degree of
obliquity gives a good silhouette of
the left main coronary artery; but
this is not visible in a solid cast (figs.
7.23 & 7.24). The anterior descending
branch is much foreshortened
proximally until the first diagonal
and first septal branches have taken
origin. The rest of the artery is well
profiled. If the degree of obliquity is
well chosen, septal branches are seen
to pass backwards (left) while
diagonal branches pass forwards
(right). Right ventricular branches of

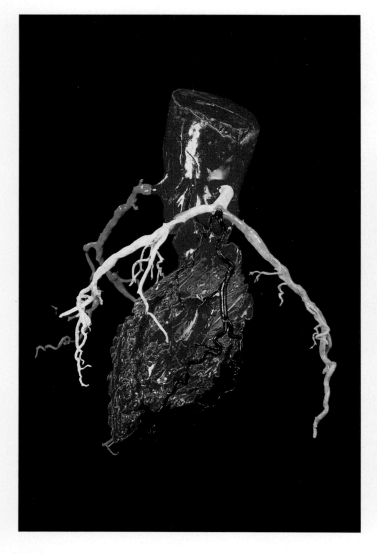

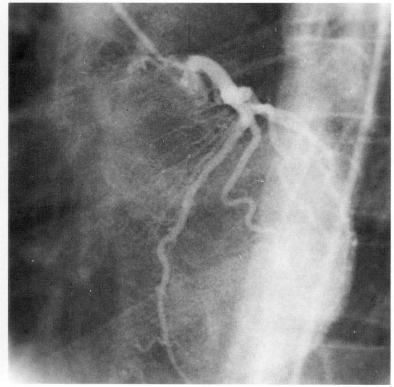

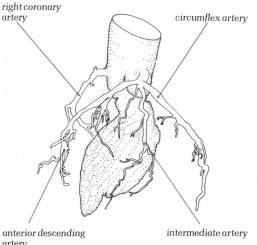

right coronary
artery

circumflex artery

anterior descending
artery

intermediate artery

Fig. 7.25   The same cast and projection as in
fig. 7.23 but with addition of craniocaudal
tilt. Note how the bifurcation is now
visualized.

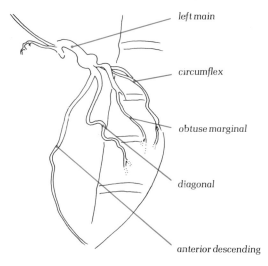

left main

circumflex

obtuse marginal

diagonal

anterior descending

Fig. 7.26   The same arteriogram as in fig. 7.24
but with craniocaudal tilt. The distal
branches lose detail due to overlap.

the anterior descending artery are not
easy to distinguish radiographically
from septal branches, except possibly
by their angle of origin (fig. 7.4).

The proximal segment of the
circumflex artery and its obtuse
marginal branch are foreshortened
and overlapped, but they become
better seen as they are better profiled
distally (fig. 7.24). A degree of
craniocaudal tilt (figs. 7.25 & 7.26)
reduces the proximal distortion and
'opens out' the bifurcation and origin
of the obtuse marginal artery.

7.15

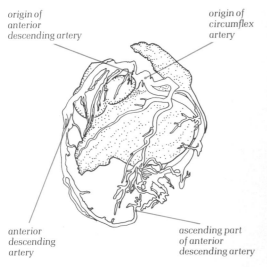

origin of
anterior
descending artery

origin of
circumflex
artery

anterior
descending
artery

ascending part
of anterior
descending artery

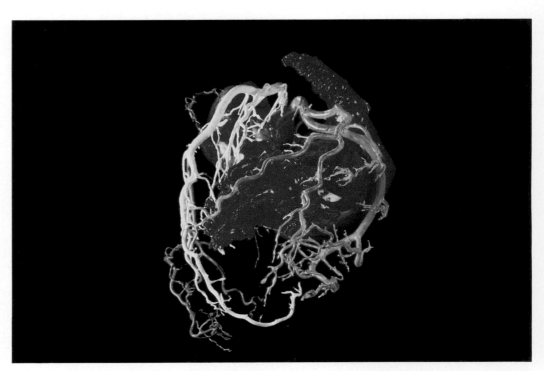

Fig. 7.27   The same cast as in figs. 7.6, 7.12 &
7.18 in left anterior oblique projection. This
individual has a dominant left coronary
artery.

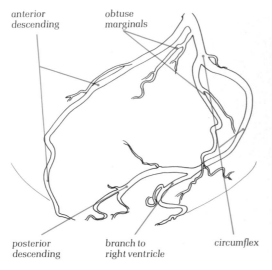

anterior
descending

obtuse
marginals

posterior
descending

branch to
right ventricle

circumflex

Fig. 7.28   Left arteriogram in a patient with
dominant left coronary artery in left anterior
oblique projection.

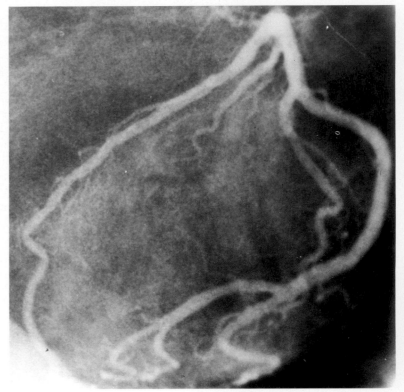

However, the branches themselves
lose detail as they overlap the spine.
   In people with left dominance, the
large size and extent of the circumflex
artery is well seen (figs. 7.27 & 7.28).
The artery forms a smooth curve, not
a 'U', as it enters the crux; but the
artery to the atrioventricular node is
seen arising vertically and the right
ventricular branches are
foreshortened as they 'recede' from
the camera.

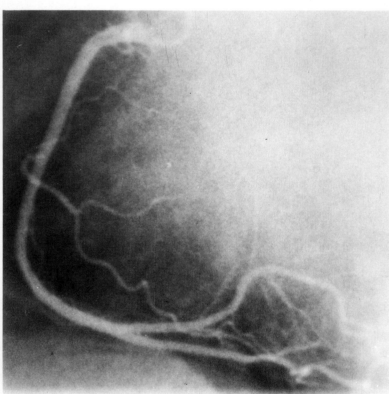

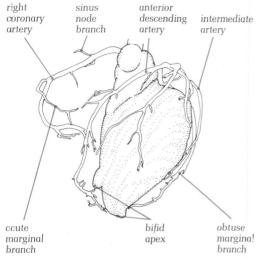

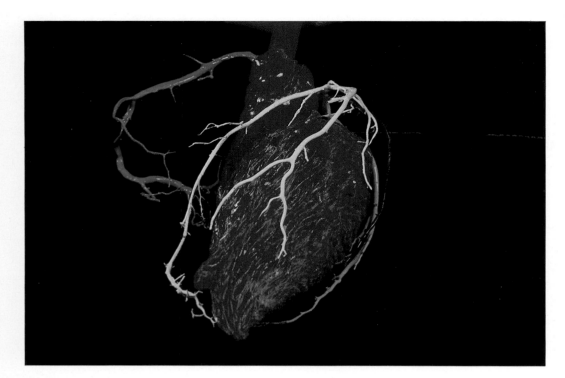

Fig. 7.29　The same cast as in fig. 7.7 in left anterior oblique projection to show the right coronary artery.

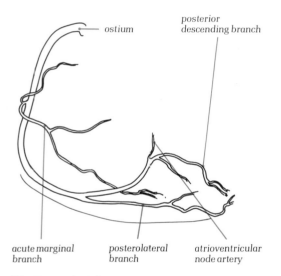

Fig. 7.30　A right coronary arteriogram in left anterior oblique projection.

Left Anterior Oblique Projection –
The Right Coronary Artery

The ostium and early passage of the right coronary artery are best profiled in this projection (figs. 7.29 & 7.30). The large silhouette is maintained as the artery passes in the right atrioventricular sulcus and enters the crux of the heart. The loop is 'opened out', but the artery to the atrioventricular node is well seen. The posterior descending and posterolateral branches are foreshortened. Because they pass in or parallel to the inferior interventricular sulcus and also overlap the spine (fig. 7.30), they are but poorly visualized.

right atrial
appendage

pulmonary
valve

infundibulum

right
atrium

tricuspid
valve

right
ventricle

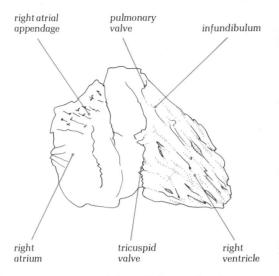

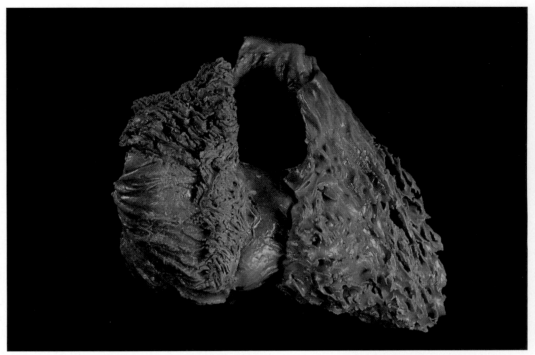

Fig. 7.31 Cast of the right heart chambers in anteroposterior projection.

right pulmonary
artery

pulmonary
bifurcation

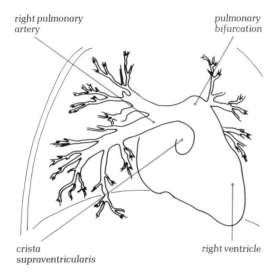

crista
supraventricularis

right ventricle

Fig. 7.32 A right ventricular angiocardiogram in anteroposterior projection. There is slight reflux of contrast through the tricuspid valve into the right atrium.

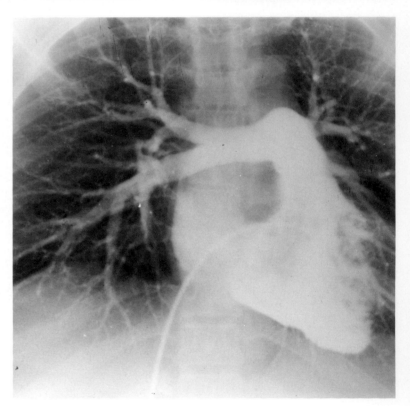

The Cardiac Chambers

The Right Heart – Anteroposterior Projection

In the anteroposterior projection, the characteristic triangular shape of the right ventricle is apparent (figs. 7.31 & 7.32). The right atrial appendage slightly overlaps the pulmonary outflow tract and, for this reason, accidental opacification of the atrium is undesirable. The tricuspid valve is well profiled and is demonstrably separate from the pulmonary valve.

Left posterior oblique (figs. 7.33 & 7.34) is not a projection often chosen for the right heart; but, as most of the features of importance are on the 'inside', it approximates an oblique frontal projection but viewed from 'within' (fig. 7.34). The venae cavae enter the right atrium at its posteromedial aspect, not the upper and lower margins; hence a catheter

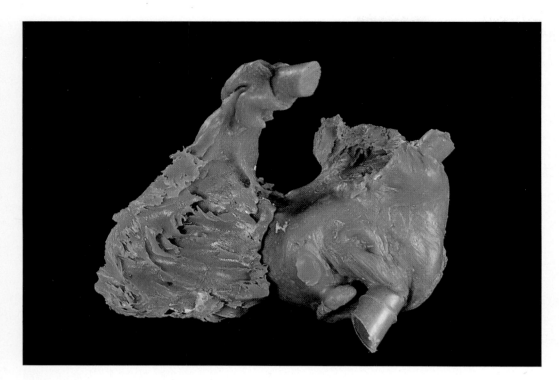

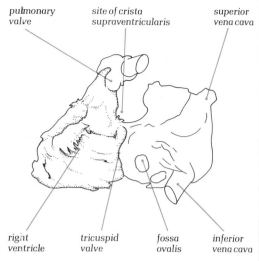

pulmonary valve | site of crista supraventricularis | superior vena cava

right ventricle | tricuspid valve | fossa ovalis | inferior vena cava

Fig. 7.33   The same cast as in fig. 7.31 in left posterior oblique projection.

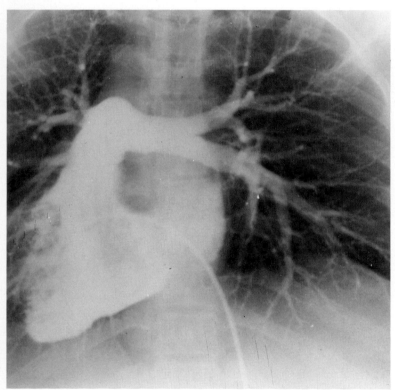

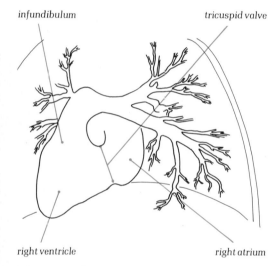

infundibulum   tricuspid valve

right ventricle   right atrium

Fig. 7.34   The same study as in fig. 7.32 photographically reversed. Its projection is less oblique than the cast in fig. 7.33.

may appear at frontal fluoroscopy to be in the atrium when it is actually still in a caval vein. The fossa ovalis 'faces' the camera. It is directed posteriorly, upwards and leftwards, indicating the route for a transseptal needle. The coronary sinus enters the chamber at the apex of the triangle formed by it, the fossa ovalis and the inferior vena cava.

The inlet (tricuspid valve), trabecular and outlet portions of the right ventricle are well seen. The tricuspid valve is in profile and its diameter is indicated (fig. 7.32). The smooth impression left by the trabecula septomarginalis is evident (figs. 7.33 & 7.34). This structure does not make a specific impression on a normal right ventricle when filled with contrast.

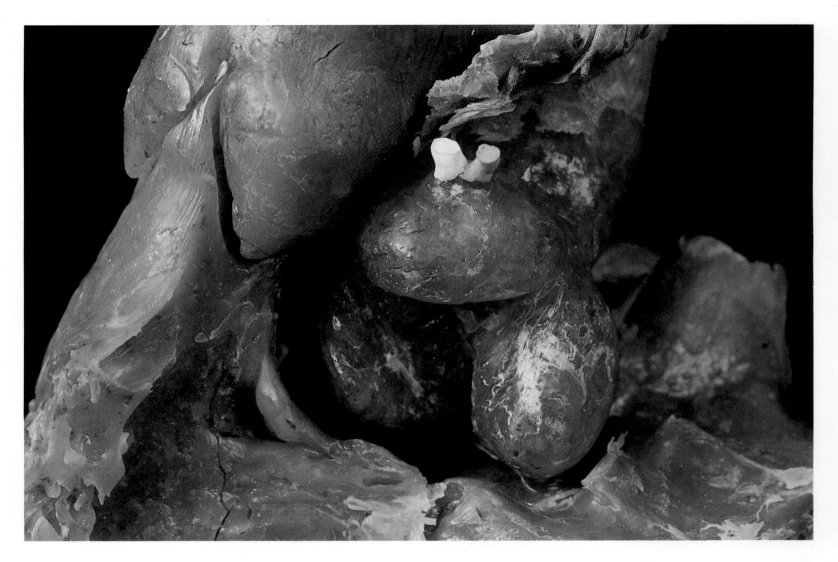

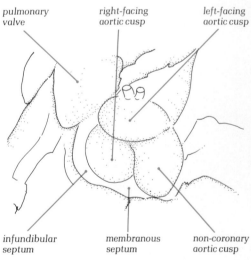

pulmonary valve   right-facing aortic cusp   left-facing aortic cusp

infundibular septum   membranous septum   non-coronary aortic cusp

Fig. 7.35 Cast of the right ventricle and aortic valve in left posterior oblique projection. Note absence of a left main coronary artery.

The area occupied by the membranous septum is very small (fig. 7.35). Defects of the septum in this region are sometimes called 'infracristal defects' because they lie beneath the ventriculo-infundibular fold and infundibular septum, while defects of the infundibular septum are sometimes called 'supracristal' or 'subpulmonary' (Baron et al., 1968). However, both types lie beneath the aortic valve and are both 'subaortic' (fig. 7.35).

The Right Heart – Lateral Projection

When examined from the lateral projection (figs. 7.36 & 7.37), the anterior position of the right ventricle

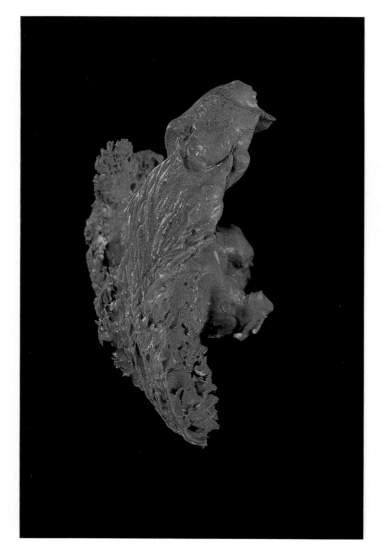

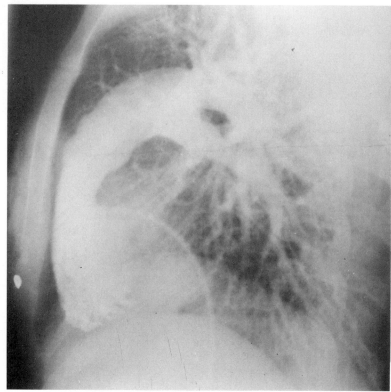

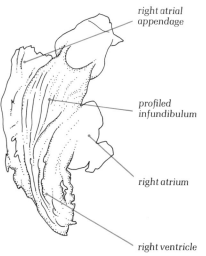

right atrial
appendage

profiled
infundibulum

right atrium

right ventricle

Fig. 7.36   The same cast as in figs. 7.31 & 7.33
in lateral projection.

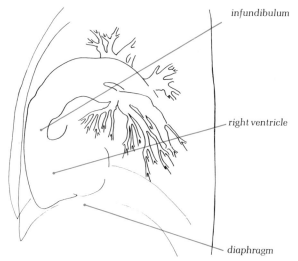

infundibulum

right ventricle

diaphragm

Fig. 7.37   Right ventricular angiocardiogram
in lateral projection.

is obvious; but it loses its triangular shape due to foreshortening. The pulmonary infundibulum is excellently profiled; but, in normal individuals, the sinuses of the pulmonary valve and the fibrous ring of the valve are invisible at angiography. A mild degree of pulmonary valve stenosis (fig. 7.38) indicates the position of the valve cusps by the unopacified blood trapped in the sinuses. The trabecular pattern of the chamber is well seen as is the transition from the trabecular pattern of the body of the ventricle to the smooth musculature of the infundibulum.

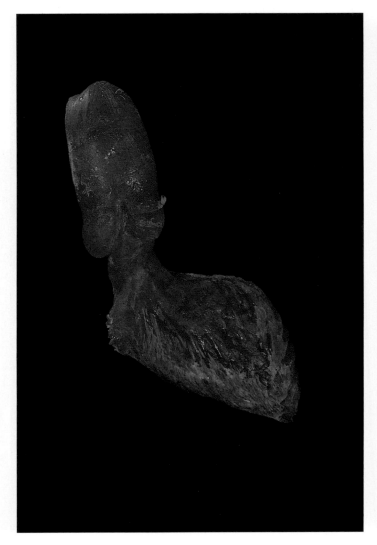

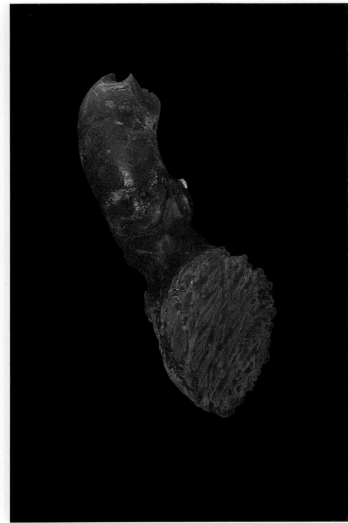

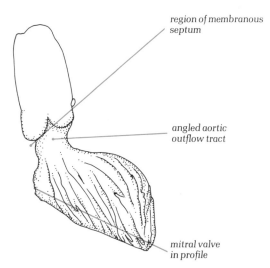

region of membranous
septum

angled aortic
outflow tract

mitral valve
in profile

Fig. 7.42   The same cast as in figs. 7.39 & 7.40
in right anterior oblique projection.

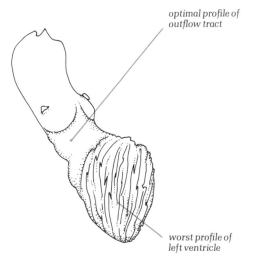

optimal profile of
outflow tract

worst profile of
left ventricle

Fig. 7.43   The same cast as in figs. 7.39, 7.40
& 7.42 in left anterior oblique projection.

The Left Heart – Right Anterior Oblique Projection

In this view, the conical shape of the left ventricle is seen in its best profile (fig. 7.42); but the area occupied by the membranous septum is not particularly well silhouetted. However, the jet passing through a defect would be very easy to locate accurately in this view. The characteristically smooth outflow tract muscle is well seen on the septal surface, facing the camera; the mitral valve is well profiled. This projection is optimal for an overall view of the left ventricle (Gorlin et al., 1967).

The Left Heart – Left Anterior Oblique Projection

As this view is angled along the long axis of the chamber, the body of the ventricle is maximally foreshortened (fig. 7.43). In contrast, the outflow tract is well profiled and the degree of angulation can bring both coronary ostia into profile. The membranous septum is in profile and, as in the lateral view (fig. 7.40), the angulation of the outflow tract is well marked. The mitral valve is invisible in this view and even a mild degree of left ventricular enlargement would obscure the aortic outflow tract and aortic valve.

8 Clinical Cardiac Anatomy II

Echocardiographic and
Scintigraphic Anatomy

Cardiac Anatomy for the Surgeon

Echocardiographic and Scintigraphic Anatomy

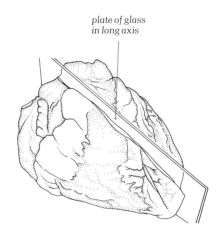

plate of glass
in long axis

Fig. 8.1 *Plate of glass inserted into the heart shows the long axis plane from the apex towards the right shoulder.*

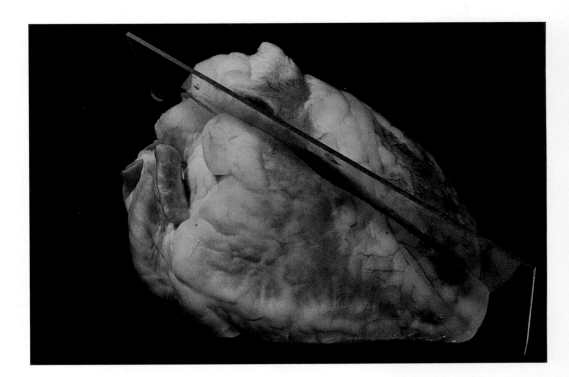

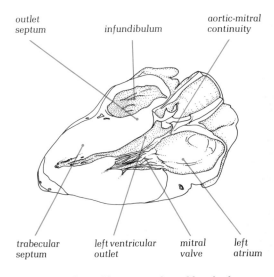

outlet
septum   infundibulum   aortic-mitral
continuity

trabecular   left ventricular   mitral   left
septum   outlet   valve   atrium

Fig. 8.2 *Slice of heart produced by the long axis cut orientated with the cardiac apex pointing to the left.*

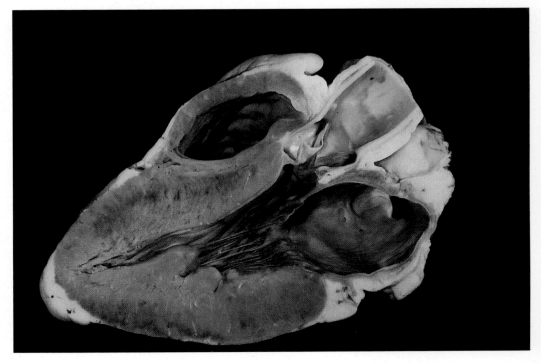

Echocardiographic Anatomy

The echocardiographer cuts the heart in a single plane and must therefore have a sound knowledge of cardiac anatomy in order to interpret his findings. With the advent of two-dimensional echocardiography, this knowledge is even more essential, since the data may be presented in very unusual orientations by the echocardiographic machine (*Tajik et al., 1978*). In this section, therefore, we will illustrate the anatomy underlying the most common echocardiographic cuts.

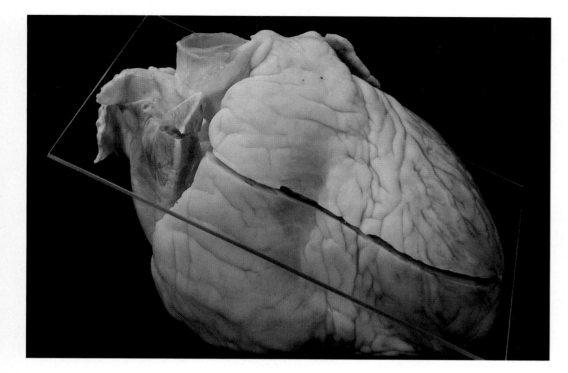

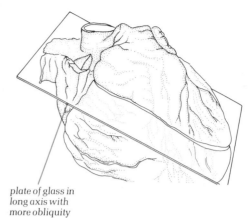

plate of glass in
long axis with
more obliquity

Fig. 8.3   Plate of glass inserted in the long
axis with more obliquity relative to the
midline.

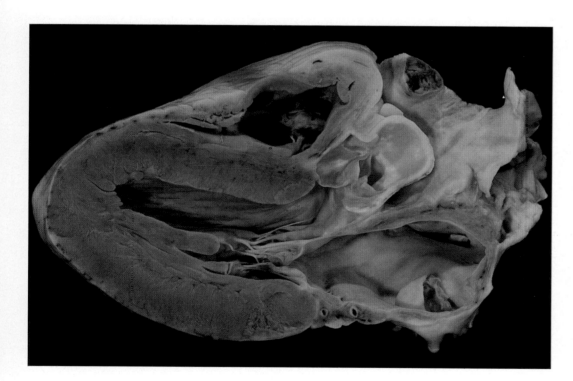

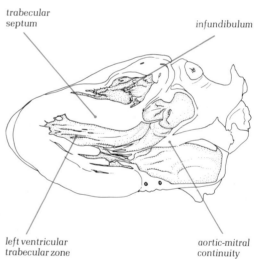

trabecular
septum

infundibulum

left ventricular
trabecular zone

aortic-mitral
continuity

Fig. 8.4   Long axis slice produced is little
different from that shown in fig. 8.2.

With single beam examination of the left ventricle, the long axis approach is usually employed. The beam is swept from the apex towards the right shoulder *(fig. 8.1)* and the slice obtained is usually presented with the cardiac apex to the left *(fig. 8.2)*. In this position, the infundibulum of the right ventricle is seen anterior to the left ventricular outlet and the aorta which, in turn, are anterior to the left ventricular inlet and the left atrium *(fig. 8.2)*. The long axis view can be obtained by varying the obliquity of cut; angling the axis of cut more towards the left as it enters the heart produces comparable results (compare *figs. 8.1 & 8.2* with *8.3 & 8.4*). When the

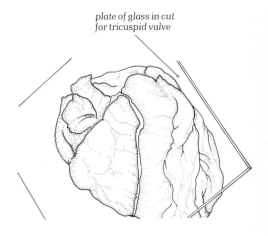

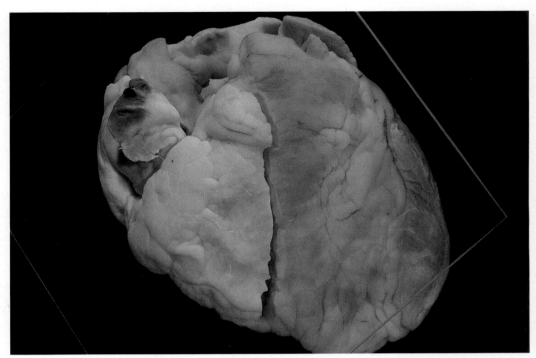

Fig. 8.5 Plate of glass inserted into the heart in its in situ position showing the plane necessary to transect the tricuspid valve.

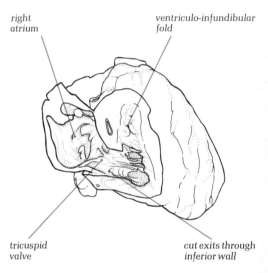

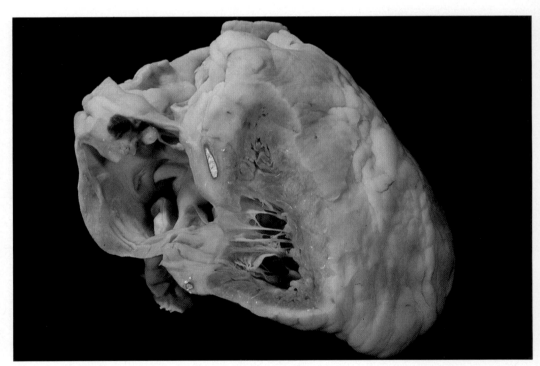

Fig. 8.6 Anatomy produced by the cut illustrated in fig. 8.5.

right ventricle is examined with a single beam technique from the anterior chest wall, the separation of pulmonary and tricuspid valves prevents their simultaneous recording. Similarly, the position of the valves relative to the transducer makes it impossible to record right ventricular structures in the same fashion as they are recorded in the left ventricle (fig. 8.5). Instead, the tricuspid valve is cut obliquely as the beam passes from the anterior chest wall through the posterior part of the

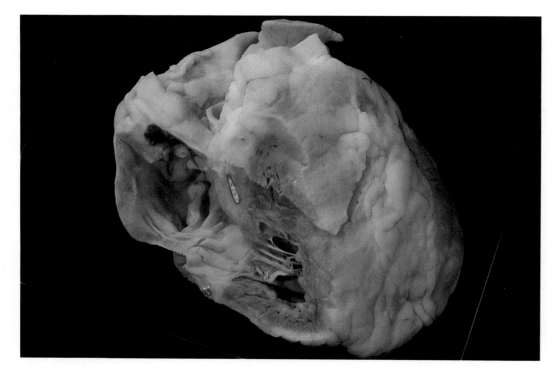

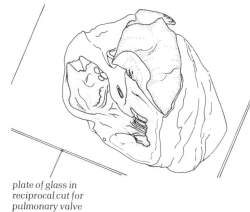

plate of glass in
reciprocal cut for
pulmonary valve

Fig. 8.7   Plate of glass inserted in the same
heart as in fig. 8.5 showing the reciprocal cut
needed to visualize the pulmonary valve.

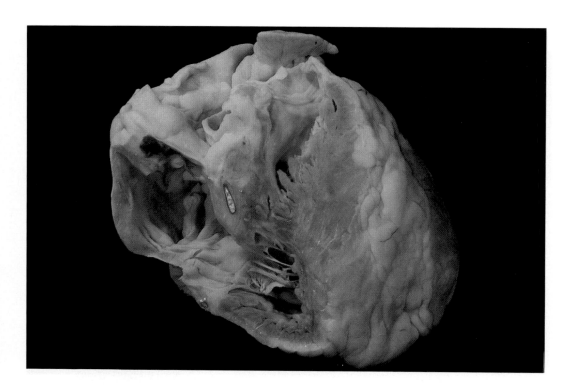

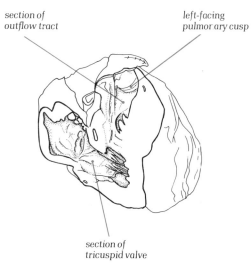

section of   left-facing
outflow tract   pulmonary cusp

section of
tricuspid valve

Fig. 8.8   Anatomy produced by the reciprocal
cut shown in fig. 8.7.

right ventricle. It rarely cuts the
septum (fig. 8.6). The angle of cut to
visualize the pulmonary valve reveals
only its facing cusps (fig. 8.7 & fig. 8.8).
However, use of two-dimensional
techniques enables the tricuspid
valve to be seen at the same time as
the mitral valve and to be compared
with it. This is done by cutting the
heart from the apex, angling the beam
towards the right shoulder but with
the plane of the beam at right angles

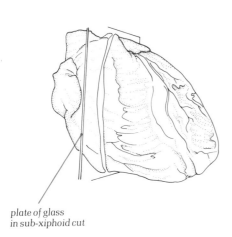

Fig. 8.13 Plate of glass inserted through the heart in the plane produced by a sub-xiphoid cut.

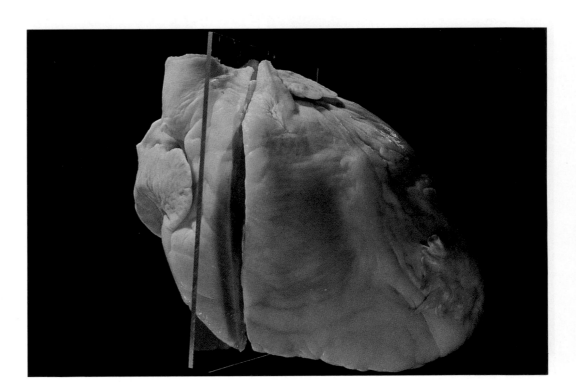

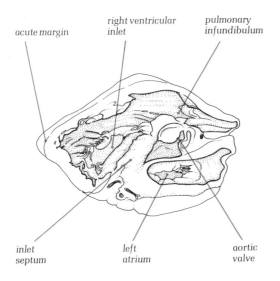

acute margin right ventricular inlet pulmonary infundibulum

inlet septum left atrium aortic valve

Fig. 8.14 Anatomy produced by the sub-xiphoid cut orientated with the acute margin of the heart to the left.

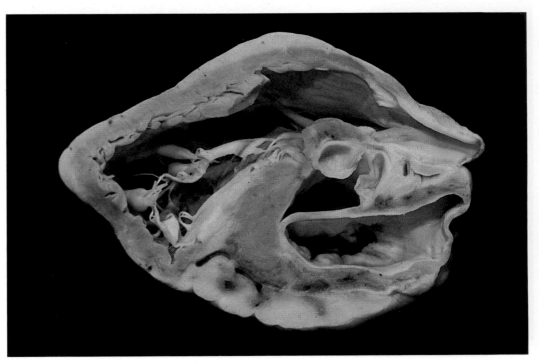

through the atria, in which case the inferior vena cava, atrial septum and pulmonary veins may be visualized; or they can be taken into the outlet of the right ventricle. This cut is usually presented echocardiographically with the pulmonary valve in inferior position but is actually obtained with the pulmonary valve far from the point of entrance of the beam (figs. 8.13 & 8.14).

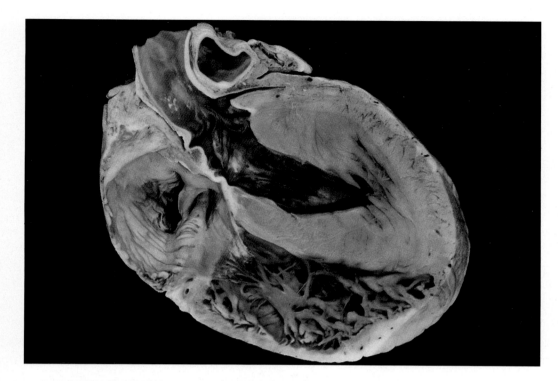

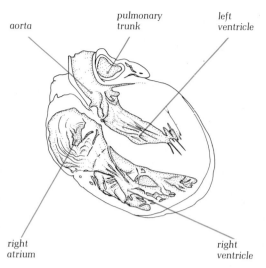

Fig. 8.15 Anatomy produced by a section through the heart in the frontal plane with the heart in its in situ position.

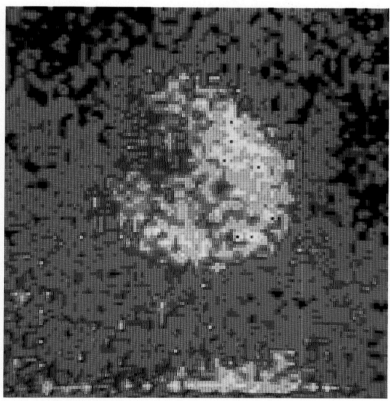

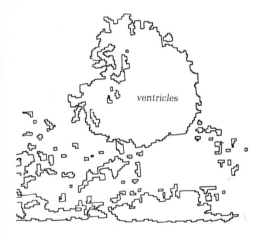

Fig. 8.16 Scintigram obtained in anteroposterior projection comparable to the anatomy shown in fig. 8.15.

Scintigraphic Anatomy

Visualization of the myocardial wall and chambers with radiographic material has attracted increasing interest of late, in particular for evaluation of the patient with signs and symptoms of myocardial ischaemia. For those techniques which visualize cardiac chambers, particularly the Technetium scanning methods, the anatomy and

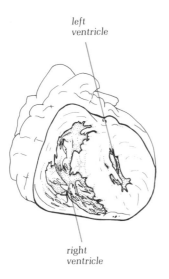

left ventricle

right ventricle

Fig. 8.17 *Anatomy produced by a section through the heart in left anterior oblique projection at 45°.*

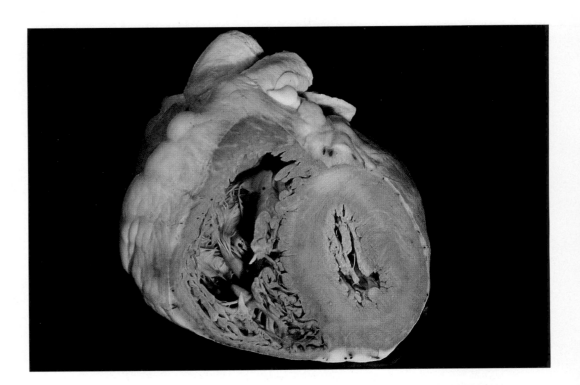

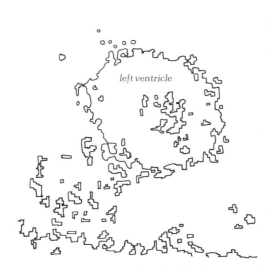

left ventricle

Fig. 8.18 *Scintigram obtained in the projection illustrated in fig. 8.17.*

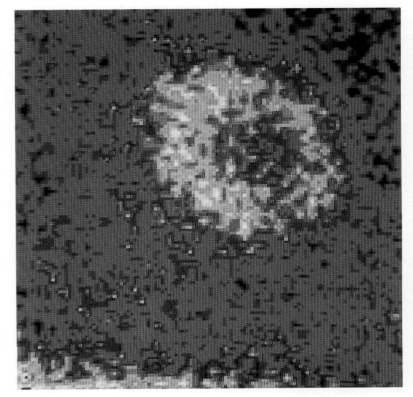

projections are as described for angiography (see *Chapter 7*). Myocardial imaging with radioactive thallium, on the other hand, gives a different image from those in echocardiography. The reason for this is that standard angiographic views are used but only the ventricular walls are visualized. The projections employed are not difficult

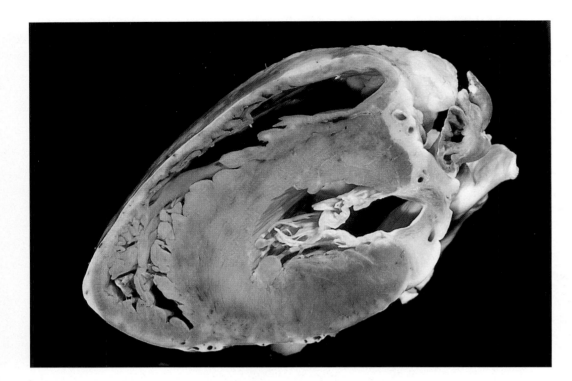

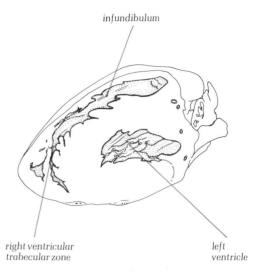

Fig. 8.19 Anatomy produced by a section through the heart in the sagittal plane with the heart in its in situ position.

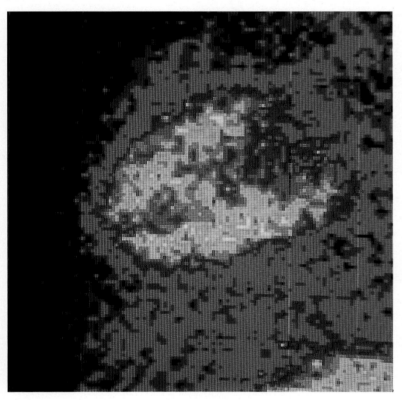

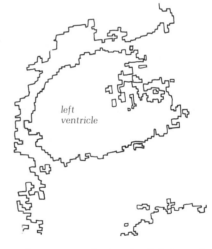

Fig. 8.20 Scintigram obtained in left lateral projection producing comparable anatomy to that in fig. 8.19.

to understand, being the anteroposterior projections, the left anterior oblique projection taken at 45° from the anteroposterior position, and the left lateral projection taken at a right angle to the anteroposterior view. The anatomy of these sections and their corresponding scintigraphic silhouettes are shown in figs. 8.15-8.20.

Cardiac Anatomy for the Surgeon

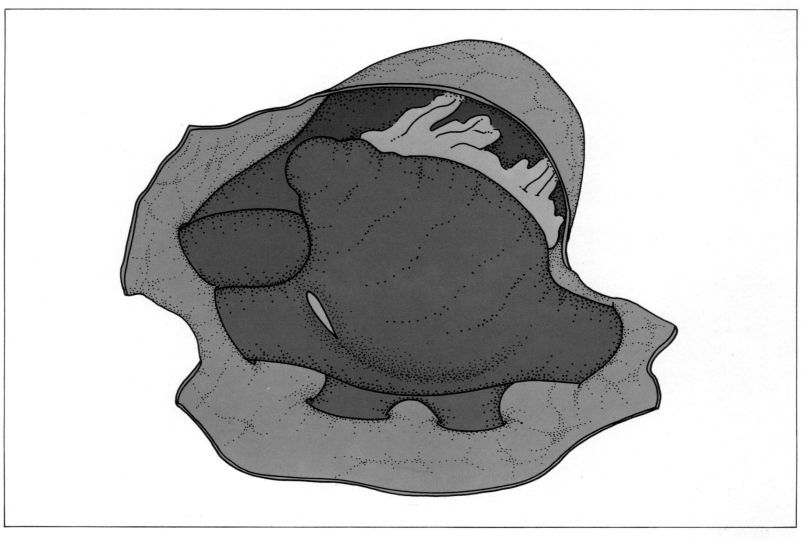

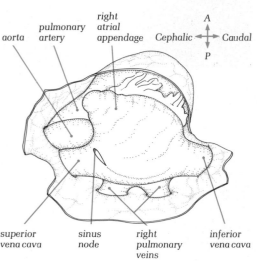

aorta — pulmonary artery — right atrial appendage — Cephalic — Caudal — A — P

superior vena cava — sinus node — right pulmonary veins — inferior vena cava

Fig. 8.21   *Diagram of the heart in situ showing the usual orientation viewed by the surgeon.*

The surgeon suffers a great disadvantage compared with the morphologist in that he has to deal with the heart *in situ*. In order to obtain access to chambers such as the left atrium or ventricle or the aortic valve, he must use routes which present a different perspective of the cardiac structures from those illustrated in standard anatomical displays. Furthermore, since he usually operates, if right-handed, with the head of the patient to the left and the feet to the right, he sees the heart at an angle of 90° compared with the anatomic position. In this chapter, we will briefly review the anatomy of the heart as seen using these approaches.

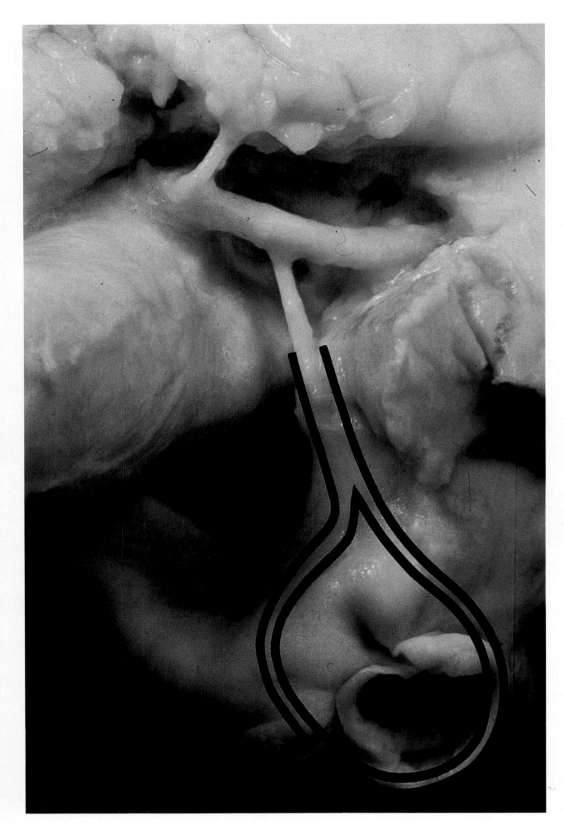

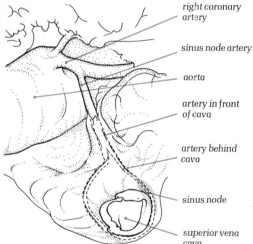

right coronary
artery

sinus node artery

aorta

artery in front
of cava

artery behind
cava

sinus node

superior vena
cava

Fig. 8.22   Dissection showing the artery to
the sinus node. Its course relative to the
superior vena cava is variable as indicated,
and a circle round the orifice is possible.

When the surgeon gains access to
the heart in the standard approach,
the superior vena cava is to be left and
the inferior vena cava to the right
(fig. 8.21). The sulcus terminalis runs
horizontally in this orientation and it
must be remembered that the sinus
node lies immediately subepicardially
in this sulcus and that its arterial
supply may come either in front of or
behind the superior vena cava (fig.
8.22). The entire area of the superior
cavo-atrial junction may, therefore,
be at risk and should be avoided when
inserting cannulae or making
incisions in the right atrium.

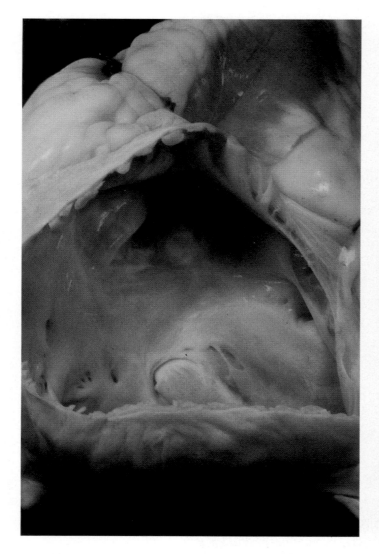

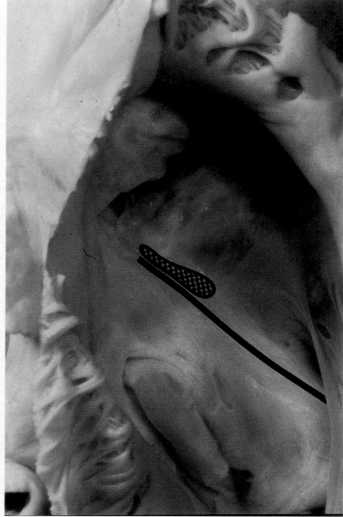

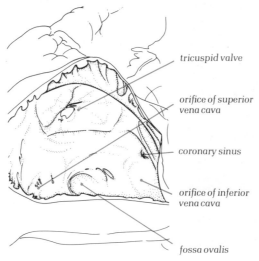

tricuspid valve

orifice of superior
vena cava

coronary sinus

orifice of inferior
vena cava

fossa ovalis

Fig. 8.23   The internal landmarks of the right
atrium as might be viewed by the surgeon.
The incision is somewhat generous!

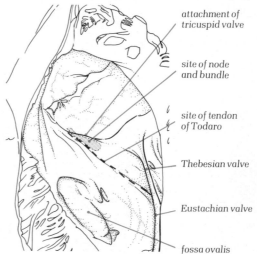

attachment of
tricuspid valve

site of node
and bundle

site of tendon
of Todaro

Thebesian valve

Eustachian valve

fossa ovalis

Fig. 8.24   The landmarks of the triangle of
Koch as viewed by the surgeon.

The internal features of the right
atrium will obviously reflect the right
angle change in orientation produced
by the surgical approach (fig. 8.23).
A feature worthy of re-emphasis,
however, is the position of the
triangle of Koch as viewed through
the right atrium. If tension is placed
on the Eustachian valve or its
remnant, in most hearts the tendon of
Todaro springs into prominence,

running from a right inferior to left
superior relationship towards the
central fibrous body. Here it meets the
annulus of the tricuspid valve septal
leaflet rising from right to left, and the
junction of the two indicates the
position of the penetrating bundle
(fig. 8.24). Even if a Eustachian valve
is not present, the sinus septum can
be taken as one border of the triangle
of Koch.

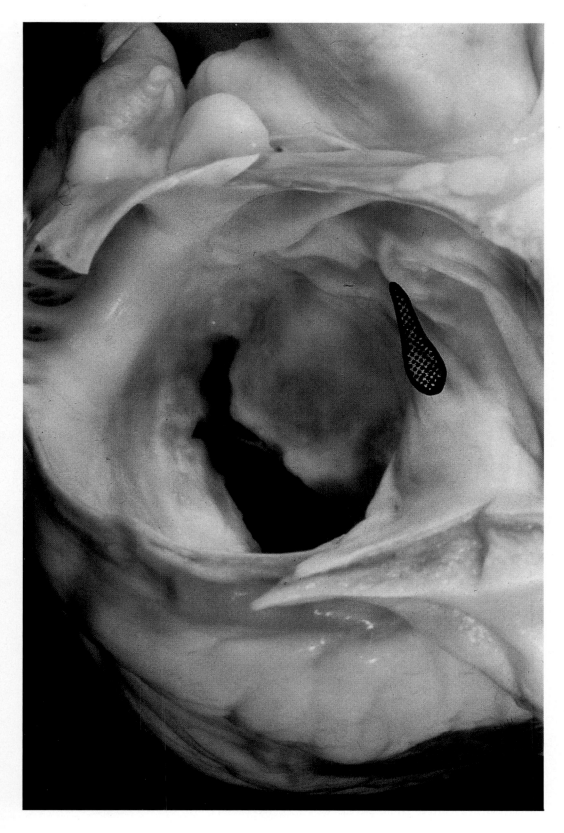

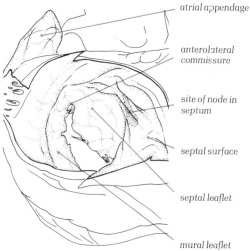

Fig. 8.25   *The orientation of the mitral valve with the heart in approximately surgical position. The roof of the left atrium is removed and the site of the conduction tissue in the septum is marked.*

atrial appendage

anterolateral commissure

site of node in septum

septal surface

septal leaflet

mural leaflet

Since one approach to the left atrium may be through the atrial septum, it must be remembered that not all the 'septal surface' seen in the floor of the right atrium is true atrial septum. Thus, incisions through the superior limbus or anterior limbus may take the surgeon into the transverse sinus or into the groove between the superior vena cava and the right pulmonary veins (see *figs.*

2.34 & 2.35). In this position, it may not be immediately apparent that this is the outside of the heart. The other usual approach to the left atrium is through the groove between the right pulmonary veins and the superior vena cava. This provides good access to the mitral valve, which is seen with its anterior leaflet in a superior position and the posterior leaflet in an inferior one (*fig. 8.25*). The danger

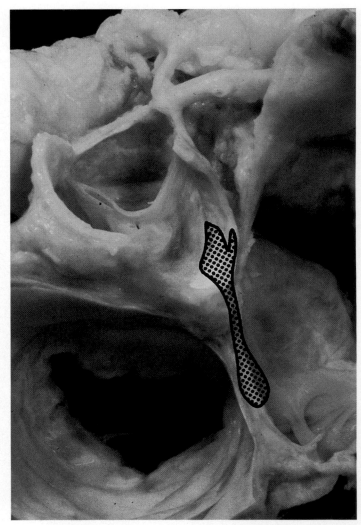

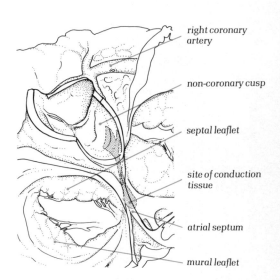

right coronary
artery

non-coronary cusp

septal leaflet

site of conduction
tissue

atrial septum

mural leaflet

Fig. 8.26   The heart seen in Fig. 8.25
dissected to show the relations of the mitral
valve to the aortic valve, the atrial septum and
the conduction tissues.

area regarding the conduction tissue
is the quadrant of the valve
immediately above the posteromedial
commissure, seen to the right of the
operative field. The conduction tissue
is, of course, hidden from the operator,
being on the ventricular outlet aspect
of the mitral valve, but its position can
be shown by a dissection which
removes the atrial septum (fig. 8.26).
The circumflex coronary artery is also
a potential danger area during mitral
valve surgery, lying as it does in the
left atrioventricular sulcus. As
indicated previously (see figs. 6.16 &
6.17), this is particularly so when the
left coronary artery is dominant,
since the circumflex artery is then

more closely related to the anterior
and posterior parts of the
atrioventricular groove. The aortic
valve is usually approached by an
oblique or transverse incision into its
right wall above the right sinus. The
aortic valve is then visualized with the
right coronary cusp superiorly and
to the right, the left coronary cusp to
the left, and the non-coronary cusp
inferiorly (fig. 8.27). The plane of the
valve is oblique so that the area to the
right will be furthest from the
operator. This is the major danger
area, since the penetrating
atrioventricular bundle is found
beneath the commissure of the non-

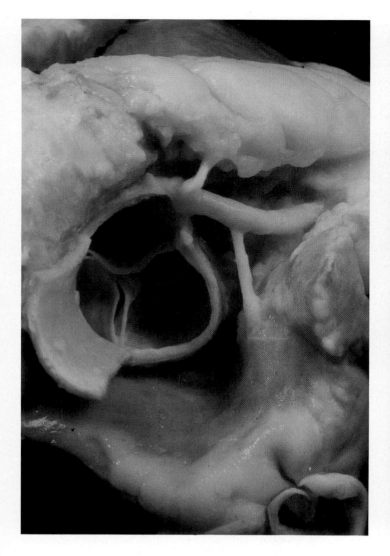

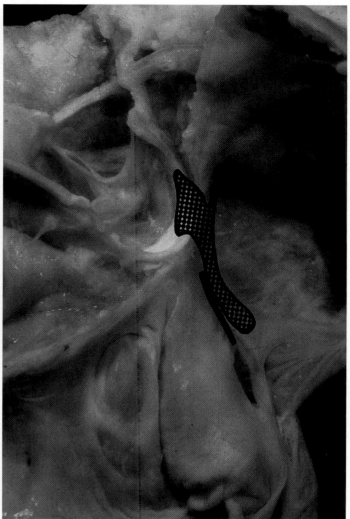

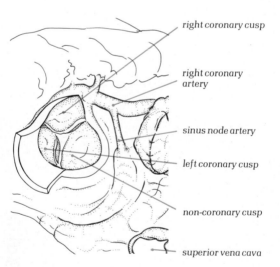

right coronary cusp

right coronary
artery

sinus node artery

left coronary cusp

non-coronary cusp

superior vena cava

Fig. 8.27   The heart in a more or less surgical
position dissected to show the relations of the
aortic valves.

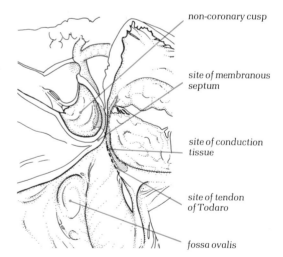

non-coronary cusp

site of membranous
septum

site of conduction
tissue

site of tendon
of Todaro

fossa ovalis

Fig. 8.28   Dissection of the heart shown in
fig. 8.27 illustrating the relations of the aortic
valve to the right atrium and the conduction
tissues.

coronary and right coronary cusps,
and the branching bundle is
immediately beneath the
interventricular component of the
membranous septum (fig. 8.28). The
multiple relationships of the aortic
valve to all cardiac chambers must be

kept in mind (see figs. 4.32-4.34).
   When making incisions into the
ventricles, care must always be taken
to avoid both papillary muscles and
major arterial branches. A right
ventricular infundibulotomy is a
relatively safe procedure. The main

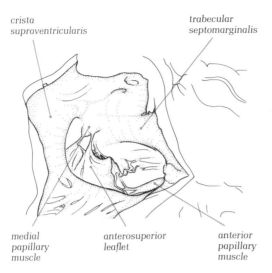

crista supraventricularis   *trabecular septomarginalis*

medial papillary muscle   *anterosuperior leaflet*   *anterior papillary muscle*

Fig. 8.29   *A generous incision in the infundibulum showing the right ventricular outflow tract as might be viewed by the surgeon.*

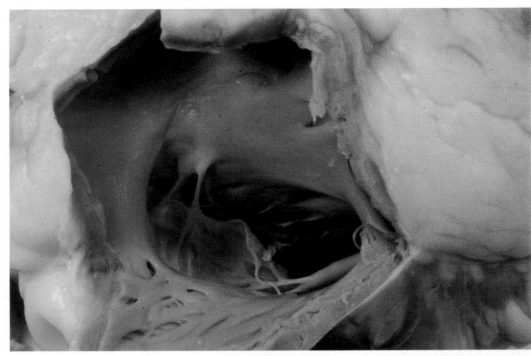

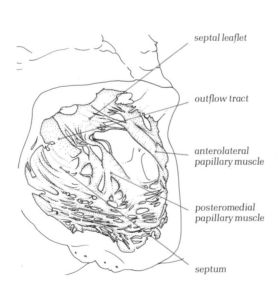

septal leaflet

outflow tract

anterolateral papillary muscle

posteromedial papillary muscle

septum

Fig. 8.30   *An exceedingly large incision between the anterior descending coronary artery and the anterolateral papillary muscle showing the access to the left ventricular outflow tract.*

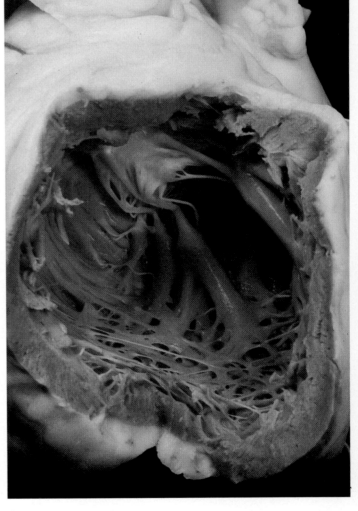

arteries at risk are the infundibular branches of the right coronary artery and the anterior descending artery, which may not be readily visible if pericardial adhesions are present. The immediate tricuspid valve tension apparatus in danger is the medial papillary muscle taking origin from the infundibular septum. This also marks the position of the right bundle branch. The anterior papillary muscle is usually well to the operator's right (fig. 8.29), but a high take-off of the moderator band must always be considered as a possible hazard. A left ventricular incision is more hazardous, since it must avoid both the important coronary branches, such as the anterior descending and its diagonal branches, and the anterolateral papillary muscle of the mitral valve. If these are avoided, good access can be obtained to the left ventricular outflow tract (fig. 8.30).

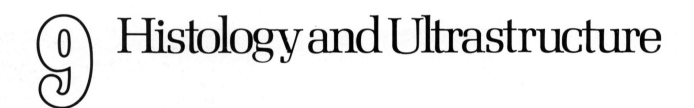

9 Histology and Ultrastructure

Histology and Ultrastructure

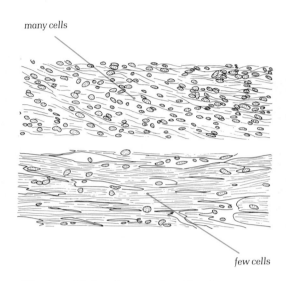

many cells

few cells

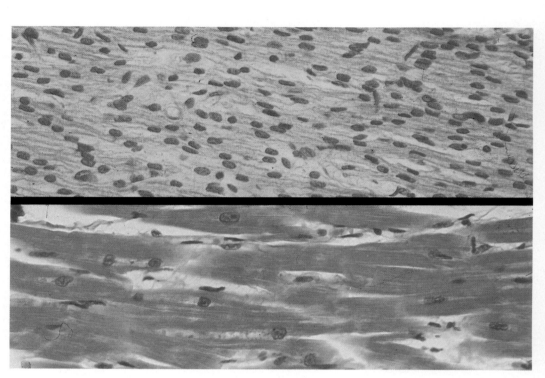

Fig. 9.1 *Light micrographs of fetal (upper) and adult (lower) myocardium taken at the same magnification. Haematoxylin and eosin stain.*

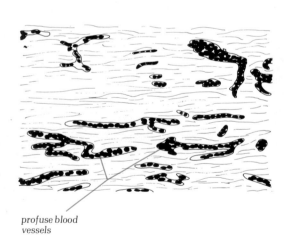

profuse blood vessels

Fig. 9.2 *Light micrograph of congested newborn myocardium demonstrating the dense capillary network intermingling with the myocytes. Haematoxylin and eosin stain.*

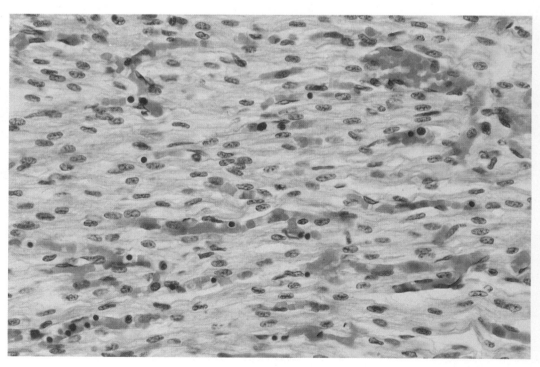

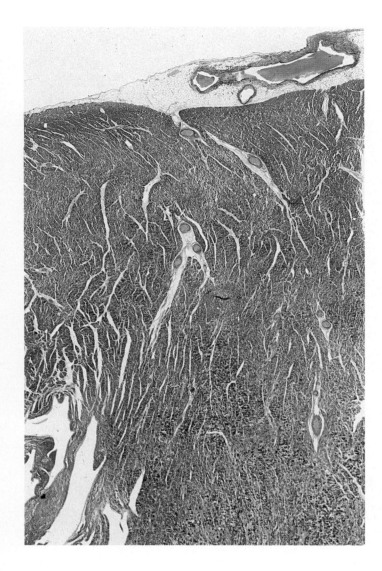

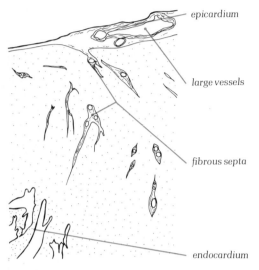

Fig. 9.3　A detail of a cross-section of the heart wall. Branches from the larger calibre epicardial vessels penetrate into the myocardium in stalks of connective tissue and taper out towards the endocardium. Trichrome stain.

Histology of Myocardium

It is beyond the scope of this book to write an all-encompassing account of the microscopical anatomy of the myocardium. It is our purpose to present a brief but comprehensive description with particular emphasis on functional correlation.

Light Microscopy

The myocardium is composed of myocardial cells or fibres, the so-called myocytes or cardiocytes. These are aggregated into fibre bundles which themselves show a particularly intricate arrangement, this varying in different parts of the heart (see *Chapter 5*). Cell boundaries are not readily identified with the light microscope and it has long been thought that the myocardium formed a true syncytium of cells. However, ultrastructural studies have shown that boundaries between the cells do exist, but that they themselves are of a complex nature (*vide infra*). For this reason, it has become fashionable to describe the myocardium in terms of a 'functional' syncytium.

In the fetus and newborn, the myocardium has a highly cellular and vascular appearance because the myocytes are still small (*fig. 9.1 upper*). With growth, the cytoplasm increases in size and the myocardium becomes apparently less cellular (*fig. 9.1 lower*), this being spurious since the basic architecture has not altered. It is important to be familiar with this change so as not to interpret pathology where one is dealing with an as yet immature tissue.

The myocardium contains a vast network of capillaries of such an extent that almost every myocardial fibre is surrounded by approximately 3-4 capillaries (*fig. 9.2*). Stalks of connective tissue traverse the myocardium containing larger calibre muscular arteries and arterioles, in addition to veins, lymphatics and nerve fibres. These structures penetrate the myocardium from the epicardium inwards and usually taper out towards the endocardial lining (*fig. 9.3*). The intramyocardial arterioles are of a muscular type but may occasionally show luminal smooth muscle cell proliferations, interlaced with elastin lamellae. Such changes are particularly frequent within the papillary muscles. It has been proposed that this arrangement of vascular smooth muscle relates to the rhythmic longitudinal stretch to which these arteries are continually subjected.

Myocytes in the normal mature heart have a length of approximately $50\text{-}100\mu$ and a fibre diameter of $5\text{-}20\mu$. The cells are enclosed by an outer membrane, the sarcolemma, which separates the cell from its extracellular environment. It plays an important role in the interchange of ions between the intra- and extracellular spaces and in the spread of electrical activity from cell to cell (*vide infra*).

9.3

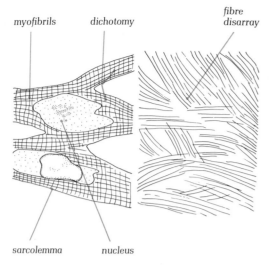

myofibrils   dichotomy   fibre disarray

sarcolemma   nucleus

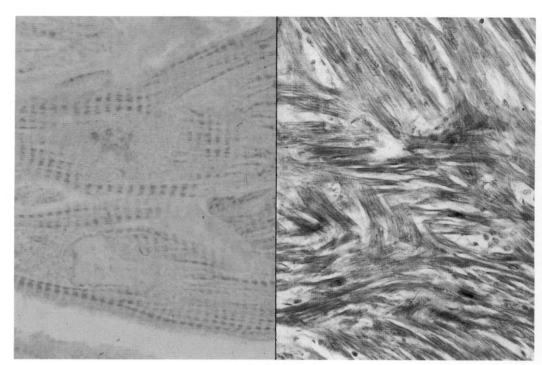

Fig. 9.4   Photomicrographs showing the distinct pattern of branching of myocytes. The left panel shows part of a cardiac muscle cell with dichotomy of its cytoplasm. The right panel shows an area of ventricular myocardium where this particular feature has led to 'disarray' of fibres which does not necessarily indicate a state of pathology. Left panel: PTAH stain; Right panel: trichrome stain.

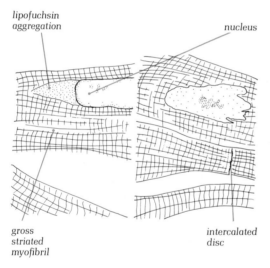

lipofuchsin aggregation   nucleus

gross striated myofibril   intercalated disc

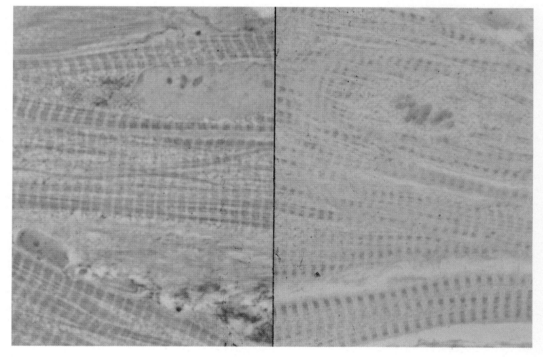

Fig. 9.5   High power micrographs illustrating the features of cardiac muscle cells. The left panel shows the centrally-positioned nucleus with juxtanuclear deposition of lipofuchsin pigment. The right panel shows parts of neighbouring myocytes with an intercalated disc. Left panel: haematoxylin and eosin stain. Right panel: PTAH stain.

The myocytes differ from skeletal or voluntary muscle cells by exhibiting a distinct pattern of branching, characterized by dichotomy (fig. 9.4, left). This may in places present an intricate lace-like fibre arrangement as seen at microscopy (fig. 9.4, right). This phenomenon of lace-like fibre arrangement has attracted much

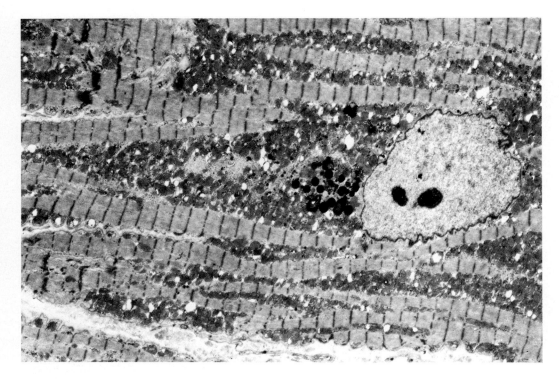

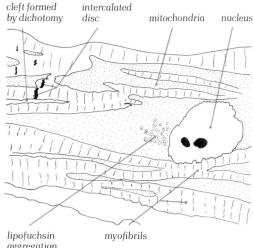

cleft formed by dichotomy   intercalated disc   mitochondria   nucleus

lipofuchsin aggregation   myofibrils

Fig. 9.6 *Low power electron micrograph of a longitudinal section of parts of normal myocytes showing the nucleus, cross-striated myofibrils with interposed mitochondria and illustrating dichotomy at several sites, with clefts appearing between the 'branches'. ×3,800.*

attention in recent years, since a microscopical disarray of fibres (fibre dysplasia) has been promoted as the 'specific' underlying histopathology in the myocardium of patients with the condition variously described as asymmetrical septal hypertrophy, hypertrophic obstructive cardiomyopathy or idiopathic hypertrophic subaortic stenosis and has also been noted in conditions with myocardial dysfunction of unknown nature (*Ferrans et al., 1972; Becu et al., 1976; Feizi et al., 1978*). But great care must be taken in this respect since normal myocardium may display a similar architecture (*Bulkley, 1977*) and hypertrophy, of whatever cause, accentuates this appearance.

As seen with the light microscope, the myocytes display a centrally-positioned nucleus, often with a perinuclear lighter zone that may contain lipofuchsin pigment (*fig. 9.5,*

left). The cytoplasm exhibits distinct cross-striations which occur at regular intervals.

In places, a different sort of cross-line can be recognized, often alternating in position through neighbouring cells, the intercalated disc (*fig. 9.5, right*). It is the intercalated disc which has been shown by electron microscopy to represent the site of intercellular connexion, being formed by interdigitating opposing membranes of the adjacent cells (*vide infra*).

Electron Microscopy*

Ultrastructural studies of the myocardium have greatly contributed to the understanding of cardiac function. As stated, it has shown that the myocardium constitutes a 'functional syncytium', characterized by end-to-end connexions via intercalated discs (*fig. 9.6*). The cell

*All electron micrographs were prepared by Dr. K. P. Dingemans, Wilhelmina Gasthuis, Amsterdam, and are reproduced with his permission.

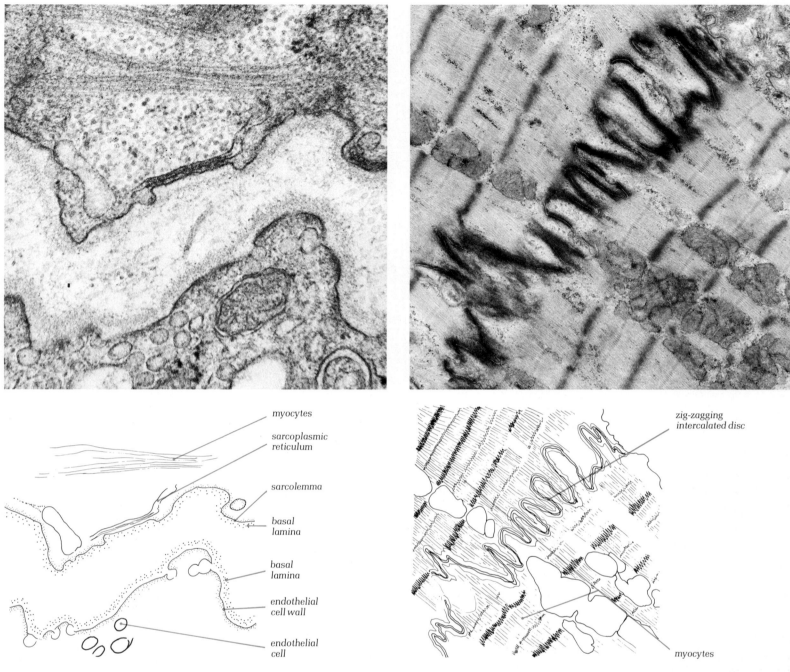

Fig. 9.7   An electron micrograph showing a detail of the cell surface of a myocyte adjacent to an endothelial cell. Note the coating of the sarcolemma by the basal lamina. At one site, sarcoplasmic reticulum lies in close apposition to the sarcolemma. ×87,000.

Fig. 9.8   Electron micrograph showing an intercalated disc connecting two adjoining myocytes. The zig-zagging 'disc' contains various types of specialized junctions. ×23.000.

surface is formed by a distinct membrane, the sarcolemma, coated on its outer aspect by the basal lamina (fig. 9.7). The intercalated disc is a continuum of the sarcolemma, which takes an intricate zig-zag course with multiple indentations and various specializations in structure along its length (fig. 9.8). One of these is termed the nexus or gap junction (fig. 9.9). It represents an area of membrane specialization where the two adjoining membranes close their interstitial gap from 300-200Å to 30-20Å. These particular regions are considered to represent sites of low electrical impedance, enabling rapid spread of electrical activity from one cell to the next. It is of interest, in this respect, that nexus were initially considered to be virtually absent among the specialized cells of the sinus node. Recent studies, however, have disclosed that this is not the case, thus shedding light upon the concept of spread of excitation within the pacemaker itself (Masson-Pevet et al., 1978).

A special derivative of the sarcolemma is the system of transverse tubules, also termed T-system or T-tubules. This system consists of invaginations of the sarcolemma which enable

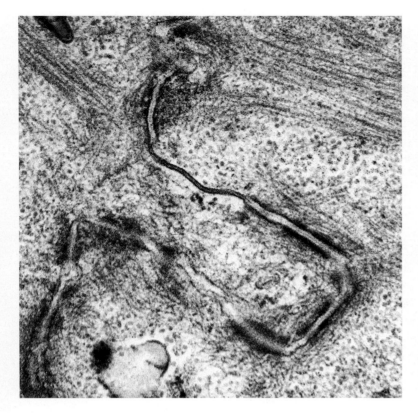

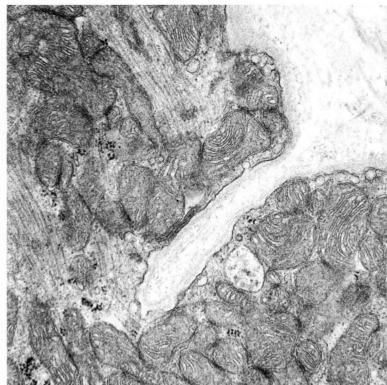

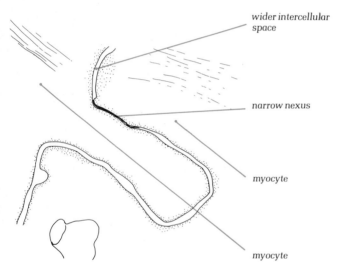

wider intercellular space

narrow nexus

myocyte

myocyte

Fig. 9.9 Electron micrograph showing a detail of an intercalated disc with a nexus where the two membranes of the disc abruptly narrow to approximately 20Å. ×86,000.

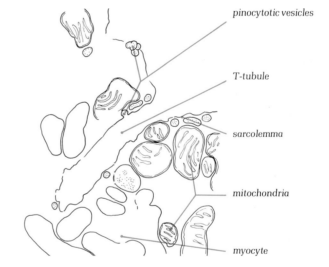

pinocytotic vesicles

T-tubule

sarcolemma

mitochondria

myocyte

Fig. 9.10 Electron micrograph showing a detail of the surface of a myocyte with the origin of a T-tubule. Pinocytotic vesicles are noted in the lateral sarcolemma and in the sarcolemma of the T-tubule. ×43,500.

extracellular 'fluid' to penetrate deep within the cytoplasm of the myocytes (fig. 9.10). The T-tubules do not actually open into the cytoplasm. Their precise functional role is as yet not fully understood, but it seems most likely that they fulfil a transport function between the interior and the exterior of the cells. T-tubules do not occur in the specialized cells of the sinus node and the specialized

atrioventricular junctional area. Moreover, the greater part of atrial cells are devoid of this system. The variation in formation of the T-tubule system underscores other morphological and electrophysiological experiences that atrial myocardium is composed of a heterogeneous cell population.

Another membranous system of major functional significance is

formed by the sarcoplasmic reticulum. It is composed of a fine network of tubules that surrounds the myofibrils and has a main orientation in the longitudinal axis of the cell. In contrast to the T-tubule system, the sarcoplasmic reticulum has no open communication with the extracellular space. It is the equivalent of the endoplasmic reticulum which is encountered in most other tissue cells. However, the sarcoplasmic reticulum

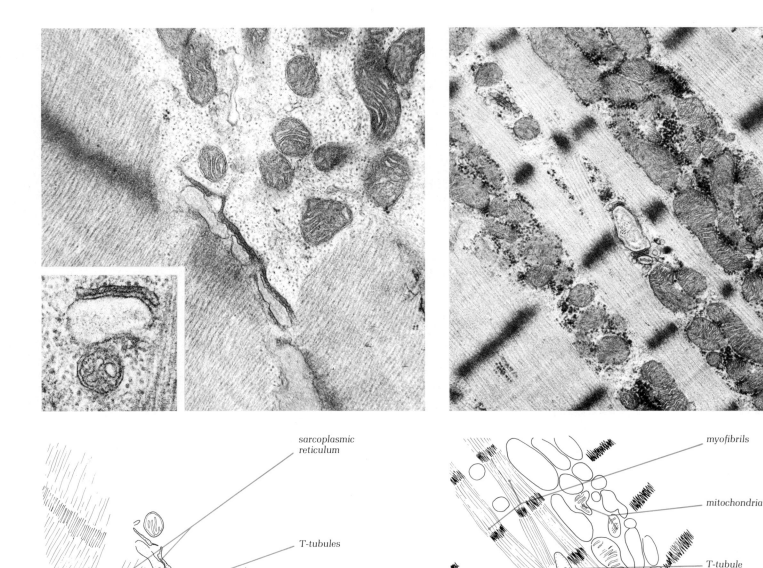

Fig. 9.11   Electron micrograph showing details of the close relationship between T-tubules and sarcoplasmic reticulum. ×43,500. The insert shows an enlargement of a minute 'vesicle' which can be recognized as a transsected T-tubule because of the presence of basal lamina material and its close association with sarcoplasmic reticulum. ×87,000.

Fig. 9.12   Electron micrograph showing a detail of the peripheral part of a myocyte with interposition of myofibrils and mitochondria. Because the muscle was fixed in a state of contraction, A and I-bands cannot be identified. The sarcomere is delineated by Z-lines. ×35,500.

is specialized in the sense that it abuts by way of discrete cisternae, the so-called junctional sarcoplasmic reticulum, on both the sarcolemma and the T-tubules (fig. 9.11). The junctional sarcoplasmic reticulum is considered the most likely site from which calcium ions are liberated to initiate contraction of the cardiocytes (vide infra).

The contractile material of the myocyte consists of myofibrils, themselves composed of myofilaments. The functional unit, in this respect, is the sarcomere (fig. 9.12). The pump function of the heart depends heavily upon integrated action of these individual units. It is the sarcomere that gives the myofibril its striated appearance. The striations in the cells are themselves formed by a series of lines and spaces with alphabetical designations. The sarcomere is defined as the contractile elements confined between two Z-lines (fig. 9.12), and is composed of two sets of interdigitating myofilaments. The Z-lines are attached to the sarcolemma and are largely responsible for producing the cross-striations (fig. 9.13). The myofilaments themselves are composed of rods of contractile proteins which through a process of cross-bridging may shorten (contraction) or lengthen (relaxation) the total length of the sarcomere. One set of myofilaments is thin and is made of actin, whereas the other set

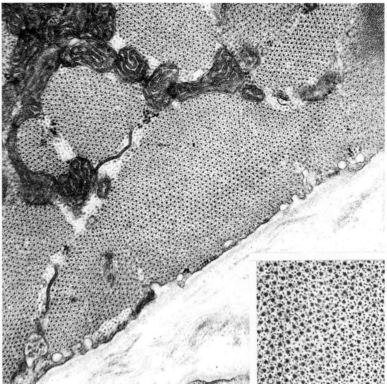

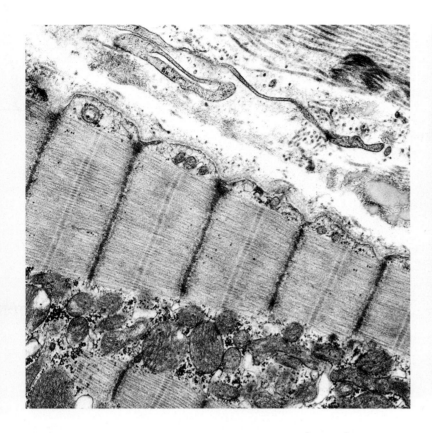

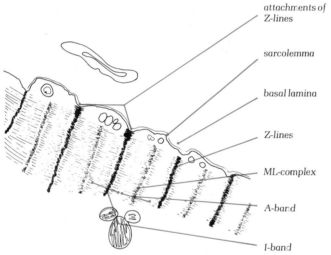

Fig. 9.13   Electron micrograph of a detail of the peripheral part of a myocyte showing the intricate attachments of the Z-lines to the scalloping sarcolemma. ×27,500.

attachments of Z-lines

sarcolemma

basal lamina

Z-lines

ML-complex

A-band

I-band

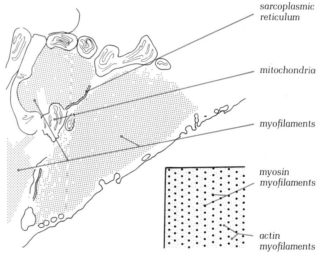

Fig. 9.14   Electron micrograph of a cross-section of a myocyte showing the large areas composed of myofilaments. ×55,000. The insert shows a detail of interposing thin (actin) and thick (myosin) myofilaments. ×105,000.

sarcoplasmic reticulum

mitochondria

myofilaments

myosin myofilaments

actin myofilaments

is thick, being composed of myosin (fig. 9.14). The actin filaments originate from the Z-line which thus provides a zone of insertion for the actin filaments of two abutting sarcomeres. The actin filaments extend between the thick myosin filaments but do not reach the centre of the area occupied by myosin. Thus because the middle area contains only myosin, the end parts of the sarcomere only actin and the intermediate area only interdigitating rods, there is a

difference in electron density that gives the sarcomere its characteristic appearance. The area of actin filaments alone forms the I-band in the centre part of which the Z-line is present. The A-band in the centre of the sarcomere is formed mainly by myosin filaments but the outer parts of this band contain both myosin and actin. The central part of the A-band, and thus of the sarcomere, which contains only myosin filaments is called the ML-complex (fig. 9.13). It

will be clear that depending on the state of contraction at the time of fixation, the ultrastructural appearance of the sarcomere will change and the lengths of these different bands will vary.

Myocytes are rich in mitochondria, which are located in between the myofibrils (fig. 9.6). They represent the main energy source for myofibrillar contraction and their large quantity further underlines the heart's dependence on oxidative metabolism.

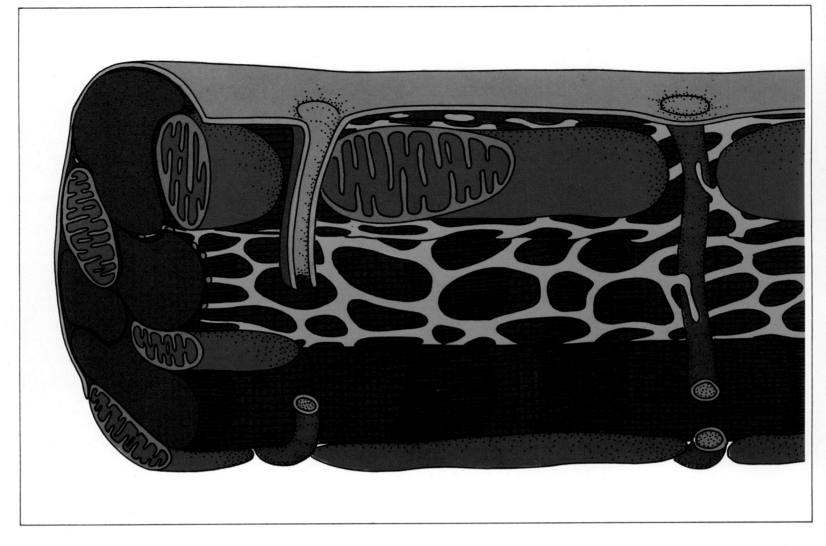

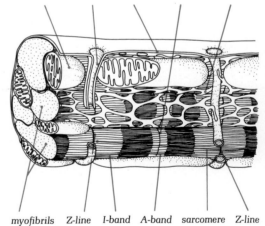

Fig. 9.15 Diagram illustrating the main ultrastructural features of cardiac muscle cells.

How do these ultrastructural features relate to the contractile activity of the heart? The intricate architecture of the myocardial 'functional syncytium' ensures a strong mechanical and electrical coupling of cells (fig. 9.15). During activation, the structural characteristics of the intercalated disc ensure rapid spread over adjoining cells and in a preferential direction. Moreover, the changes in membrane potential and ion shifts are transmitted rapidly through the T-system to reach deep into the cell.

A release of calcium from the storage areas in the junctional sarcoplasmic reticulum may activate the contractile elements of the sarcomere. Through a process of cross-linking, the actin and myosin filaments slide along each other, thereby shortening the sarcomere. Integrated and coordinated interaction will thus lead to myocardial contraction. Subsequent reabsorption of calcium by the sarcoplasmic reticulum will restore the initial situation and lead to relaxation.

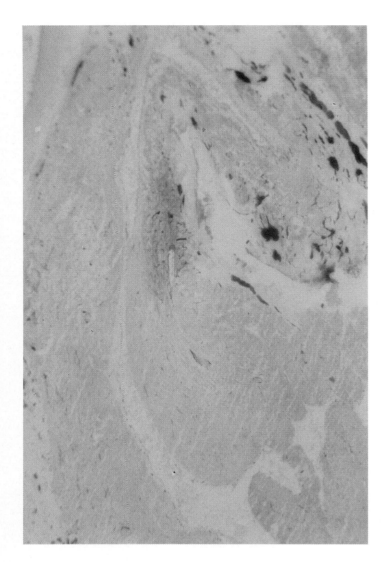

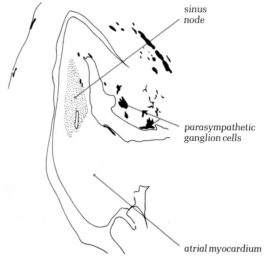

sinus
node

parasympathetic
ganglion cells

atrial myocardium

Fig. 9.16   Low power photomicrograph of
the atrial tissues of a mid-term human fetus
processed to show cholinesterase activity.
It shows the ganglia related to the sinus node.
Gomori technique.

Microscopic Innervation

The precise extent of the innervation of the heart and the type of innervation in different parts of the heart remains uncertain. There are discrepancies between results obtained by physiological, pharmacological and anatomical techniques and there are further discrepancies between results of given techniques in given disciplines. There are several possible reasons for these apparently conflicting findings. Firstly, it is known that there is considerable species variation in the pattern of innervation of the heart. Secondly, the sensitivity of techniques varies from discipline to discipline. Results obtained using anatomical techniques are relatively crude in many respects. Finally, the specificity of techniques is frequently questionable, making the interpretation of results difficult. Thus, even with the wealth of investigations on cardiac innervation, it is still not possible to state with certainty how the different chambers

of the human heart are innervated. Certainly more information is becoming available concerning animal species with the use of sophisticated ultrastructural techniques. But because of difficulties in obtaining suitable tissue, these techniques are not feasible in the human heart, except possibly for examination of fetal tissues. Then the difficulty arises that we cannot be sure that the innervative pattern of the fetal heart is the same as in the adult, there being considerable evidence that the development of nerve plexuses, particularly the sympathetic fibres, continues well after birth (James, 1970; Finlay & Anderson, 1974). Thus, at best we can give only an imprecise picture of the innervation of the human cardiac structures. We can generalize more with respect to innervation of the mammalian heart (Yamauchi, 1969) but these observations must be interpreted with much caution in respect to the human heart.

It is certainly known that the heart contains parasympathetic effector nerves, sympathetic effector nerves and sensory nerves. In common with other visceral muscle receiving autonomic effector innervation, the cardiac muscle does not receive its innervation through discrete motor end-plates as does voluntary muscle. Instead, the cardiac muscle is innervated by a terminal or ground plexus. The ground plexus in the atrial chambers contains both parasympathetic and sympathetic fibres, the two frequently running adjacent to each other. In contrast, in the ventricles and in relation to the coronary arteries, most, if not all, of the fibres in the ground plexus are sympathetic. Evidence from anatomic studies have mostly been interpreted to suggest that the ventricles do not receive a parasympathetic innervation. Thus, all the ganglion cells of the parasympathetic nerves are found within the atrial chambers (fig. 9.16) or else in the

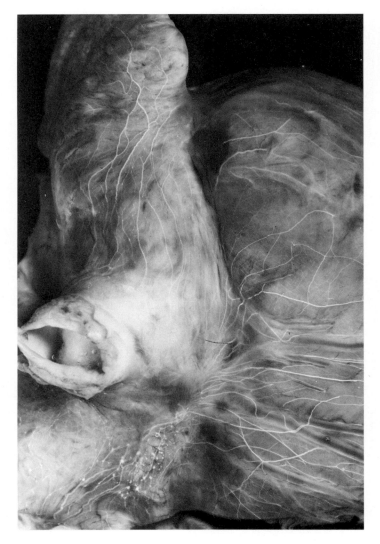

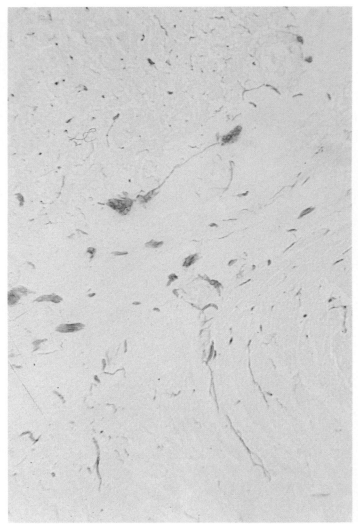

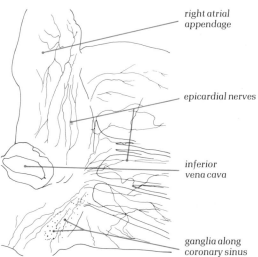

right atrial
appendage

epicardial nerves

inferior
vena cava

ganglia along
coronary sinus

atrial myocardium

parasympathetic
ganglion cells

atrioventricular
sulcus

ventricular
myocardium

Fig. 9.17   The atrioventricular sulcus of a
three-year-old child showing the
parasympathetic ganglia and nerves. The
whole heart was processed for cholinesterase
using the Lewis & Shute technique. Courtesy
of Dr. J. Tranum-Jensen.

Fig. 9.18   Low power photomicrograph of
ganglia in the atrioventricular sulcus of a
mid-term human fetus. Gomori's
cholinesterase technique. Note the nerves
extending into the ventricle.

atrioventricular sulci (figs. 9.17 &
9.18). But physiological studies have
shown that vagal stimulation does
influence the ventricles. Is this
influence from direct parasympathetic
effector innervation? Microscopic
preparations of animal hearts show
that the density of innervation of

atrial myocardium is considerably
higher than that of ventricular
myocardium.

Using an histochemical technique
for sympathetic nerves (the formalin
fluorescence technique), this
propensity for innervation in the
atria is easily shown (fig. 9.19), but

sympathetic fibres are unequivocally
present in the ventricular myocardium
and in relation to coronary arteries.
But what of the parasympathetic
innervation? It is known that the
enzyme acetylcholinesterase is
located in parasympathetic nerves
and that specific inhibitors can be

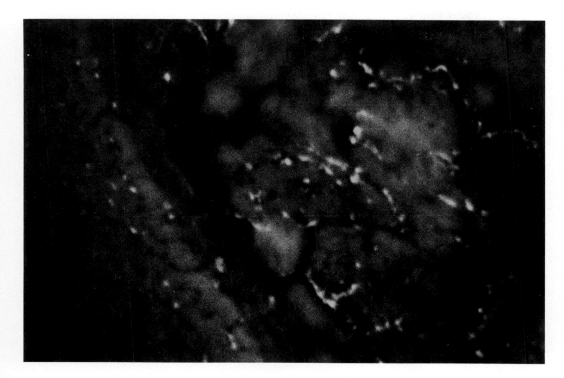

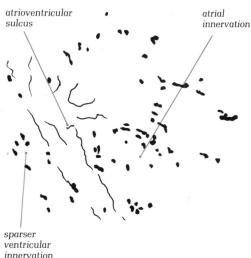

Fig. 9.19 Photomicrograph illustrating the sympathetic innervation of the rabbit heart. It is more profuse in the atria than the ventricles. Formol fluorescence technique. Courtesy of Prof. J. A. Gosling.

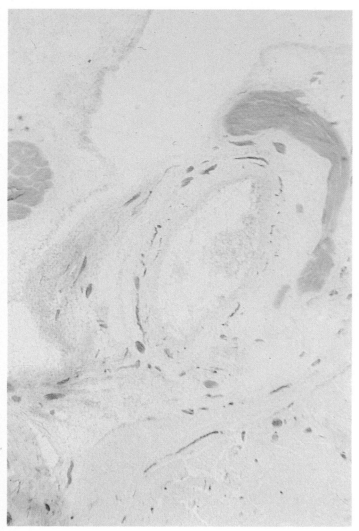

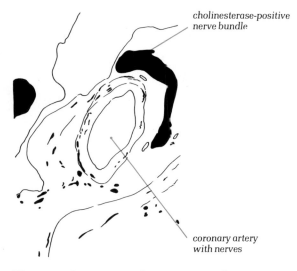

Fig. 9.20 Low power photomicrograph showing the cholinesterase-positive nerves accompanying a large coronary artery in a mid-term human fetus. Gomori technique.

used in histochemical techniques to demonstrate only this enzyme. It is then a fact that in the guinea pig heart, the acetylcholinesterase-containing nerves are confined to atrial myocardium and to the ventricular conduction tissues (*Anderson, 1972*). In other species however, such as rats, rabbits and the human fetus, some acetylcholinesterase-containing nerves are observed in the ventricular myocardium and in relation to the coronary arteries (fig. 9.20). Does this indicate a parasympathetic ventricular innervation in these species, or does it suggest lack of specificity of the so-called 'specific' inhibitors? Ultrastructural investigations can help in unravelling this dilemma. It is known that the final end-organ of the autonomic innervation is varicosities along the length of the terminal plexus. These varicosities are well visualized in

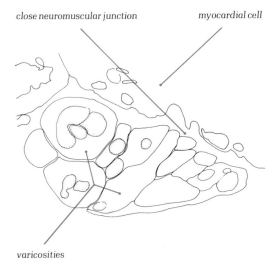

close neuromuscular junction   myocardial cell

varicosities

Fig. 9.21   Electron micrograph illustrating a neuromuscular contact in the rabbit atria. Note that the varicosities lose their Schwann cell sheath as they approach the muscle. Permanganate fixation, × 35,200. Courtesy of Dr. J. Dixon.

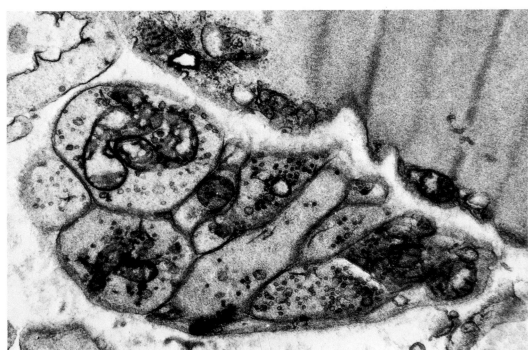

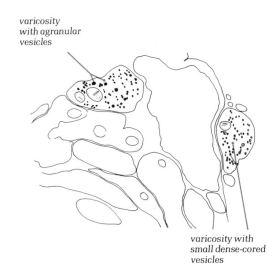

varicosity with agranular vesicles

varicosity with small dense-cored vesicles

Fig. 9.22   Electron micrograph of sympathetic (with dense-cored vesicles) and parasympathetic (with agranular vesicles) varicosities from the ground plexus of rabbit atrium. Permanganate fixation, × 35,200. Courtesy of Dr. J. Dixon.

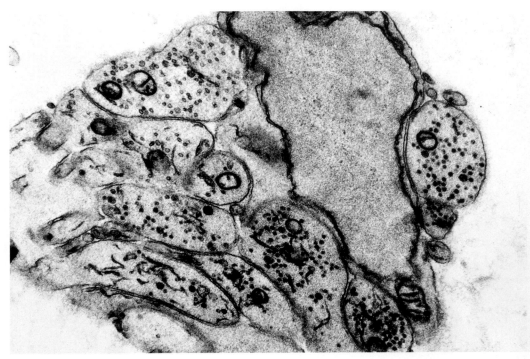

formalin fluorescence preparations. Ultrastructural studies show that the nerve fibres at the site of the varicosities lose their neurilemmal covering and come close to the surface membrane of the larger organ cell (cardiocyte or smooth muscle cell in a coronary artery) but that the larger cell membrane remains unspecialized (fig. 9.21). Furthermore, the varicosities themselves contain multiple vesicles and the type of vesicle permits differentiation of the sympathetic and parasympathetic nerves. Sympathetic nerves have varicosities containing numerous small dense-cored vesicles (fig. 9.22) whereas parasympathetic nerves contain a few large dense-cored vesicles and numerous agranular vesicles (fig. 9.22). Ultrastructural studies based on these criteria show that the ventricular myocardium

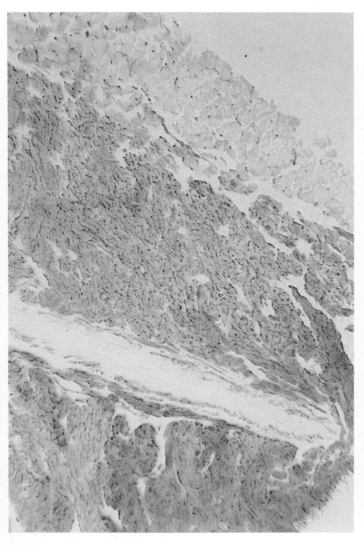

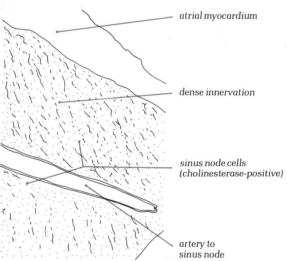

atrial myocardium

dense innervation

sinus node cells
(cholinesterase-positive)

artery to
sinus node

sinus node with
dense innervation

sinus node artery
with fluorescing
nerves

Fig. 9.23   Lower power photomicrograph
showing the profuse cholinesterase-positive
innervation of the dog sinus node. The nodal
cells are themselves cholinesterase-positive.
Gomori technique.

Fig. 9.24   Low power photomicrograph
showing the profuse sympathetic innervation
of the minipig sinus node. Formol
fluorescence technique. Courtesy of Dr. J.
Tranum-Jensen.

itself (apart from the conduction
tissues – *vide infra*) contain few if any
parasympathetic fibres.

Although both ultrastructural and
light microscopic studies show that
the atrial myocardium receives a rich
dual innervation, there is little doubt
that the most densely innervated part

of the heart is the conduction tissues.
But again there is considerable
species variation in the innervation
pattern. The sinus node generally
receives an exceedingly rich dual
innervation. Indeed, the node can be
easily distinguished by its innervation
pattern (*figs. 9.23 & 9.24*). It is

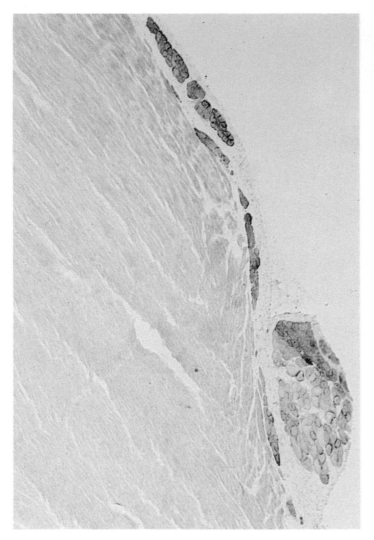

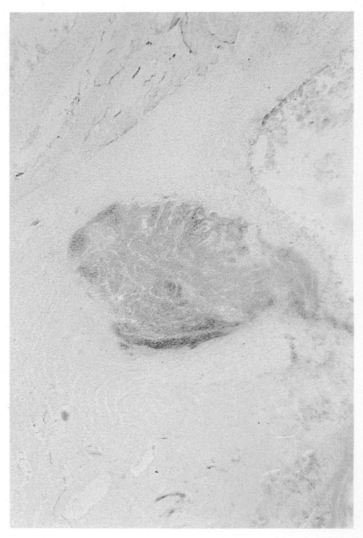

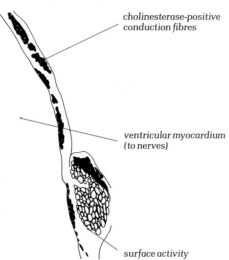

cholinesterase-positive
conduction fibres

ventricular myocardium
(to nerves)

surface activity

Fig. 9.25   Low power photomicrograph
showing the sarcolemmal activity of dog
ventricular conduction fibres which gives the
spurious appearance of innervation. Gomori
technique.

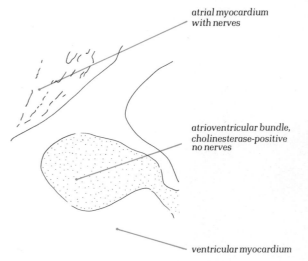

atrial myocardium
with nerves

atrioventricular bundle,
cholinesterase-positive
no nerves

ventricular myocardium

Fig. 9.26   Low power photomicrograph
showing the cholinesterase-positive
penetrating atrioventricular bundle of a
mid-term human fetus. Although itself
cholinesterase-positive, it is not associated
with any cholinesterase-positive nerves.
Gomori technique.

significant that while the node itself
is particularly well innervated, the
internodal atrial myocardium is
innervated only to the same extent as
the myocardium of the appendages,
still further evidence pointing to the
lack of 'specialized internodal tracts'.

The atrial part of the atrioventricular
node is similarly generously
innervated from both
parasympathetic and sympathetic
sources. But the most striking species
variation is found in the pattern of
innervation of the ventricular

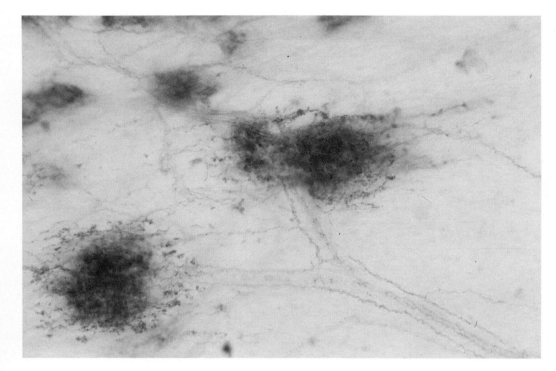

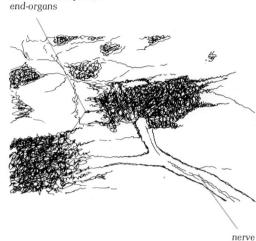

Fig. 9.27   Low power photomicrograph showing cholinesterase-positive end-organs in the endocardium of the minipig left atrium. Lewis & Shute technique. Courtesy of Dr. J. Tranum-Jensen.

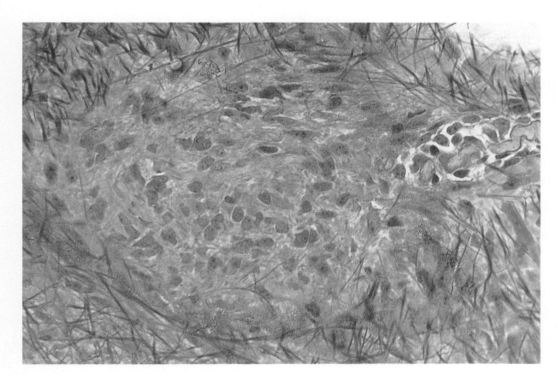

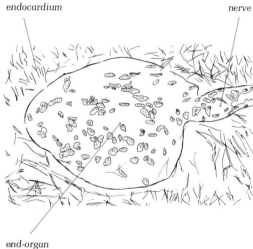

Fig. 9.28   Photomicrograph of thin (1µ) Epon section of one of the end-organs illustrated in fig. 9.27. Methylene blue stain. Courtesy of Dr. J. Tranum-Jensen.

conduction tissues. In the guinea pig, these tissues receive a surprisingly rich supply of acetylcholinesterase-containing nerves but are devoid of nerves demonstrable by formalin fluorescence. The rabbit ventricular conduction tissues receive rich plexuses from both sympathetic and parasympathetic sources, but the rat tissues, while receiving sympathetic innervation, are devoid of acetylcholinesterase-containing nerves despite the fact that the conduction tissue cells themselves are

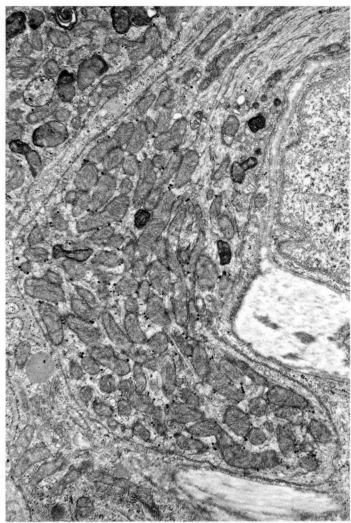

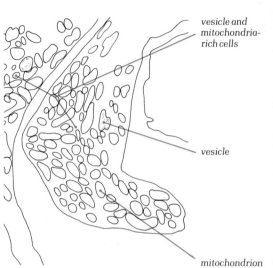

vesicle and
mitochondria-
rich cells

vesicle

mitochondrion

Fig. 9.29   Electron micrograph of the
mitochondria-rich and varicosity-packed
cells from the end-organ illustrated in fig.
9.28, × 10,000. Courtesy of Dr. J.
Tranum-Jensen.

cholinesterase-positive. In this
respect it is important to distinguish
between sarcolemmal activity
demonstrated by cholinesterase
staining and true innervation. In the
dog, for example, our studies have
shown rich surface activity on the
membranes of the cells of the
ventricular conduction tissues (fig.
9.25) but others have, we believe,
interpreted this same activity as being
contained within nerves (Kent et al.,
1974). This point is vital in
considering the innervation pattern
of human conduction tissues. Our
studies (fig. 9.26), confined to the
fetus, show that activity is confined to
the cells of the ventricular conduction
tissue themselves, a parasympathetic
innervation being absent.
Ultrastructural studies have
confirmed the rich dual innervation of
both sinus and atrioventricular nodes
and equally point to the confusing
species variation in innervation of the
ventricular conduction tissues.

In addition to the nerve plexuses
found in the myocardium and in
relation to the coronary arteries,
further extensive nerve plexuses are
to be found in both the epicardial and
endocardial layers of the heart as well
as in the parietal pericardium. These
plexuses are demonstrable by both
fluorescence and cholinesterase
techniques. It is therefore likely that
these rich nerve networks subserve
a sensory function. Discrete sensory
endings were described in the various
membranes of the heart by earlier
workers and the existence of such
discrete endings has recently been
unequivocally proven by
ultrastructural and histochemical
techniques, particularly in the atrial
chambers (Tranum-Jensen, 1975).
The endings are easily seen in
cholinesterase preparation (fig. 9.27).
Ultrastructural sections show their
complex nature (figs. 9.28 & 9.29).

10 The Development of the Heart

The Development of the Heart

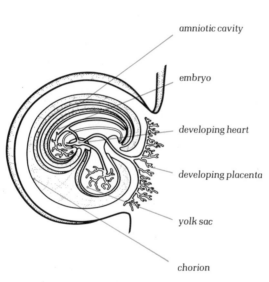

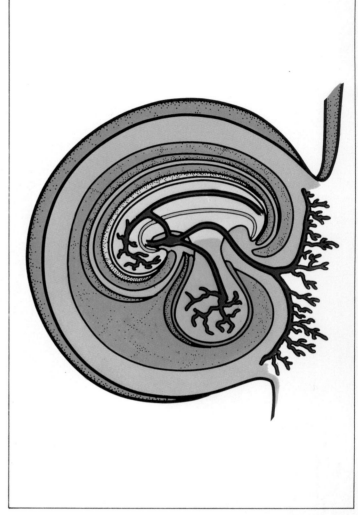

amniotic cavity

embryo

developing heart

developing placenta

yolk sac

chorion

Fig. 10.1   *The relationship of the developing venous plexus in the young embryo to the fetal membranes (chorion and yolk sac) and to the embryo itself.*

Knowledge of the development of the heart can be a great aid to the understanding of the morphology of not only the normal heart but of congenitally malformed hearts. Similarly, awareness of the origin and formation of the conductive tissues helps in the comprehension of their disposition in normal and abnormal hearts. However, there is no consensus regarding the events which occur during cardiac development. Much disagreement centres upon the choice of terms used to describe the different components of the heart while it is not yet known with certainty what is formed from these developmental components. That there should be disagreement is hardly surprising, since the cardiac

embryologist has previously attempted to reconstruct a three-dimensional structure from microscopic study of two-dimensional sections, the whole problem being compounded by the fourth dimension of time. Recent developments such as scanning electron microscopy (*Pexieder, 1978*) and sophisticated marking techniques (*de la Cruz et al., 1977*) used in developing animal hearts have alleviated some of the problems, but all features are not clarified as yet to the satisfaction of all. In this section, we will give our own simplified account of cardiac development, based on the study of serially-sectioned embryos but aided by many deductions made from

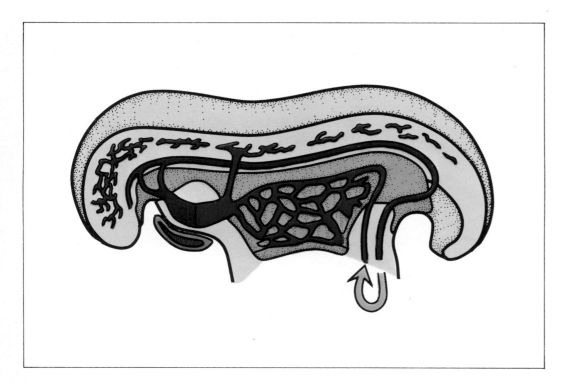

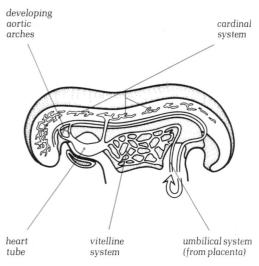

developing
aortic
arches

cardinal
system

heart
tube

vitelline
system

umbilical system
(from placenta)

Fig. 10.2   The relationship of the venous
systems to the young embryo itself.

examination of congenitally malformed hearts. The dangers implicit in this exercise are fully recognized and our account is presented simply as one interpretation of the events occurring during cardiac development, and similarly is presented within the strictures imposed by our primitive methodology.

Early Formation of the Heart Tube

The human embryo grows at a pace which rapidly exceeds the possibilities of nutrition provided by simple diffusion. Early establishment of a circulation and a means of gas and waste exchange is, therefore, an immediate requirement of the mammalian fetus. The embryonic vessels of the fetus and its membranes are consequently developed as soon as the third week, being first seen in the yolk sac. Additional channels develop in the chorion and in the embryo itself (fig. 10.1). Three sets of channels are formed on both right and left sides of the developing embryo, joining together at the developing connecting stalk of the embryo proper. More distally, the chorionic vessels establish contact with the maternal circulation and form the placenta. Within the embryo itself, the three systems run into the venous end of the developing heart tubes, bilateral structures formed on the undersurface of the embryo. These in turn connect with primordial bilateral arterial channels formed alongside the growing backbone. However, fusion of the anterior heart tubes occurs exceedingly early in development so that cardiac development can be considered from a stage following formation of the head fold, when the three venous systems enter the inferior end of the tube as bilaterally symmetrical structures (fig. 10.2); and the arterial

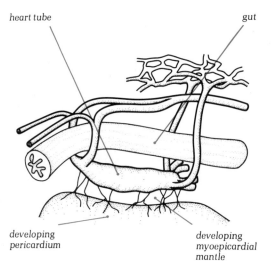

Fig. 10.3   Initially, the heart tube is placed between the gut and an anterior portion of the intraembryonic coelom which will form the pericardial cavity.

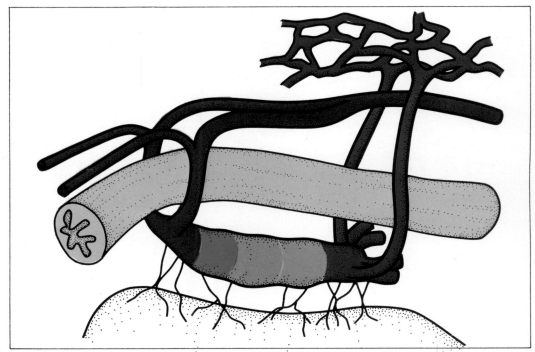

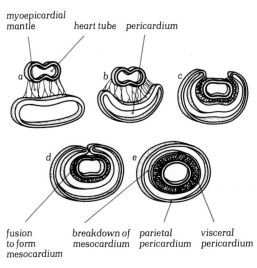

Fig. 10.4   The series of processes which occur as the heart tube sinks into the anterior pericardium. The myoepicardial mantle forms the myocardial part of the heart.

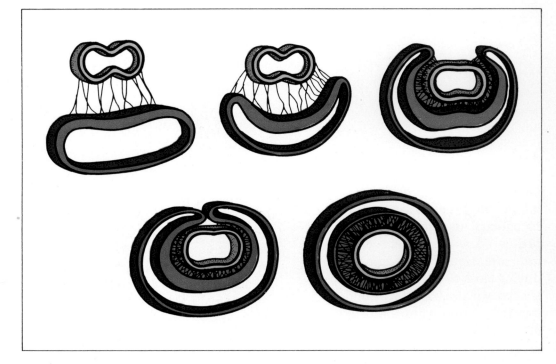

channels leave the superior end of the tube, showing bilateral symmetry as they arch round the pharynx to enter the posterior descending aortae (fig. 10.3).

The initial heart tube itself forms only the endocardial lining of the heart. This endocardial tube is invaginated into the pericardial cavity, part of the embryonic coelom and the myocardial and pericardial tissues are derived from the coelomic mesenchyme. Initially, the fused central part of the heart tube is suspended within the pericardium on a mesopericardial fold (fig. 10.4), and the pericardium is reflected at venous and arterial poles of the heart

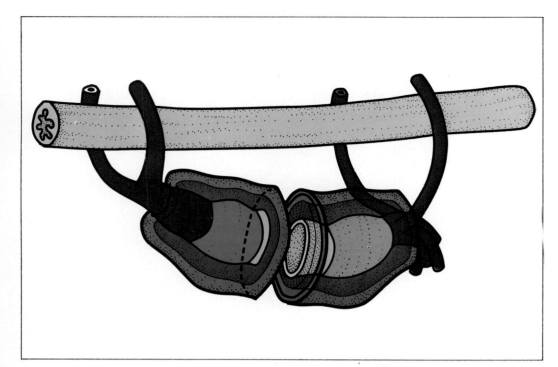

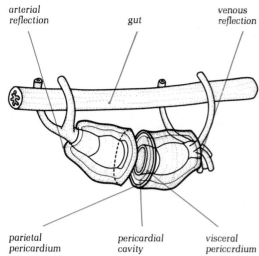

Fig. 10.5 *The visceral and parietal layers of the pericardial cavity are continuous at the venous and arterial poles of the heart.*

tube *(fig. 10.5).* Soon, the mesopericardium breaks down, leaving the endocardial heart tube suspended within a sleeve of visceral pericardium, this, in turn, being reflected at either pole into the parietal pericardium. The myocardium itself is formed by migration of a myoepicardial mantle from the inner aspect of the visceral pericardium. The visceral pericardium then becomes the epicardium, the mantle becomes the myocardium, and the initial heart tube persists as the endocardial lining *(fig. 10.4).*

During these events, the heart tube itself undergoes considerable bending. Initially, it is a straight tube extending from the venous pole (where it is bilaterally symmetrical and receives the venous systems) to the arterial pole (where it is again bilaterally symmetrical). The tube shows at this early stage a series of constrictions along its length. These enable it to be divided into segments which have been variously named by different investigators. Five segments are present *(fig. 10.6).* The segment receiving the venous return is generally termed the sinus venosus, and itself shows symmetry, the two extensions being the right and left sinus horns. The sinus venosus

drains to the atrial primordium, which again is generally recognized as the primitive atrium. It is the next three segments which give problems in nomenclature. For this reason, we prefer to use descriptive rather than nominative terms, and describe them as the inlet and outlet portions of the ventricular segment of the tube and the arterial segment *(fig. 10.6).* The four constrictions between these five dilated areas of the primary heart tube are, therefore, the sinuatrial junction, the atrioventricular canal, the inlet-outlet junction and the ventriculo-arterial junction. Bending of the heart tube occurs at the atrioventricular canal and between the inlet and outlet components of the ventricular segment. The atrioventricular bend is through a right angle, the venous and atrial part of the tube moving to the posterior aspect of the pericardial cavity so that the inlet part of the ventricular segment drops down in front of it. The ventricular segment itself bends through 180°, producing a rightward loop and bringing the arterial part of the tube directly in front of the atrioventricular canal *(fig. 10.6).* This process in itself confers a long outer curvature and a much shorter inner curvature upon the ventricular segment. The short inner curve is

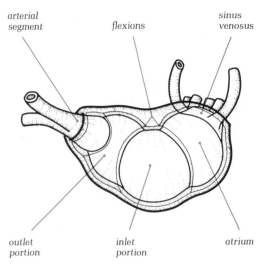

Fig. 10.6 *Bending of the heart tube occurs between the atrial segment and inlet and outlet portions of the ventricular loop.*

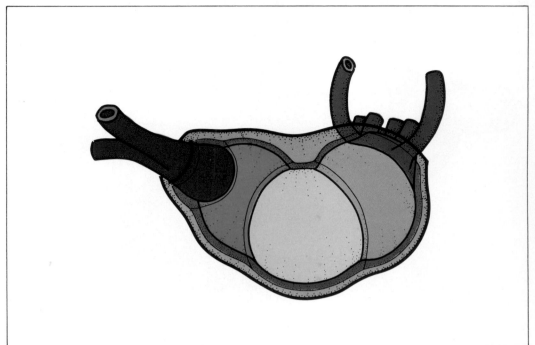

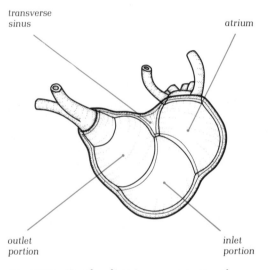

Fig. 10.7 *Further looping accentuates the transverse sinus at the site of the inner curvature.*

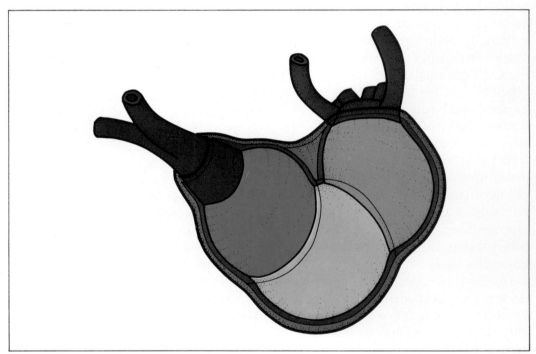

between the anterior aspect of the atrium and the posterior aspect of the arterial segment. It is lined throughout by epicardium, and the space between its floor (the roof of the ventricular segment) and the pericardial reflection is the transverse sinus of the pericardium (*fig. 10.7*).

Following this bending process, frequently termed 'looping', the heart tube achieves a 'cardiac' contour. The atrioventricular canal at this stage empties in its entirety to the inlet part of the ventricular loop, while the arterial segment is supported by the outlet component. Consequently, the atrioventricular and ventriculo-arterial junctions are separated by the inner heart curvature (*fig. 10.7*). Transformation of this single-streamed structure into the dual circulations of the definitive heart then depends on septation of the tube, together with transfer of parts of the segments relative to one another to permit septation. These processes occur simultaneously or in close succession; but for descriptive purposes, it is convenient to consider them separately.

10.6

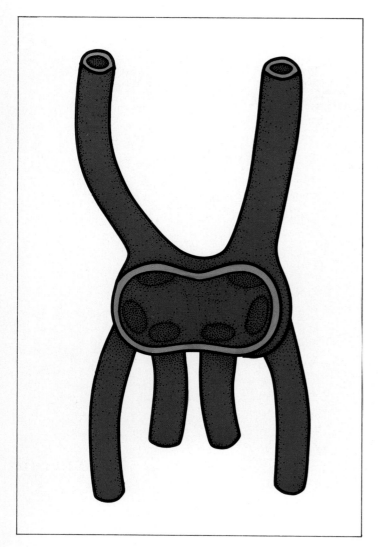

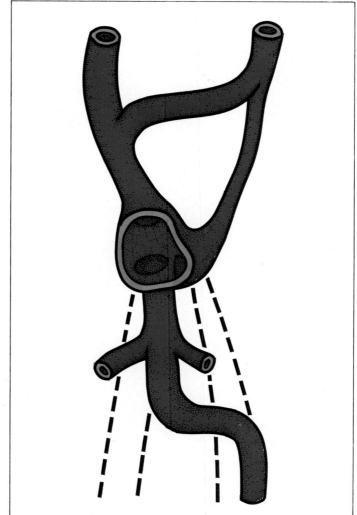

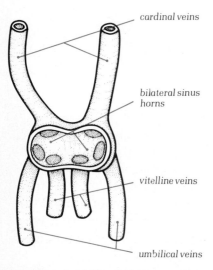

cardinal veins

bilateral sinus horns

vitelline veins

umbilical veins

Fig. 10.8   Initially, the sinus venosus is a bilaterally symmetrical structure receiving on each side cardinal, vitelline and umbilical veins.

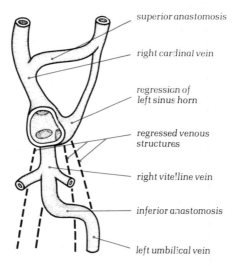

superior anastomosis

right cardinal vein

regression of left sinus horn

regressed venous structures

right vitelline vein

inferior anastomosis

left umbilical vein

Fig. 10.9   Development of left-to-right anastomoses in the cardinal and umbilical systems result in growth of the sinus horn and regression of the left sinus horn.

Septation of the Atria

Atrial septation demands transfer of systemic venous return to the right side of the primitive atrium together with establishment of pulmonary venous circulation. The three systems of venous tributaries which drain to the sinus venosus have no connexion with the pulmonary circulation. This develops *in situ* in the developing lung buds, themselves formed posterior to the heart as growths (via the trachea) of the foregut. Initially, therefore, the intrapulmonary venous system is in communication with the veins developed along the gut (the splanchnic venous plexus) rather than with the venous pole of the heart tube *(vide infra)*. All venous tributaries entering the heart tube are systemic veins, draining the yolk sac (vitelline veins), the placenta (umbilical veins) and the embryo itself (cardinal veins). As described, in early stages, these vessels drain symmetrically to each sinus horn in the order of, from lateral to medial, cardinal vein, umbilical

10.7

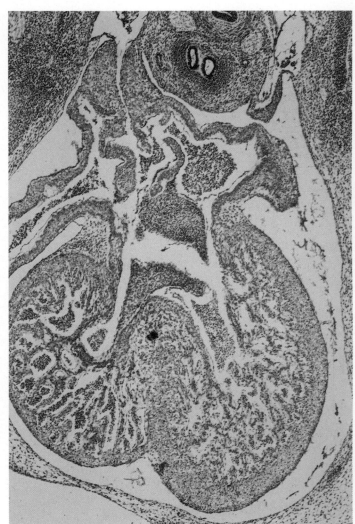

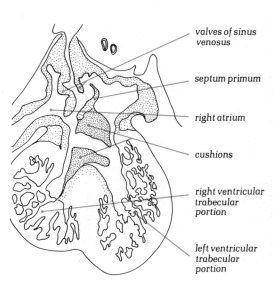

valves of sinus venosus

septum primum

right atrium

cushions

right ventricular trabecular portion

left ventricular trabecular portion

Fig. 10.10   *Frontal section of a 13mm crown-rump length human embryo showing the prominent state of the valves of the sinus venosus at this early stage of development.*

vein and vitelline vein *(fig. 10.8)*. During early development, however, there is drastic reorganization of the venous channels so that most left-sided blood is diverted to right-sided veins. This is accomplished by formation of anastomotic channels. One in the head, the left brachiocephalic vein, transfers all left-sided cardinal blood to the right cardinal vein. Another in the trunk, the ductus venosus, transfers blood from the left umbilical vein to the termination of the right vitelline vein. Concomitant with this, there is regression of both distal vitelline systems and the proximal left vitelline vein along with the distal right umbilical vein and both proximal umbilical veins. The end result is that only two channels remain draining blood to the sinus venosus, the right cardinal vein and the right vitelline vein *(fig. 10.9)*. Because both are right-sided structures, there is a shift of the sinuatrial junction to the right side of the primitive atrium *(fig. 10.9)* which, in the meantime, has evaginated pouches, the appendages, to either side of the newly-centralized arterial segment of the heart tube. With shift of the sinuatrial junction, there is a decrease in size of left sinus horn, which regresses to become the coronary sinus. Following this venous reorganization, therefore, the sinuatrial junction opens to the right side of the primitive atrium. The complete junction invaginates itself into the primitive atrium, the bilaminate funnel thus formed becoming the prominent right and left valves of the sinus venosus *(fig. 10.10)*. A new structure, the primary pulmonary vein, then grows out from the left posterior wall of the atrium, growing between the enlarged right sinus horn and the regressing left sinus horn *(fig. 10.11)*. The primary pulmonary vein extends towards the developing lung buds, where it establishes contact with the intrapulmonary venous plexus and enables pulmonary venous blood to drain to the left side of the primitive atrium. The stage is now set for atrial septation; but in the meantime, septation has already commenced in the atrioventricular canal. This is achieved by growth of two opposing masses of mesenchymal tissue at the superior and inferior borders of the canal. These endocardial cushions fuse to septate the canal. At the same time, a crescentic ingrowth develops from the roof of the primitive atrium just to the left of the superior commissure of the valves of the sinus venosus. This ingrowth, the septum primum, grows down through the cavity of the primitive atrium; and as

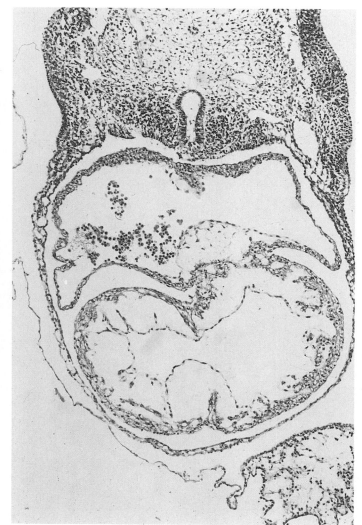

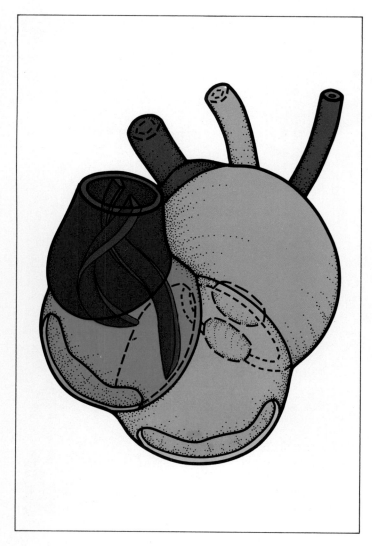

outlet segment

inlet segment

site of left
ventricular pouch

site of right
ventricular pouch

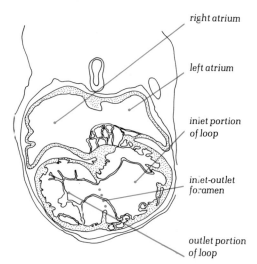

right atrium

left atrium

inlet portion
of loop

inlet-outlet
foramen

outlet portion
of loop

Fig. 10.17   Development of the ventricles is
dependent upon growth of the trabecular
zones which grow from the inlet and outlet
segments of the loop.

Fig. 10.18   Histological section of an early
human embryo showing the ventricular
component of the primary heart tube.

earlier investigators (Kramer, 1942;
Van Mierop et al., 1963; Los, 1968;
Goor et al., 1972). The latter cushions
are continuous with yet other
cushions developing in the arterial
segment of the tube, termed truncal
cushions by earlier investigators
(Van Mierop et al., 1963). While this

reorganization of cushion tissue has
been occurring at the extremities of
the ventricular loop, dispersion of
cushion tissue occurs along the
greater curvature of the loop in two
areas, one in the inlet and the other in
the outlet component (fig. 10.17).
Pouches grow outwards from both of

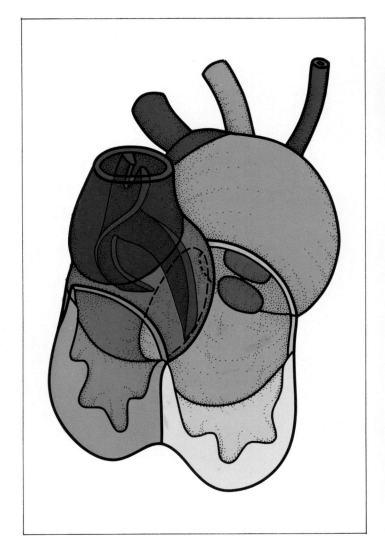

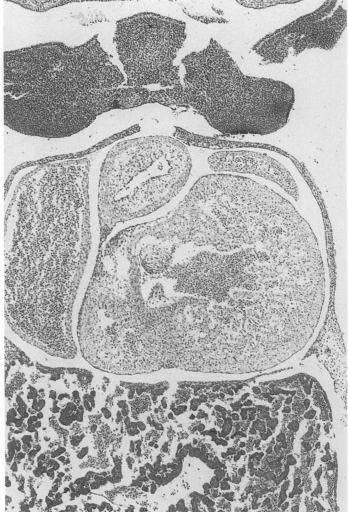

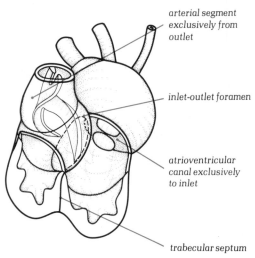

arterial segment
exclusively from
outlet

inlet-outlet foramen

atrioventricular
canal exclusively
to inlet

trabecular septum

Fig. 10.19   After trabecular pouch formation,
the atrioventricular canal communicates
exclusively with the inlet portion of the
ventricular loop while the arterial segment is
supported entirely above the outlet portion.

arterial segment

primary heart
tube

right ventricular
pouch

trabecular septum

left ventricular
pouch

Fig. 10.20   Histological section of a human
embryo after commencement of pouch
formation.

these areas to either side of the lower edge of the inlet-outlet foramen (figs. 10.19, 10.20). The pouch growing from the inlet component will eventually form the trabecular component of the left ventricle, while that growing from the outlet component will form the trabecular component of the right ventricle.

Following pouch formation, which also produces the trabecular septum between the pouches, the atrioventricular canal and the inlet component drain into the inlet trabecular pouch while the outlet component and arterial segment are supported above the outlet trabecular pouch. Already, however, septation

has commenced in the atrioventricular canal and outlet component. To produce a normal heart, it is therefore necessary for the new right atrioventricular orifice (formed by division of the atrioventricular canal), together with part of the inlet component of the primary heart tube, to be transferred to a position draining

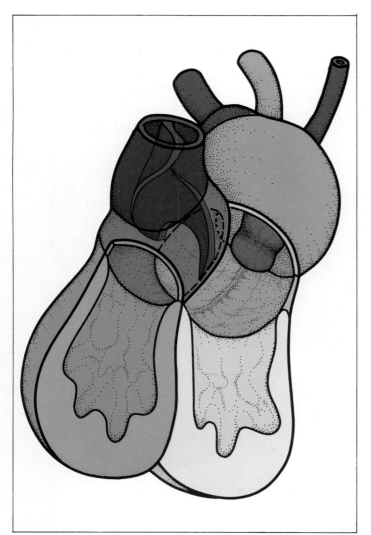

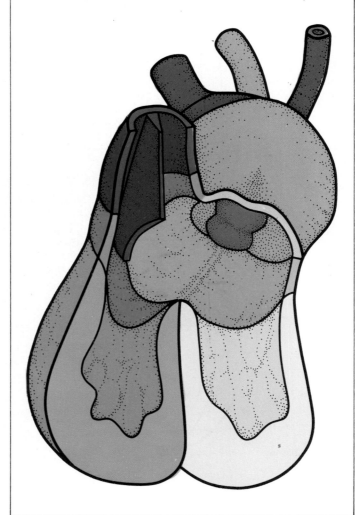

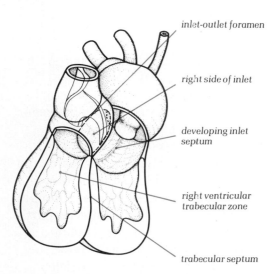

inlet-outlet foramen

right side of inlet

developing inlet septum

right ventricular trabecular zone

trabecular septum

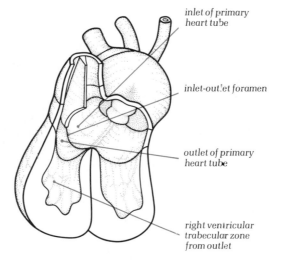

inlet of primary heart tube

inlet-outlet foramen

outlet of primary heart tube

right ventricular trabecular zone from outlet

Fig. 10.21   The commencement of transfer of the right side of the atrioventricular canal, together with part of the inlet of the primary tube, to the right ventricular trabecular zone.

Fig. 10.22   A later stage of transfer, showing how part of the inlet of the primary heart tube contributes to the right ventricle.

into the outlet trabecular pouch. Similarly, part of the outlet component supporting the developing aorta must be transferred to a position above the inlet trabecular pouch. The precise mechanics underlying these transfers are controversial and, to a great extent, of little consequence to understanding development. Suffice it

to say that the transfer processes involve considerable moulding and reorganization of the inlet-outlet foramen.

As the right atrioventricular orifice and its supporting inlet component achieve a position draining into the outlet trabecular pouch (fig. 10.21), they expand towards the trabecular pouch, 'pushing' the posterior and

rightward rim of the inlet-outlet foramen before them (fig. 10.22). When this transfer is achieved, whatever its mechanics, a new septum is formed between the right and left inlet components which extends apically to fuse distally with the posterior border of the trabecular septum and proximally with the

10.15

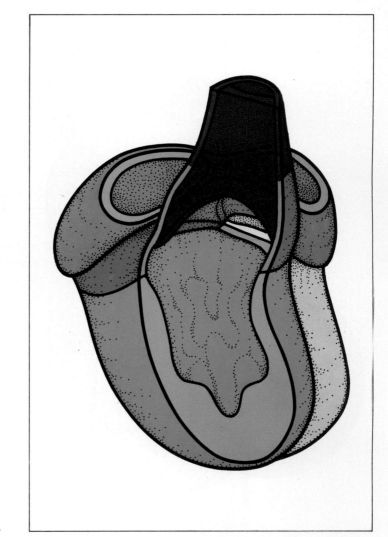

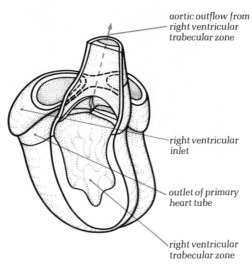

aortic outflow from
right ventricular
trabecular zone

right ventricular
inlet

outlet of primary
heart tube

right ventricular
trabecular zone

*Fig. 10.23   Initially the aortic outflow tract
is above the right ventricular trabecular zone.*

underside of the atrioventricular
endocardial cushions. This new
septum is, from its position, the inlet
septum. The foramen through which
the inlet trabecular pouch now
communicates with the arterial
segment, for convenience considered
as though still above the outlet
component, is no longer the inlet-
outlet foramen. It is only the left half
of this foramen, the rightward and
posterior edge of the new exit from the
inlet trabecular pouch being the
newly-formed inlet septum and the
fused atrioventricular endocardial
cushions. Following this
development, the outlet trabecular
pouch now has its own inlet, the right
atrioventricular orifice. The left
ventricular pouch, which grew from
the inlet portion of the heart tube and
always possessed an inlet, still lacks
a direct arterial outlet because the
entire arterial segment is committed
to the outlet trabecular pouch.
Consequently, the final event in
ventricular development must be
transfer to the inlet trabecular pouch

of the developing aortic component
of the arterial segment together with
its supporting outlet component of
primary heart tube. Again, the precise
mechanics of transfer are
controversial, but effective
attenuation of the inner curvature of
the primary loop occurs during the
transfer *(Asami, 1969; Goor et al.,
1972; Anderson et al., 1974)*. Whether
this is a consequence of active
resorption of tissue, or excessive
growth of the areas adjacent to the
inner curve, is as yet undetermined;
and, for the purpose of understanding,
it is unimportant. The vital point for
comprehension is to appreciate that
this process also involves
reorientation of the initial inlet-outlet
foramen, this time taking its anterior
and leftward rim above the inlet
trabecular pouch. This necessitates
further moulding in the area of exit
from the inlet trabecular pouch.
Initially, this exit is roofed by the
inner heart curvature *(fig. 10.23)*. As
the aortic outlet component is

transformed, so the central part of the
inner heart curve is taken to a
position above the inlet trabecular
pouch, sinking into position between
the newly-formed right and left
atrioventricular orifices *(fig. 10.24)*.
Simultaneously with this transfer, the
endocardial cushion septum formed
between the arterial outlets is brought
into alignment with the anterior part
of the trabecular septum, leaving a
small foramen between the now
completed right and left ventricles
(fig. 10.24). This foramen is then
closed by further growth of
endocardial or sulcus tissue, the
origin of which is once more
controversial *(Odgers, 1938; Wenink,
1974)*. Yet again, the precise origin of
this tissue is of minor importance, the
important conceptual fact to be
grasped being that the
interventricular foramen cannot be
closed until each trabecular pouch
has its own inlet and outlet *(fig. 10.25)*.
Only then does the foramen not serve
as either an entrance or exit for one or

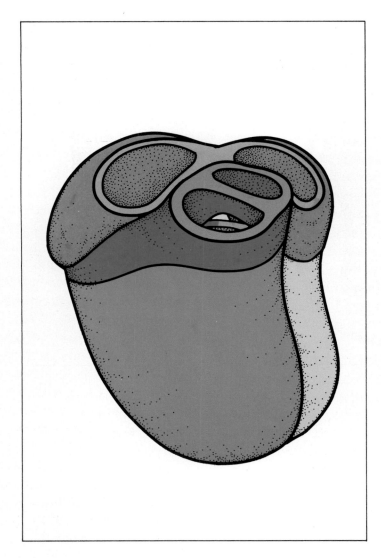

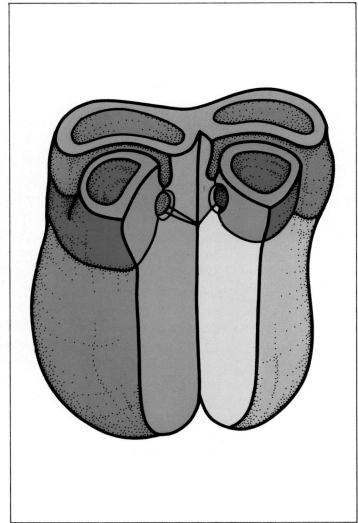

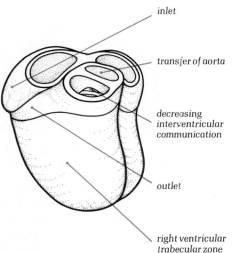

inlet

transfer of aorta

decreasing
interventricular
communication

outlet

right ventricular
trabecular zone

Fig. 10.24 Associated with transfer of the
aortic outflow component to the left ventricle
there is attenuation of the inner heart
curvature.

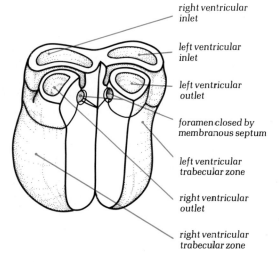

right ventricular
inlet

left ventricular
inlet

left ventricular
outlet

foramen closed by
membranous septum

left ventricular
trabecular zone

right ventricular
outlet

right ventricular
trabecular zone

Fig. 10.25 The foramen between the
definitive right and left ventricles, each with
three components, which will be closed by the
membranous septum.

other pouch, and only then can it be
closed by mesenchymal tissue. The
initial inlet-outlet foramen is never
closed. Its right and posterior part is
reorientated to form the junction of
the right ventricular inlet component
with the rest of the chamber; its left
anterior part is reorientated to form
the junction of the aortic outlet

component with the remainder of the
left ventricle. Following these various
changes, each ventricle has three
developmental components that have
joined together (*Van Mierop &
Gessner, 1972*; fig. 10.25). The
definitive left ventricle comprises the
inlet trabecular pouch, the left half of
the atrioventricular canal and its

adjacent ventricular inlet component,
and the aortic component of the
outlet part of the ventricular loop.
The definitive right ventricle is made
up of the outlet trabecular pouch, the
right half of the atrioventricular canal
and its adjacent inlet component, and
the pulmonary component of the
ventricular loop outlet (fig. 10.25).

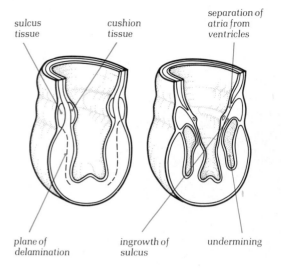

sulcus tissue   cushion tissue   separation of atria from ventricles

plane of delamination   ingrowth of sulcus   undermining

Fig. 10.26 *Formation of the atrioventricular valves by a process of undermining and delamination of the endocardial layer with ingrowth of tissue from the atrioventricular sulcus, before (left) and after (right).*

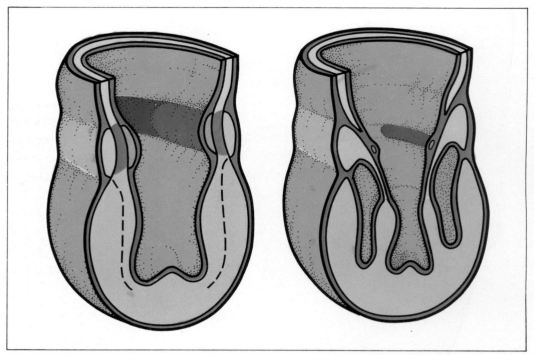

Completion of this ventricular septation occurs by the end of the sixth week of intrauterine life, when the embryo is less than 2cms in length. However, at this early stage, there are no atrioventricular or arterial valves. It is probable that the endocardial cushions function as temporary valves during this period, as well as serving to 'glue' the opposing parts of the heart tube together. It is very likely that the cushions contribute very little to the definitive valves or to definitive septal structures. The atrioventricular valves are instead formed by a process of undermining of the superficial layer of the ventricular inlet portions, the attached parts persisting as the papillary muscles and the liberated superficial sheets becoming infiltrated with ingrowing atrioventricular sulcus tissue to form the valve leaflets *(fig. 10.26)*. The valve annuli are also formed by ingrowth from the epicardial atrioventricular sulcus tissue, this ingrowth severing the atrioventricular muscular continuities which still exist at the completion of septation *(fig. 10.27)*. Maturation of both the annuli and valve leaflets is a relatively late development, occurring from the sixth week of intrauterine life and being largely completed by mid-term,

although development of the annuli continues on after birth, especially in the region of the central fibrous body. Nonetheless, in the normal heart at birth, only the atrioventricular conduction system connects the atrial and ventricular musculatures *(vide infra)*.

The morphological differences between the ventricles are well explained from their developmental history. Because the aorta is transferred into the left ventricle, its outlet loses its initially complete mesenchymal annulus. Following this, the aortic valve develops in fibrous continuity with the atrioventricular valves, the continuity with the right valve occurring via the membranous septum. In contrast, the pulmonary artery retains its embryonic position above the trabecular pouch of the right ventricle. It retains its mesenchymal infundibulum, the inner heart curvature continuing to separate the pulmonary valve from the tricuspid valve while the outlet septum separates the pulmonary valve from the aortic valve. The prominent septal trabeculation of the right ventricle, termed by us the trabecula septomarginalis, is seen early in

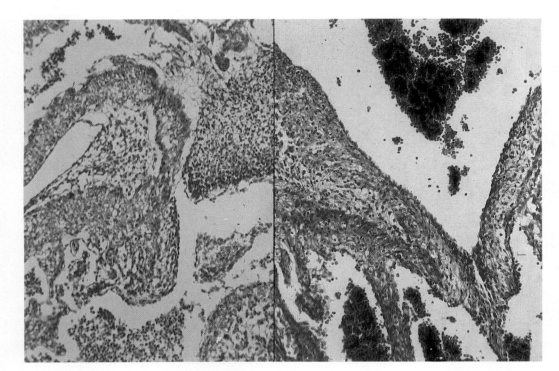

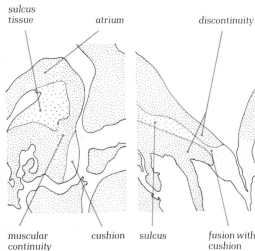

muscular
continuity   cushion   sulcus   fusion with
cushion

Fig. 10.27   *Histological sections showing the
atrioventricular junction before (left) and
after (right) the ingrowth of the sulcus tissue.*

development and is intimately
connected with the development of
tension apparatus of the tricuspid
valve. Its precise origin remains
obscure. Finally, it should be
remembered that when the
membranous septum closes the
interventricular foramen, the
tricuspid valve leaflets are at that
time undifferentiated. Development of
atrioventricular and interventricular
components of the septum is,
therefore, dependent upon
undermining of the septal leaflet of
the tricuspid valve. This is a late event
and in many instances is still not
completed at birth (*Allwork &
Anderson, 1979*). The development of
the arterial valves is considered after
an account has been given of the
development of the great arteries.

Formation of the Great Arteries

The arterial segment of the primary
heart tube is initially an undivided
structure connected to six pairs of
aortic arches which encircle the
developing pharynx to drain into
paired posterior aortae, those two, in
turn, fusing to form a single posterior
aortic channel (fig. 10.27).
Transformation of this aortic arch
system into the aortic and pulmonary
circulation is dependent upon
septation of the arterial segment of

the heart tube, regression of some of
the aortic arches and division of the
proximal arch system.

Opposing endocardial cushions are
formed in the arterial segment of the
primary heart tube at the same time as
they develop in the distal part of the
outlet portion of the ventricular loop.
There is disagreement as to whether
the cushions in the two segments are
the same continuous structures
('bulbotruncal' cushions of Los, 1968),
or separate and discrete entities
('bulbar' cushions in the ventricular
loop, 'truncal' cushions in the arterial
segment of Van Mierop et al., 1963).
From the standpoint of normal
development, the distinction is
immaterial, since the cushions
develop at the same time and as a
continuous septum to divide the
aortic and pulmonary outflow tracts.
The arterial valves are formed at the
junction of the arterial segment of the
primary tube with its ventricular loop
portion. The skeleton of the facing
cusps of both aortic and pulmonary
valves is derived from the opposing
endocardial cushions. The non-facing
cusp of each valve is formed on the
basis of a separate, intercalated
endocardial swelling (*Kramer, 1942*).
Whether the definitive valve leaflets

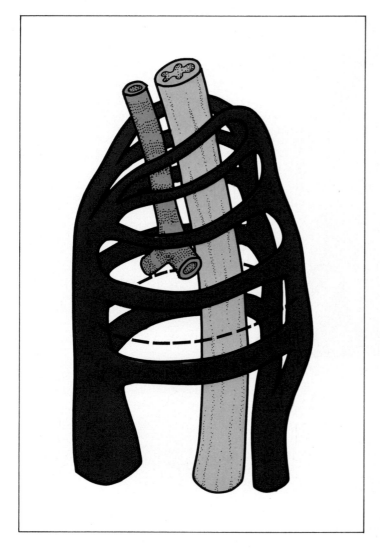

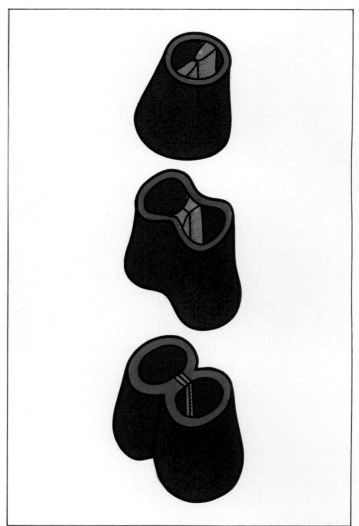

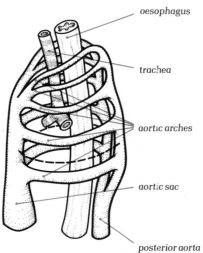

oesophagus

trachea

aortic arches

aortic sac

posterior aorta

Fig. 10.28   An hypothetical drawing of the six aortic arches. These arches never exist at the same time and there is doubt concerning the existence of the fifth pair.

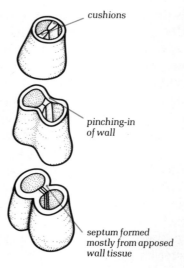

cushions

pinching-in of wall

septum formed mostly from apposed wall tissue

Fig. 10.29   The definitive outlet septum is formed in only a small part by the endocardial cushions which initially septate the outlet and arterial segment.

are derived from the cushions is uncertain. It is likely that the outlet septum and proximal arterial septum are derived not from cushion tissue but by apposition of arterial and outflow tract wall (fig. 10.29). It is therefore unlikely that the final valve leaflets are formed from endocardial cushion tissue.

The arterial segment of the primary heart tube forms only the proximal part of the ascending portions of the aorta and pulmonary artery. The remainder of the circulation is derived from the aortic sac and the aortic arch system. As indicated, six pairs of arches are formed, which initially connect the aortic sac to the

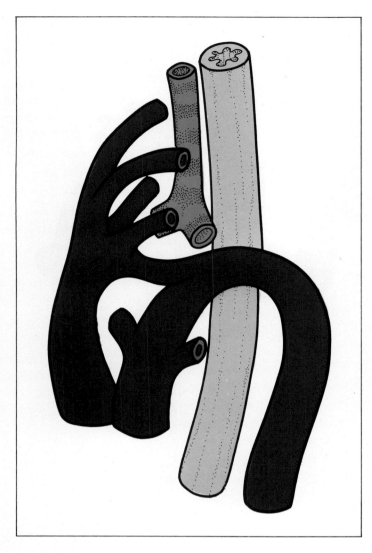

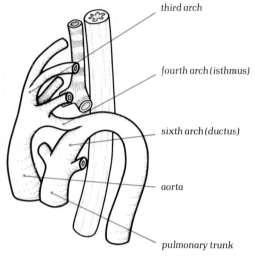

third arch

fourth arch (isthmus)

sixth arch (ductus)

aorta

pulmonary trunk

Fig. 10.30   The definitive aortic arches and arteries contain persisting portions of the third, fourth and sixth pairs of arches, mostly on the left side.

descending aorta, although the existence of discrete fifth arches is another controversial topic. Be that as it may, the greater part of the definitive circulation is formed from the fourth and sixth arches (fig. 10.30). The first and second arch structures largely disappear, persisting only as small arteries related to the cavity of the middle ear. The third arch system is incorporated into the carotid arteries, but the left side of the fourth arch persists as the definitive aortic arch and descending thoracic aorta. The fifth arch disappears in its entirety (if indeed it ever exists), while the sixth arch forms the right and left main pulmonary arteries within the pericardial cavity. The right-sided connexions of the fourth and sixth arches to the descending aorta also disappear, but the connexion between the left sixth arch and the descending left aortic arch becomes the ductus arteriosus.

The intrapulmonary arteries, as with the intrapulmonary veins, develop *pari passu* with the growing lung bud. Initially, the developing lung buds have arterial connexions both with the anterior arch system and the posterior descending aortic arch (*Congdon, 1922*). The posterior connexions normally disappear, leaving the intrapulmonary arteries in communication anteriorly with the sixth aortic arches. Because of the diversion of flow away from the lungs during intrauterine life, the pulmonary arteries between the sixth arch and the lung are small structures in comparison to the calibre of the left sixth arch until after birth.

The carotid arteries are derived from the third aortic arch system. In contrast, the subclavian arteries are derived from the seventh cervical intersegmental arteries. Initially, these arteries attach to the descending aorta well below the final level of the subclavian arteries. Considerable moulding and migration is needed to place these arteries in their definitive positions. In the case of the right subclavian, this involves regression and disappearance of the right aortic

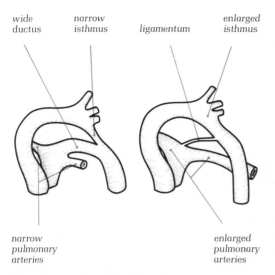

Fig. 10.31 *Considerable changes are required after birth to convert the fetal arrangement of blood vessels (left) to the definitive form (right).*

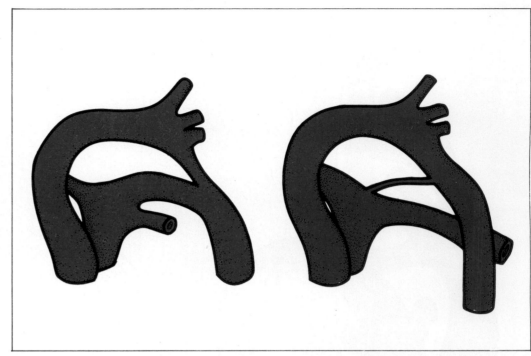

arch, while on the left side, the process involves a reversal of the position of the subclavian relative to the isthmus, a process which Bruins *(1973)* has descriptively likened to the castling movement in chess. In addition to this castling movement, further moulding is required in the region of the isthmus during development. In intrauterine life, the ascending aorta carries blood mostly for the head and neck while blood reaches the descending aorta mostly from the ductus. The isthmus at this stage inserts into the mainstream of sixth arch and descending aorta *(fig. 10.31)*. At birth, the ductus closes and, almost immediately, it is necessary for the isthmus to expand so that the mainstream is from the fourth arch to the descending aorta *(fig. 10.31)*. The final remoulding is a more gradual process; but certainly by three months of age, the ductus should be converted into a ligament and the isthmus widened so that no

gradient exists across it between upper and lower limbs.

Thus far, the junction of the aortic sac to the arterial segment of the primary heart tube has been ignored. Great play is made in certain accounts of development concerning the spiral disposition of the outflow endocardial cushions in producing the characteristic spiralling of the great arteries. Certainly, at the time of looping of the primary heart tube and immediately afterwards, the cushions are disposed in spiral fashion as they ascend into the arterial segment. However, at this time the cushions are not joined across the lumen. The careful reconstructions of Los *(1968)* show that as they fuse, they fuse to form a straight septum. Indeed, examination of the definitive heart will show that the outlet septum and the proximal walls of the aorta and pulmonary artery are basically straight structures. The spiralling of the great arteries occurs in their

ascending portions. The reconstructions of Los *(1968)* show that this part of the aortic arch system is separated by growth of a wedge of tissue towards the heart from the junction of the fourth and sixth arches with the aortic sac. This wedge of mesenchyme is called the aortico-pulmonary septum. As the heart tube cushions fuse, it joins with their distal edge so as to connect the sixth arch to the anterior pulmonary outflow tract and the fourth arch to the posterior aortic outflow tract. Thereafter, moulding and formation of the ascending aorta and pulmonary trunk to either side of the aortico-pulmonary septum produce the characteristic spiralling of the arteries.

Development of the Coronary Arteries

The septation of the cardiac chambers and great arteries is complete by the time the embryo is

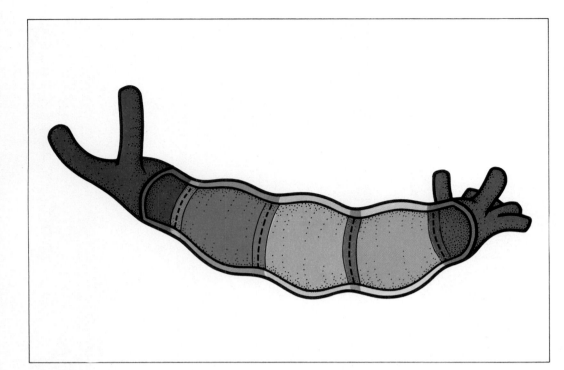

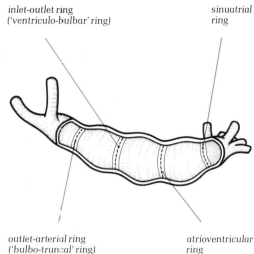

inlet-outlet ring
('ventriculo-bulbar' ring)

sinuatrial
ring

outlet-arterial ring
('bulbo-truncal' ring)

atrioventricular
ring

Fig. 10.32   Initially the segments of the
primary heart tube are separated by
junctional rings of histologically specialized
tissue.

2cms long, that is, by the end of the
second month of development.
Thereafter, considerable growth and
moulding of the heart occurs up to
term, including determination and
formation of the atrioventricular
valves as described. During the same
period as the valves are formed, the
coronary circulation is established by
coalescence and growth of the
coronary arteries and veins.
Primordia of major coronary arteries
are developed in relation to the
sinuses of both the aorta and the
pulmonary trunk (Hackensellner,
1956) but normally, the definitive
coronary arteries persist only in
relation to the facing sinuses of the
aortic root.

Development of the Conduction System and Fibrous Skeleton

The development of these two
systems, one of conduction tissue and
the other of fibrous tissue, is
inextricably linked. Initially, the

myoblastic tissue of the heart tube
segments is in continuity across all
the junctions between them. In the
definitive heart, this continuity is
retained except at the atrioventricular
junction. At this latter junction, the
atrial and ventricular myocardial
segments are totally separated by the
fibrous skeleton. This skeleton is
pierced only by the atrioventricular
bundle. It is pertinent that in lower
animals there is considerable
evidence to indicate that rings of
specialized tissue exist as the
connecting tissue between the cardiac
segments (Benninghoff, 1923).
Certainly, in the human embryo, there
is strong evidence to show that such
a ring of atrioventricular specialized
tissue initially connects the atrial
and ventricular musculatures
(Anderson & Taylor, 1972). It is
tempting, therefore, to speculate that
the human conduction system is
derived from a series of junctional
rings of specialized tissue (Wenink,

1976), particularly since the sinus
node is a sinuatrial junctional
structure and the ventricular bundle
branches originate astride the septum
between inlet and outlet portions of
the primary heart tube (fig. 10.32).
However, the only true annular
conduction tissue structure we have
encountered is the atrioventricular
ring, the provenance of the other
structures from specialized rings still
requiring proof, although evidence is
accumulating that the ventriculo-
bulbar ring is also a reality. In our
experience, the sinus node is first
recognized as a specialized structure
at about the time of completion of
septation (Anderson et al., 1978). It is
a wedge of distinct cells set into the
angle between the superior vena cava
and the primitive atrium, its body
being lateral to the junction but
extensions running both medially
into the interatrial groove and
inferiorly towards the opening of the
inferior vena cava (fig. 10.33). When

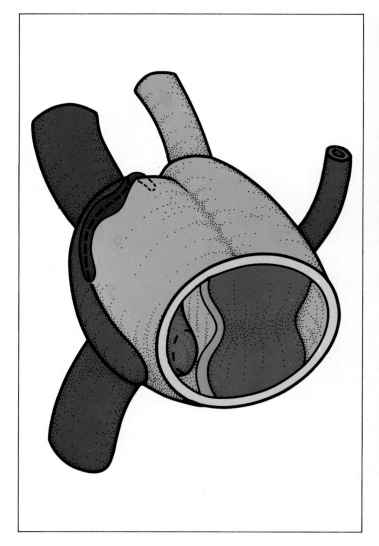

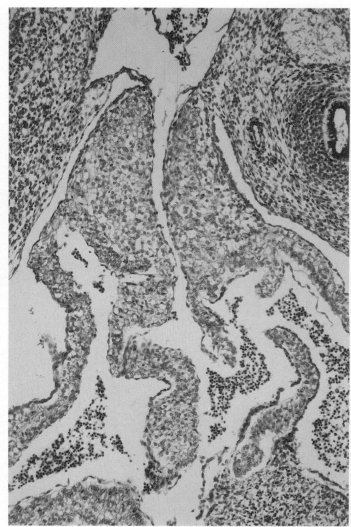

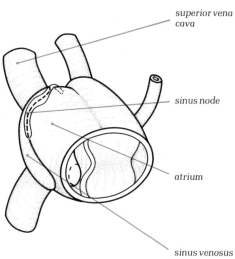

superior vena cava

sinus node

atrium

sinus venosus

Fig. 10.33   The sinus node is a sinuatrial junctional structure and is initially more extensive than in the definitive heart.

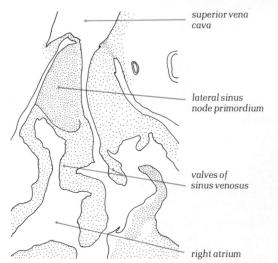

superior vena cava

lateral sinus node primordium

valves of sinus venosus

right atrium

Fig. 10.34   Histological section of the sinus node primordium when first seen in an early human embryo. Note it is a lateral structure.

first seen, it is a prominent structure but is not related to a prominent artery (fig. 10.34). This establishes itself within the nodal primordia as the coronary arterial system itself develops. Subsequently, there is a diminution in size of the node relative to the remainder of the atrium and, at term, it occupies its definitive position in the sulcus terminalis lateral to the cavo-atrial junction.

Although we have found no evidence to show that the sinus node is derived from a sinuatrial ring of specialized tissue, a ring of sorts certainly exists in the valves of the sinus venosus, which early in development are prominent muscular structures extending between the sinuatrial and atrioventricular junctions. This ring has been implicated as one possible specialized internodal tract and indeed, in definitive animal hearts, remnants of the ring can be discovered. However, the sinuatrial ring bundle is made of small cells (Tranum-Jensen & Bojsen-Moller, 1973), and has been shown to conduct slowly rather than as a rapid tract

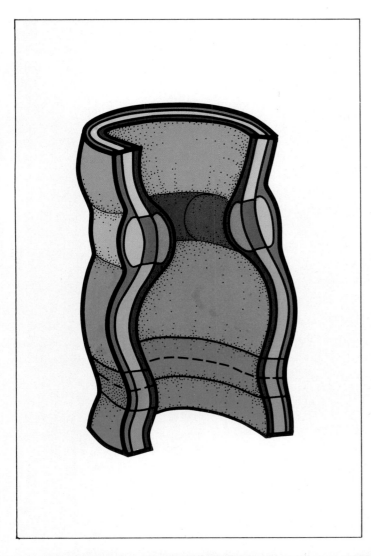

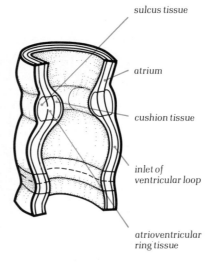

Fig. 10.35 *There is a complete ring of histologically specialized tissue at the atrioventricular junction which is sandwiched between atrioventricular, sulcus and cushion tissue.*

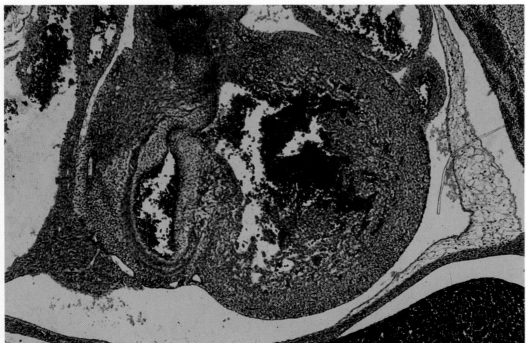

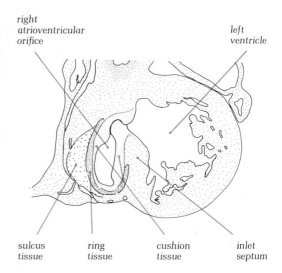

Fig. 10.36 *Transverse section of the human right atrioventricular junction just after the completion of septation showing the sandwiched atrioventricular ring specialized tissue.*

(Masuda & Paes de Carvalho, 1975). Furthermore, in human hearts, there is no evidence of this ring, the valves of the sinus venosus becoming fibrous structures and tending to disappear, although cellular structures in this position have been identified in two fetal hearts *(Gittenberger de Groot & Wenink, 1978).*

The atrioventricular junction is the one area where a ring of specialized tissue can be implicated with a fair degree of certainty in the development of the definitive conduction system. At early stages, prior to septation of the atrioventricular canal, a complete ring of specialized tissue surrounds the canal connecting atrial and ventricular muscles. At this stage, the specialized tissue is sandwiched between developing cushion tissue inside the canal and atrioventricular sulcus tissue outside the canal *(figs. 10.35 & 10.36).* As the trabecular

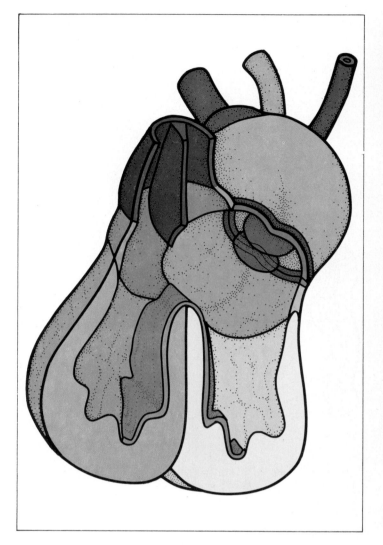

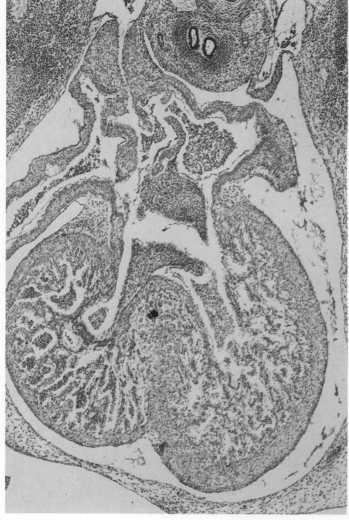

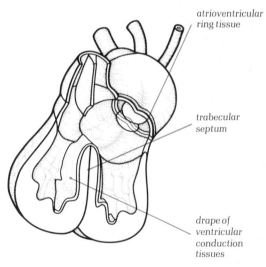

atrioventricular
ring tissue

trabecular
septum

drape of
ventricular
conduction
tissues

Fig. 10.37   The atrioventricular specialized
tissue is a ring during development, but the
ventricular conduction tissues when first
seen are a drape across the developing
trabecular septum.

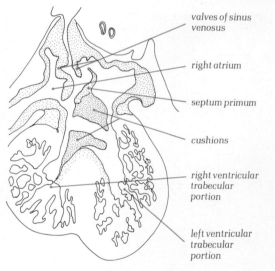

valves of sinus
venosus

right atrium

septum primum

cushions

right ventricular
trabecular
portion

left ventricular
trabecular
portion

Fig. 10.38   Frontal section of a human
embryo prior to the completion of septation
showing the drape of ventricular conduction
tissue on the trabecular septum.

pouches grow from the ventricular
loop, a further source of specialized
tissue is seen, this time on the crest of
the septum formed between the
pouches. However, this second source
is not a ring but a drape, the tissue on
the crest being continuous with

subendocardial sheets of specialized
tissue which extend into the
developing trabecular pouches
(figs. 10.37 & 10.38). During transfer of
the right side of the inlet portion of the
primary heart tube, the
atrioventricular ring tissue becomes

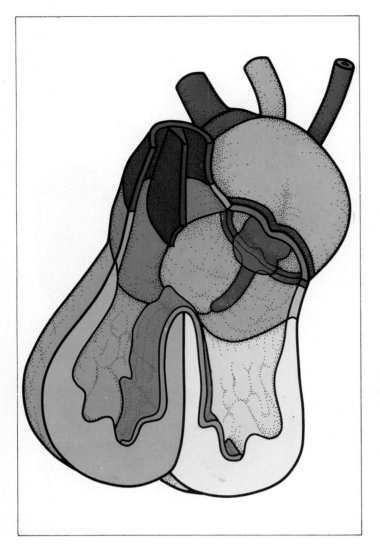

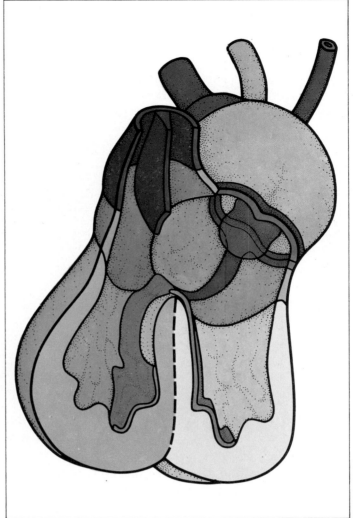

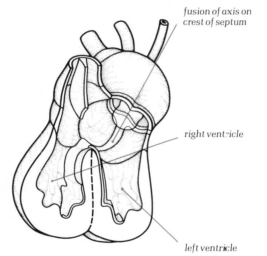

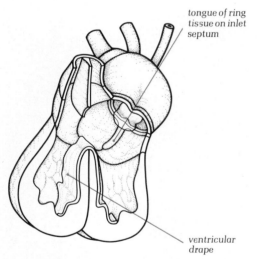

tongue of ring
tissue on inlet
septum

ventricular
drape

Fig. 10.39   Growth of the inlet septum
carries with it a tongue of tissue from the
posterior part of the atrioventricular ring
towards the ventricular drape.

fusion of axis on
crest of septum

right ventricle

left ventricle

Fig. 10.40   Fusion of the inlet and trabecular
septa establishes a continuous axis of
atrioventricular conduction tissue carried on
the crest of the newly-formed muscular
ventricular septum.

connected to the trabecular drape
tissue. It seems likely that this occurs
by evagination of the posterior part of
the ring on the inlet septum which
develops beneath the inferior
endocardial cushion (fig. 10.39). This
growth of the inlet septum creates

an axis of tissue between atrium
and ventricle which is still
separated from the atrium by the
endocardial cushion and at this stage
is in contact only with the posterior
atrial wall (fig. 10.40). This axis

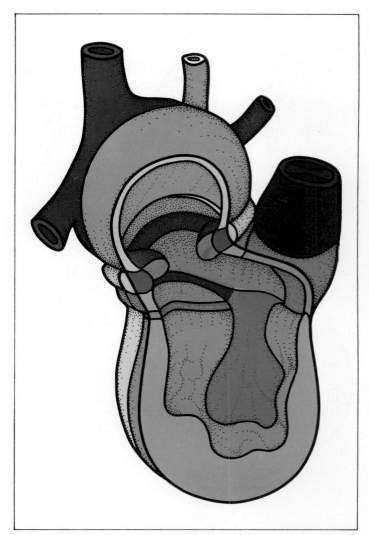

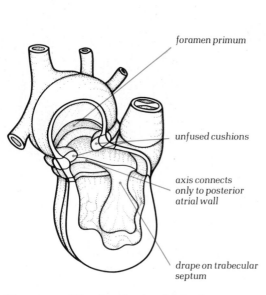

foramen primum

unfused cushions

axis connects
only to posterior
atrial wall

drape on trabecular
septum

Fig. 10.41   Viewing the developing heart
from the right shows how at first the newly-
formed axis connects the ventricular drape
only to the posterior atrial tissues.

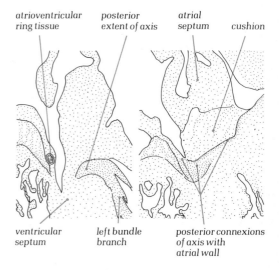

atrioventricular
ring tissue

posterior
extent of axis

atrial
septum

cushion

ventricular
septum

left bundle
branch

posterior connexions
of axis with
atrial wall

Fig. 10.42   Further sections of the human
embryo illustrated in Fig. 10.38 showing the
posterior connexions of the conduction axis
with the posterior atrial wall.

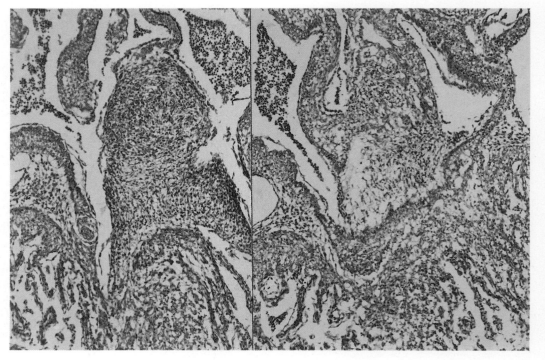

becomes the nodal-bundle axis, and
its initial evagination explains well
its two posterior prong-like
extensions towards the tricuspid and
mitral rings (figs. 10.41 & 10.42). The
connexions between the axis and the
atrial septum are developed later

because the axis is developed prior to
formation of the atrial septum. Thus,
the septum primum grows down to
the cushion (fig. 10.43). Only after
recession of the cushion are
connexions established between the
myocardium of the inferior limbus

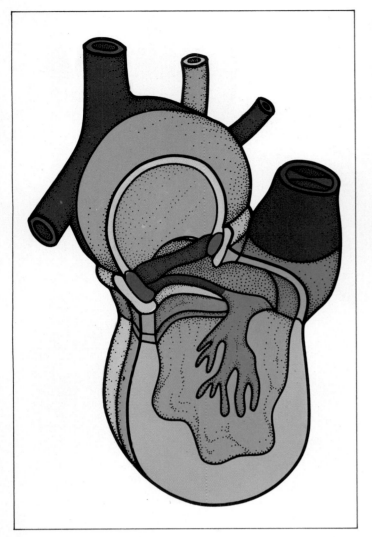

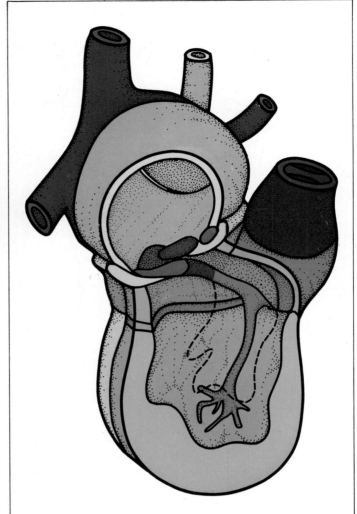

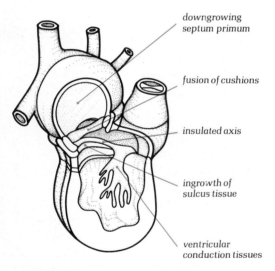

downgrowing
septum primum

fusion of cushions

insulated axis

ingrowth of
sulcus tissue

ventricular
conduction tissues

Fig. 10.43   With growth of the inlet septum,
the sulcus tissue grows inwards to insulate
the conduction axis from the ventricular
septum.

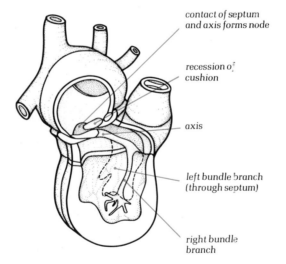

contact of septum
and axis forms node

recession of
cushion

axis

left bundle branch
(through septum)

right bundle
branch

Fig. 10.44   With further growth, the cushion
tissue recedes, permitting the atrial septal
structure to make contact with the
conduction axis.

and the axis (fig. 10.44), producing the
circumferential anterior transitional
cells. The node, therefore, becomes the
penetrating bundle at the point at
which it passes beneath the part of
the central fibrous body derived from
the fused endocardial cushions.

The cushions themselves do not
form the annulus fibrosus. As
indicated, initially atrial and
ventricular myocardial fibres are
continuous throughout the canal.

10.29

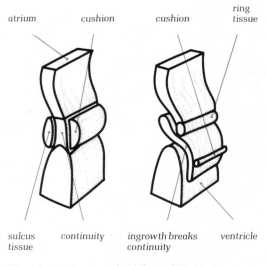

Fig. 10.45 Ingrowth of the sulcus tissue elsewhere round the junctions produces ablation of the atrioventricular continuity.

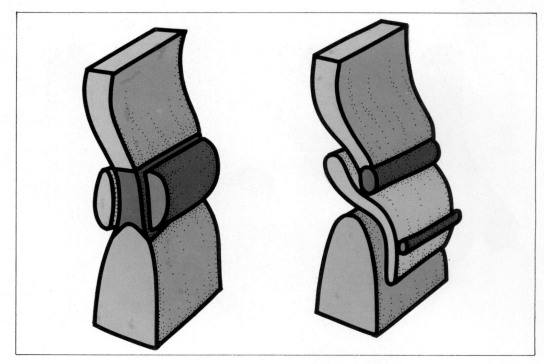

This continuity is destroyed by ingrowth of atrioventricular sulcus tissue, growing in such a way as to sequestrate the atrioventricular ring specialized tissue on the atrial side of the newly-formed annulus (fig. 10.45). In the region of the septum, the sulcus tissue also grows in to insinuate itself between the nodal-bundle axis and ventricular myocardium. The axis enters a tunnel of fibrous tissue to become the penetrating bundle, the superior part being derived from cushion tissue and the inferior part from sulcus tissue. More anteriorly, the nodal-bundle axis becomes continuous with the branching bundle derived from the trabecular drape tissue. This tissue is also separated from the ventricular myocardium by a fibrous sheath which is continuous with the sulcus

sheath, the latter forming the septal annulus fibrosus. Thus, contact between the ventricular conduction tissue derived from the trabecular drape and the ventricular myocardium is not established until the tissue reaches the ventricular apices. It would seem that, as with the sinus node, there is regression of the ventricular conduction tissues, since the extensive trabecular drape eventually becomes the more localized bundle branches, particularly in the right ventricle where the proximal right bundle branch is a narrow cord. The mechanics of this process remain to be elucidated, but it is significant that ventricular conduction tissue is never found on the ventricular surfaces of the inlet septum (although carried on its atrial aspect) and is never observed in the outlet septum.